Diagnostic and Therapeutic Advances in Pediatric Oncology

Cancer Treatment and Research

STEVEN T. ROSEN, M.D., *Series Editor*

Robert H. Lurie Cancer Center, Northwestern University Medical School

Surwit, E.A., Alberts, D.S. (eds.): Endometrial Cancer. 1989. ISBN 0-7923-0286-9.
Champlin, R. (ed.): Bone Marrow Transplantation. 1990. ISBN 0-7923-0612-0.
Goldenberg, D. (ed.): Cancer Imaging with Radiolabeled Antibodies. 1990. ISBN 0-7923-0631-7.
Jacobs, C. (ed.): Carcinomas of the Head and Neck. 1990. ISBN 0-7923-0668-6.
Lippman, M.E., Dickson, R. (eds.): Regulatory Mechanisms in Breast Cancer: Advances in Cellular and Molecular Biology of Breast Cancer. 1990. ISBN 0-7923-0868-9.
Nathanson, L. (ed.): Malignant Melanoma: Genetics, Growth Factors, Metastases, and Antigens. 1991. ISBN 0-7923-0895-6.
Sugarbaker, P.H. (ed.): Management of Gastric Cancer. 1991. ISBN 0-7923-1102-7.
Pinedo, H.M., Verweij, J., Suit, H.D. (eds.): Soft Tissue Sarcomas: New Developments in the Multidisciplinary Approach to Treatment. 1991. ISBN 0-7923-1139-6.
Ozols, R.F. (ed.): Molecular and Clinical Advances in Anticancer Drug Resistance. 1991. ISBN 0-7923-1212-0.
Muggia, F.M. (ed.): New Drugs, Concepts and Results in Cancer Chemotherapy. 1991. ISBN 0-7923-1253-8.
Dickson, R.B., Lippman, M.E. (eds.): Genes, Oncogenes and Hormones: Advances in Cellular and Molecular Biology of Breast Cancer. 1992. ISBN 0-7923-1748-3.
Humphrey, G., Bennett, Schraffordt Koops, H., Molenaar, W.M., Postma, A. (eds.): Osteosarcoma in Adolescents and Young Adults: New Developments and Controversies. 1993. ISBN 0-7923-1905-2.
Benz, C.C., Liu, E.T. (eds.): Oncogenes and Tumor Suppressor Genes in Human Malignancies. 1993. ISBN 0-7923-1960-5.
Freireich, E.J., Kantarjian, H. (eds.): Leukemia: Advances in Research and Treatment. 1993. ISBN 0-7923-1967-2.
Dana, B.W. (ed.): Malignant Lymphomas, Including Hodgkin's Disease: Diagnosis, Management, and Special Problems. 1993. ISBN 0-7923-2171-5.
Nathanson, L. (ed.): Current Research and Clinical Management of Melanoma. 1993. ISBN 0-7923-2152-9.
Verweij, J., Pinedo, H.M., Suit, H.D. (eds.): Multidisciplinary Treatment of Soft Tissue Sarcomas. 1993. ISBN 0-7923-2183-9.
Rosen, S.T., Kuzel, T.M. (eds.): Immunoconjugate Therapy of Hematologic Malignancies. 1993. ISBN 0-7923-2270-3.
Sugarbaker, P.H. (ed.): Hepatobiliary Cancer. 1994. ISBN 0-7923-2501-X.
Rothenberg, M.L. (ed.): Gynecologic Oncology: Controversies and New Developments. 1994. ISBN 0-7923-2634-2.
Dickson, R.B., Lippman, M.E. (eds.): Mammary Tumorigenesis and Malignant Progression. 1994. ISBN 0-7923-2647-4.
Hansen, H.H., (ed.): Lung Cancer. Advances in Basic and Clinical Research. 1994. ISBN 0-7923-2835-3.
Goldstein, L.J., Ozols, R.F. (eds.): Anticancer Drug Resistance. Advances in Molecular and Clinical Research. 1994. ISBN 0-7923-2836-1.
Hong, W.K., Weber, R.S. (eds.): Head and Neck Cancer. Basic and Clinical Aspects. 1994. ISBN 0-7923-3015-3.
Thall, P.F. (ed.): Recent Advances in Clinical Trial Design and Analysis. 1995. ISBN 0-7923-3235-0.
Buckner, C.D. (ed.): Technical and Biological Components of Marrow Transplantation. 1995. ISBN 0-7923-3394-2.
Winter, J.N. (ed.): Blood Stem Cell Transplantation. 1997. ISBN 0-7923-4260-7.
Muggia, F.M. (ed.): Concepts, Mechanisms, and New Targets for Chemotherapy. 1995. ISBN 0-7923-3525-2.
Klastersky, J. (ed.): Infectious Complications of Cancer. 1995. ISBN 0-7923-3598-8.
Kurzrock, R., Talpaz, M. (eds.): Cytokines: Interleukins and Their Receptors. 1995. ISBN 0-7923-3636-4.
Sugarbaker, P. (ed.): Peritoneal Carcinomatosis: Drugs and Diseases. 1995. ISBN 0-7923-3726-3.
Sugarbaker, P. (ed.): Peritoneal Carcinomatosis: Principles of Management. 1995. ISBN 0-7923-3727-1.
Dickson, R.B., Lippman, M.E. (eds.): Mammary Tumor Cell Cycle, Differentiation and Metastasis. 1995. ISBN 0-7923-3905-3.
Freireich, E.J., Kantarjian, H. (eds.): Molecular Genetics and Therapy of Leukemia. 1995. ISBN 0-7923-3912-6.
Cabanillas, F., Rodriguez, M.A. (eds.): Advances in Lymphoma Research. 1996. ISBN 0-7923-3929-0.
Miller, A.B. (ed.): Advances in Cancer Screening. 1996. ISBN 0-7923-4019-1.
Hait, W.N. (ed.): Drug Resistance. 1996. ISBN 0-7923-4022-1.
Pienta, K.J. (ed.): Diagnosis and Treatment of Genitourinary Malignancies. 1996. ISBN 0-7923-4164-3.
Arnold, A.J. (ed.): Endocrine Neoplasms. 1997. ISBN 0-7923-4354-9.
Pollock, R.E. (ed.): Surgical Oncology. 1997. ISBN 0-7923-9900-5.
Verweij, J., Pinedo, H.M., Suit, H.D. (eds.): Soft Tissue Sarcomas: Present Achievements and Future Prospects. 1997. ISBN 0-7923-9913-7.

Diagnostic and Therapeutic Advances in Pediatric Oncology

edited by

DAVID O. WALTERHOUSE, M.D.
SUSAN L. COHN, M.D.
Northwestern University Medical School
Robert H. Lurie Cancer Center
Department of Pediatrics
Children's Memorial Hospital
Chicago, Illinois

KLUWER ACADEMIC PUBLISHERS
BOSTON / DORDRECHT / LONDON

Distributors for North America:
Kluwer Academic Publishers
101 Philip Drive
Assinippi Park
Norwell, Massachusetts 02061 USA

Distributors for all other countries:
Kluwer Academic Publishers Group
Distribution Centre
Post Office Box 322
3300 AH Dordrecht, THE NETHERLANDS

Library of Congress Cataloging-in-Publication Data

Diagnostic and therapeutic advances in pediatric oncology / edited by
    David O. Walterhouse, Susan L. Cohn.
        p.   cm. — (Cancer treatment and research; v. 92)
    Includes bibliographical references and index.
    ISBN 0-7923-9978-1 (alk. paper)
    1. Tumors in children — Congresses.   I. Walterhouse, David O.
II. Cohn, Susan L.   III. Series.
[DNLM: 1. Neoplasms — in infancy & childhood.   2. Neoplasms —
therapy.
W1 CA693 v.92 1997/QZ 275 D536 1997]
    RC281.C4D53   1997
618.92'994 — dc21
DNLM/DLC
for Library of Congress   97-25313
                                                                            CIP

Printed on acid-free paper.

PRINTED IN THE UNITED STATES OF AMERICA

Contents

Contributors

Susan L. Cohn, M.D.
Children's Memorial Hospital
Division of Hematology/Oncology, Box #30
2300 Children's Plaza
Chicago, IL 60614

Jeffrey S. Dome, M.D.
Johns Hopkins Oncology Center
Division of Pediatric Oncology
CMSC 800
600 North Wolfe Street
Baltimore, MD 21287

Edwin C. Douglass, M.D.
St. Christopher's Hospital for Children
Division of Hematology/Oncology
Front & Erie
Philadelphia, PA 19134-1095

Linda Granowetter, M.D.
Mount Sinai School of Medicine
Pediatric Hematology/Oncology Box 1208
1 Gustave L. Levy Place
New York, NY 10029-6574

Paul Grundy, M.D.
Molecular Oncology Program
Cross Cancer Institute
11560 University Avenue
Edmonton Alberta T6G1Z2, Canada

Maureen Haugen, RN, M.S., C.P.N.P.
Children's Memorial Hospital

Division of Hematology/Oncology, Box #30
2300 Children's Plaza
Chicago, IL 60614

Morris Kletzel, M.D.
Children's Memorial Hospital
Division of Hematology/Oncology, Box #30
2300 Children's Plaza
Chicago, IL 60614

Cynthia Kretschmar, M.D.
Division of Hematology/Oncology
Department of Pediatrics
The Floating Hospital for Children at the New England Medical Center
Tufts University School of Medicine
Boston, MA 02111

Kenneth L. McClain, M.D., Ph.D.
Texas Children's Cancer Center and Hematology Service
1102 Bates Street, Suite 10.010
Houston, TX 77030

Dafna Meitar, M.D.
Children's Memorial Hospital
Division of Hematology/Oncology, Box #30
2300 Children's Plaza
Chicago, IL 60614

Elaine R. Morgan, M.D.
Children's Memorial Hospital
Division of Hematology/Oncology, Box #30
2300 Children's Plaza
Chicago, IL 60614

Alberto S. Pappo, M.D.
Department of Hematology-Oncology
St. Jude Children's Research Hospital
332 North Lauderdale
Memphis, TN 38105-2729

Elizabeth J. Perlman, M.D.
The Department of Pathology
Johns Hopkins Hospital
600 North Wolfe Street
Baltimore, MD 21287-3881

Cindy L. Schwartz, M.D.
Johns Hopkins Oncology Center
Division of Pediatric Oncology
CMSC 800
600 North Wolfe Street
Baltimore, MD 21287

David N. Shapiro, M.D.
Department of Experimental Oncology
St. Jude Children's Research Hospital
332 North Lauderdale
Memphis, TN 38105-2729

Gail E. Tomlinson, M.D., Ph.D.
University of Texas Southwestern Medical Center
Department of Pediatrics
5323 Harry Hines Boulevard
Dallas, Texas 75235-9063

Joon Won Yoon, Ph.D.
Children's Memorial Institute for Education and Research
Developmental Systems Biology, Box #204
Children's Memorial Hospital
2310 North Halsted Street
Chicago, IL 60614

David O. Walterhouse, M.D.
Division of Hematology/Oncology, Box #30
Children's Memorial Hospital
2300 Children's Plaza
Chicago, IL 60614

Daniel C. West, M.D.
University of California, Davis Medical Center
Department of Pediatrics
2516 Stockton Boulevard
Sacramento, CA 95616

Preface

The purpose of *Diagnostic and Therapeutic Advances in Pediatric Oncology* for the Cancer Treatment and Research Series is to provide an up-to-date summary of how recent advances in cancer research are being applied to the care of children with solid tumors. The interface of cancer research with clinical practice in pediatric oncology has never been more intimate than today. While researchers are identifying oncogenes and tumor suppressor genes and are studying their specific functions, clinicians are using knowledge of oncogenes and tumor suppressor genes for diagnosing cancer in children, for therapeutic decision-making purposes, and for prognostic purposes. The first three chapters in this book describe models for understanding the causes of childhood cancer that were perhaps initially identified by clinicians and that are now being studied and understood by researchers. These chapters will describe research evidence that supports roles for the involvement of normal developmental regulatory genes in childhood oncogenesis, of abnormal immune regulation in childhood oncogenesis, and of heredity in childhood oncogenesis. The next eight chapters are devoted to descriptions of the application of new research developments to clinical practice with reference to the most common forms of solid tumors of childhood outside the central nervous system. The final chapter will describe late effects of childhood cancer and its therapy and the impact research is having on understanding and perhaps preventing these late effects. The emphasis on bridging research developments and clinical practice will make this book a unique resource for researchers and clinicians as the application of research developments to clinical practice increases and as clinical observations are studied with modern research tools.

David Walterhouse and Susan Cohn

I

Understanding the Causes of Tumors of Childhood

1. Embryonic development and pediatric oncogenesis

David O. Walterhouse and Joon Won Yoon

1. Introduction

In recent years, significant advances in understanding the molecular genetics of human cancer have been made. Application of these research advances to clinical practice is beginning. While researchers are identifying oncogenes and tumor suppressor genes and studying their specific functions, clinicians are using knowledge of oncogenes and tumor suppressor genes for diagnosing cancer, for therapeutic decision making purposes, and for prognostic purposes. Clearly, the future will bring new therapies based on molecular genetic advances.

Application of molecular genetic advances to clinical practice is particularly relevant to the pediatric oncologist. Major breakthroughs in understanding tumor suppressor genes have been made through the study of specific childhood tumors such as retinoblastoma, Wilms' tumor, and rhabdomyosarcoma. Identification of genes located at chromosomal translocation breakpoints and studies of the function of fusion transcripts resulting from these translocations are ongoing for rhabdomyosarcoma and Ewing's sarcoma. Finally, molecular genetic abnormalities that can be identified within childhood neuroblastoma tumor cells perhaps represent the best example of how oncologists today determine prognosis and treatment based on molecular genetics.

The field of pediatric oncology is characterized by a unique group of embryonal-type tumors that differ markedly from the more common adult tumors that typically arise in differentiated tissues. Based on the histologic embryonal nature of these tumors as well as the young age of the patients, it has been hypothesized that childhood tumors may result from dysregulation of normal developmental regulatory gene pathways during embryonic as well as postembryonic development. Greaves hypothesized that the initiating events of childhood leukemia occur in utero in cells under proliferative stress, with promoting events occurring during the early childhood years, and he argues that the solution to understanding childhood leukemia lies within the developmental biology of the cell type from which the disease arises [1]. This hypothesis suggests that our understanding of childhood oncogenesis will be enhanced by an understanding of embryonic development.

D.O. Walterhouse and S.L. Cohn (eds), DIAGNOSTIC AND THERAPEUTIC ADVANCES IN PEDIATRIC ONCOLOGY. Copyright © 1997. Kluwer Academic Publishers, Boston. All rights reserved.

Within the past decade, a great deal has been learned about the molecular genetic regulation of mammalian embryonic development. Two recurring themes of critical importance to pediatric oncologists have been demonstrated by studies of embryonic development and will be dealt with in detail throughout this chapter. First, there is significant evidence for evolutionary conservation of several of the molecular genetic pathways regulating embryonic development in organisms as diverse as fruit flies, mice, and humans. Applying principles and direct knowledge obtained from studying development in organisms such as fruit flies is significantly enhancing our progress in understanding mammalian development and oncogenesis. Second, the previously hypothesized links between childhood cancer and embryonic development of humans have been supported by the identification of developmental regulatory genes, oncogenes, and tumor suppressor genes and by showing that genes involved in pediatric oncogenesis indeed frequently function normally during development.

The purpose of this chapter is to describe molecular genetic mechanisms that have recently been shown to regulate specific aspects of mammalian embryonic development and to relate these developmental regulatory processes to what is known about childhood cancer at a molecular genetic level. It is hoped that, by more clearly understanding development, we will obtain insights into known mechanisms contributing to the development of childhood cancer as well as insight into new mechanisms that have not been previously considered.

2. Molecular genetic control of development

Central problems of developmental biology identified decades ago include cell fate specification and embryonic pattern formation. In recent years, molecular biology techniques have been applied to embryologic problems, and characterization of the central problems of developmental biology at a molecular and cellular level has begun. Following fertilization, cellular proliferation begins at an accelerated rate. The cells of the developing embryo follow four basic developmental pathways, namely, proliferation, differentiation, quiescence, or apoptosis [2]. As these cellular processes proceed and cell migration occurs, the developing embryo develops a polarity, and eventually pattern formation begins in which differentiating cells form the specific tissues and organs in a specified body plan. Peptide growth factors, extracellular matrix components, cell–cell interactions, and transcription factors all regulate these processes.

In this chapter, some of the known mechanisms regulating development will be considered in detail. First, the developmental regulatory role of the HOX gene family will be considered. This family of genes has been studied in greater detail than any other in mammalian development, and lessons learned from studying this family during development may have application to other families of genes during development as well as to understanding oncogenesis.

Central to understanding the role of HOX genes in mammalian development has been the high degree of evolutionary conservation of these genes. Second, genomic imprinting will be considered. Imprinting is a novel form of gene regulation identified during mammalian development in which expression of specific genes demonstrate parental dependency. Imprinting has already proven to have direct application to our understanding of mechanisms of oncogenesis. Finally, specification of cell fate and pattern formation during development by specific genes that have already been shown to play a role in childhood cancer will be considered.

3. HOX genes in normal development

Genes that control the early events of embryogenesis have been most intensively studied in *Drosophila melanogaster*. Homeobox genes represent the most intensively studied group of developmental regulatory genes in *Drosophila*. Since the discovery of the homeobox as a *Drosophila* developmental regulatory gene motif, increasing numbers of homeobox-containing genes have been identified in mammals [3–5]. Much of the progress in understanding the function of these genes in mammals is in fact based directly on work in *Drosophila*. Since genetic studies in *Drosophila* generally proceed at a more rapid pace than is possible in mammals, this ability to extrapolate to the mammal information learned from fruit flies has greatly accelerated our understanding of molecular genetic control of human development. Comparative biology has proven to be a critical tool in understanding development, and the experience with development suggests that comparative biology will be an important tool in understanding the genetics of human cancer. Understanding *Drosophila* development is of importance to the pediatric oncologist.

3.1. HOX genes in Drosophila development

Drosophila are segmented organisms containing a head segment, three thoracic segments, and eight abdominal segments (figure 1). Each segment of the adult fly has its own identity characterized by a specific cuticle pattern and the presence of specific structures. For example, the first thoracic segment has only legs, the second has legs and wings, and the third has legs and balancers known as *halteres*.

The stages of embryonic development in the fruit fly that lead to the segmented pattern of the adult have been well described, and classes of genes regulating these embryonic stages have also been described, including maternal-effect genes, segmentation genes, and homeotic genes. First, mRNAs of maternal-effect genes, which are present in gradients along the anterior–posterior axis in the unfertilized egg, are responsible for determining the polarity of the developing embryo. An anterior group of maternal-effect

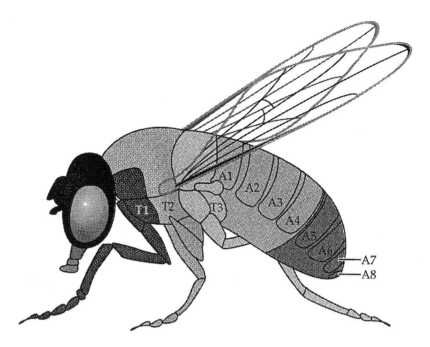

Figure 1. Illustration of an adult fruit fly, demonstrating a head segment, three thoracic segments, and eight abdominal segments, each with a unique identity. (Reprinted with permission of Sinauer Associates, Inc. from Gilbert: *Developmental Biology*, Fourth Edition, 1994.)

genes, including the homeobox gene *bicoid*, is necessary for development of head and thoracic structures, while a posterior group of maternal-effect genes, including *nanos*, is required for development of the abdomen. Maternal-effect genes encode proteins that activate or repress expression of specific zygotic genes called *segmentation genes* [6]. Segmentation genes are responsible for dividing the developing embryo into segments.

Three classes of segmentation genes have been identified based on general phenotypic patterns caused by mutations within these genes. These classes of

→

Figure 2. Expression of developmental regulatory gene products during *Drosophila* development. (**A**) Protein product of the maternal effect gene *nanos* localizes to the posterior pole of the *Drosophila* egg. (**B**) A broad band of expression of the gap segmentation gene product *Kruppel* in the fly embryo divides the embryo into three broad regions. (**C**) Expression of the protein product of the pair-rule segmentation gene *fushi tarazu* further divides the developing embryo by expression in seven stripes along the anterior–posterior axis. (**D**) The segment polarity gene product of *gooseberry* is expressed in every segment along the anterior–posterior axis of the developing embryo. Note that the posterior end of the embryo has curled toward the head. This embryonic stage is referred to as *germ band extension*. (Reprinted with permission from Patel NH. 1994. Developmental evolution: insights from studies of insect segmentation. *Science* 266: 582. Copyright 1994 American Association for the Advancement of Science.)

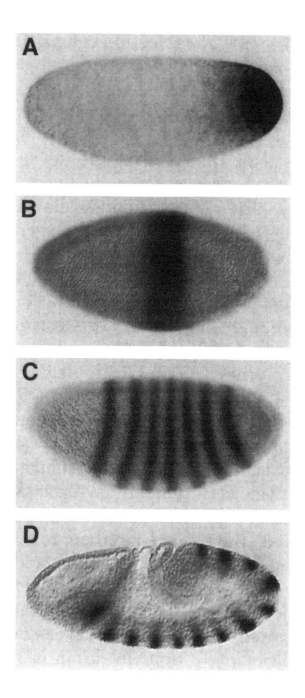

segmentation genes are called *gap genes*, *pair rule genes*, and *segment polarity genes* (figure 2) [7]. The first class of segmentation gene to be activated, the gap genes, are expressed in approximately three broad bands along the anterior–posterior axis of the embryo, dividing the developing embryo into three broad domains. Mutations within gap genes result in the loss of adjacent segments in the adult fly, or 'gaps' in the normal developmental pattern. Examples of gap genes include *Kruppel*, *knirps*, and *hunchback*. Mutations within *Kruppel* may result in loss of all thoracic and the first five abdominal segments in the adult fly.

The different concentrations of the gap gene proteins along the anterior–posterior axis cause expression of the pair rule segmentation genes, which are expressed in seven vertical bands along the anterior–posterior axis, subdividing the gap domains into smaller domains that are each about two segment primordia wide. Mutations within pair rule genes cause deletion of portions of every other body segment. Examples of pair rule genes include *hairy* (which shows sequence homology with human *N-myc*), *even-skipped*, and *fushi tarazu*.

The stripes of the pair rule gene products activate expression of the segment polarity segmentation genes. The segment polarity gene products form 14 bands across the embryo, subdividing the pair rule domains and dividing the embryo into the final segment-wide units. Mutations within segment polarity genes result in deletions within each body segment and replacement of the deleted region of the segment by a mirror-image structure from another portion of the segment. Examples of segment polarity genes include *cubitus interruptus* (which shows sequence homology with human *GLI*), *gooseberry* (which shows sequence homology with the PAX family genes), and *patched*. Mutations within *cubitus interruptus* result in loss of the posterior portion of each segment and replacement of the posterior portion with a mirror-image duplication of the anterior portion.

Gap, pair rule, and segment polarity proteins interact to activate the homeotic developmental regulatory genes. Homeotic genes determine the fate or identity of each segment. Mutations within homeotic genes result in changes in cell fate, with normal body structures appearing in inappropriate segments. *Antennapedia* is an example of a homeotic gene that specifies the fate of the second thoracic segment. *Antennapedia* directs the development of legs and wings within this segment. If *Antennapedia* is ectopically expressed in the head, then legs will grow in place of normal antennae; if *Antennapedia* is not expressed in the second thoracic segment, then antennae will grow in place of legs.

Most *Drosophila* homeotic genes are clustered, forming the *Antennapedia/Bithorax* complex of genes. Genes making up the *Antennapedia/Bithorax* complex include, from 3′ to 5′ along the chromosome, *labial*, *proboscipedia*, *deformed*, *sex combs reduced*, *antennapedia*, *ultrabithorax*, *abdominal A*, and *abdominal B*. The genes of the *Antennapedia/Bithorax* complex are the focus of this section of the chapter, since they have been extensively studied and

8

illustrate some important principles of the molecular genetic control of embryonic development.

Each gene within this complex contains a highly conserved 183-base-pair (bp) motif called the *homeobox* as well as divergent sequences outside the homeobox region [8]. Homeobox genes encode proteins containing a 61-amino-acid motif called the *homeodomain*. The amino acid sequence of the antennapedia homeodomain is RKRGRQTYTRYQTLELEK EFHFNRYLTRRRRIEIAHALCLTERQIKIWFQNRRMKWKKEN. The secondary structure of the homeodomain is a helix-turn-helix that mediates DNA binding to the 5′-TAAT-3′ core motif and allows the protein to function as a transcription factor [9–12]. Although these genes encode proteins with highly similar homeodomains and presumably similar DNA binding affinity, specificity of function may occur through specific temporal and spatial expression patterns as well as unique protein sequences lying outside of the homeodomain [13].

Expression patterns for the genes of the *Antennapedia/Bithorax* complex have been analyzed using in situ hybridization, and their expression is most prominent within the epidermis and the central nervous system. Each gene in the complex has been shown to direct cell fate during a specific developmental period within a specific region along the anterior–posterior axis of the developing embryo [14–16]. In general, genes located most 3′ in the complex, i.e., *labial, proboscipedia*, and *deformed*, are expressed earliest and specify head structures; genes located centrally within the complex, i.e., *sex combs reduced, antennapedia*, and *ultrabithorax*, are expressed next and specify thoracic segments; and genes located more 5′, i.e., *abdominal A* and *B*, are expressed last and specify abdominal segments. This organization, with the order of the genes within the complex mapping the anterior–posterior axis of the developing embryo, is referred to as *colinearity* [17]. Based on these studies in *Drosophila*, colinearity has become recognized as a fundamental mechanism for the determination of regional identity during development. In addition, based on *Drosophila* studies, it has been demonstrated that more posterior-acting genes within the complex appear to repress more anterior-acting genes. For example, *antennapedia* is repressed posteriorly by all the homeotic gene products found posterior to it, and deletion of any posterior-acting gene will result in extension of the expression domain of *antennapedia* posteriorly. To fully understand the function of these genes, downstream target genes must be identified. Identification of downstream targets is the focus of much current research in the field.

3.2. HOX genes in mammalian development

Mammalian development is poorly understood relative to development of the fruit fly because of the increased complexity of the genome as well as the complexity of the events during embryonic development. Knowledge from the fruit fly, however, has provided a framework upon which to build an understanding of the molecular genetics of mammalian development. Searches of the mammalian genome, including mouse and human, for the recurrent homeobox motifs found in the *Drosophila* homeotic genes have demonstrated evolutionary conservation of the homebox.

Mammalian homeobox genes have been identified that share a homeodomain highly related to the homeodomain of the *Drosophila Antennapedia/Bithorax* complex genes [10]. Mouse and human genes belonging to this class are called HOX genes [18,19]. As in the case of flies, the mammalian HOX genes are clustered [4,20–26]. In the mammal, four distinct clusters have been identified on four distinct chromosomes [4]. It is believed that these clusters of homeobox genes arose by duplication and divergence from a common ancestral cluster [27]. The human HOXA, HOXB, HOXC, and HOXD gene clusters are located on chromosomes 7, 17, 12, and 2, respectively. The order of the genes in each cluster is highly conserved, and genes in specific positions in the four clusters can be aligned based on maximal sequence homology (figure 3).

Relationship of *Antennapedia-Bithorax* complex and *HOX* complexes

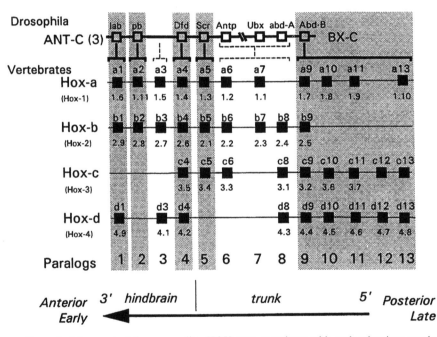

Figure 3. Alignment of the mammalian HOX gene complexes with each other into paralogous groups and with the *Drosophila Antennapedia/Bithorax* complex. Current nomenclature is shown above the boxes, and old nomenclature is listed below the boxes. As indicated, 3′ genes are expressed earliest during development and most anteriorly within the embryo, while 5′ genes are expressed later during development and most posteriorly within the embryo (Reprinted with permission of Krumlauf R. 1994. Hox genes in vertebrate development. *Cell* 78: 192. Copyright held by Cell Press.)

This alignment defines 13 'paralogous' groups of genes within the clusters [28]. None of the clusters includes genes in all 13 paralogous groups. A total of 38 HOX genes have been identified in the four HOX clusters, with each cluster containing 9 to 11 genes. The strongest homologies to the *Antennapedia/Bithorax* complex genes of *Drosophila* are between paralogous group 1 and *labial*, group 2 and *proboscipedia*, group 4 and *deformed*, group 5 and *sex combs reduced*, and groups 9–13 and *abdominal B* [27]. Group 3 has no comparable *Drosophila* gene, and groups 6–8 have comparable degrees of similarity to *antennapedia, ultrabithorax*, and *abdominal A*. Based on the similar cluster organization of the mammalian genes with the *Drosophila* genes and on significant sequence similarity not only within the homeodomain but also extending outside the homeodomain between mammalian HOX genes and *Drosophila Antennapedia/Bithorax* complex genes, it has been suggested that mammalian HOX genes may play a fundamental role during embryonic development similar to the role of the *Drosophila* genes [26,29,30].

The function of HOX genes is now being studied using loss-of-function knockout mice and gain-of-function transgenic mice. Although the phenotypes of these mice are frequently less severe than might be predicted by the expression patterns during development, early analysis of these animals has shown that HOX genes truly function as vertebrate homeotic genes, specifying segmental identity along the anterior–posterior axis of the developing embryo. Phenotypic alterations in the mice can be somewhat predictable based on the phenotype of *Drosophila*, with mutations in the corresponding paralogous gene. Several 'rules' governing HOX gene expression and function have been described.

First, HOX genes in mammals demonstrate temporal and spatial colinear expression. Within each complex, genes at the extreme 3′ end of the clusters are activated earliest temporally and have the most anterior boundaries of expression (figure 4) [31]. Temporally, transcripts are never detected from a given HOX gene before transcripts are produced by the 3′ neighbor in the complex. Spatially, restricted domains of expression have been described in the nervous system, including the neural tube, neural crest, and hindbrain segments; and within paraxial mesoderm, limbs, surface ectoderm, branchial arches, gut, and gonadal tissue. The 3′ paralogous group 1 and 2 genes are expressed starting in anterior positions within the hindbrain, and the 5′ paralogous groups 12 and 13 genes are expressed in more posterior regions, such as the genitalia [27]. In the central nervous system, the anterior border of expression of many of the HOX genes coincides with rhombomeric boundaries in the developing hindbrain, indicating the segmental organization of the brain [32]. Targeted mutagenesis of HOXA1 in mice results in delayed closure of the neural tube in the hindbrain region as well as abnormalities attributable to defects in structures derived from hindbrain rhombomeres 4–7, (including absence of several cranial nerve motor nuclei and sensory ganglia, inner ear defects, and basal skull anomalies), while HOXA3-deficient mice have a more

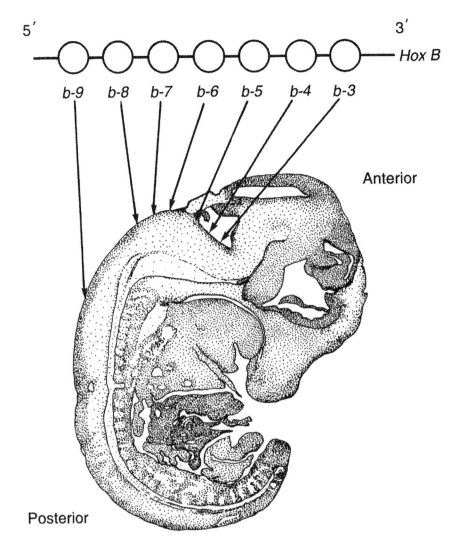

5'   3'

b-9   b-8   b-7   b-6   b-5   b-4   b-3   Hox B

Anterior

Posterior

Figure 4. The HOXB complex is illustrated in the upper part of the figure, and a sagittal section of a day 12.5 mouse embryo is drawn in the lower part of the figure. Arrows indicate the anterior boundaries of expression within the central nervous system for the HOXB complex genes. The 3' genes are expressed more anteriorly, and the 5' genes are expressed more posteriorly. (Reprinted with permission of The McGraw-Hill Companies from Kalthoff: *Analysis of Biological Development*, 1996.)

posterior distinctive pattern of craniofacial, thyroid, thymic, and cardiac anomalies [33,34].

Second, there is significant overlap in expression domains among members of paralogous groups, particularly for the HOXA and HOXD clusters, and redundant or partially redundant function of the genes makes interpretation

12

of mutations in only one gene sometimes difficult [35]. Details of the regulation of this complex coordinated expression pattern remain unknown.

Third, HOX gene expression appears to be dependent on cell proliferation, with significant HOX gene expression occurring in actively proliferating regions [36]. It has been proposed that HOX genes may function by coupling proliferation with morphogenesis [36,37].

Fourth, more HOX genes are generally expressed in posterior regions, and more posterior-acting HOX proteins appear to be dominant over more anterior-acting proteins. This finding is referred to as *posterior prevalence* and refers to the fact that a given HOX gene will exert its function in a region where it is the most posterior of the HOX genes expressed [38]. Thus, loss of HOX gene function leads to the development of anterior structures where more posterior structures should have formed, particularly within the anterior part of the expression domain. For example, targeted gene disruption of HOXC8 results in the conversion of the first lumbar vertebra into a thoracic vertebra with an additional rib, and targeted disruption of HOXB4 results in transformation of the second cervical vertebra, the axis, into a duplicate first cervical vertebra, the atlas [39]. Alternatively, ectopic anterior expression of HOX genes leads to the development of posterior structures where more anterior structures should normally be found. For example, overexpression of HOXA7 transforms the basio-occiptal bone into a proatlas structure, and overexpression of HOXD4 results in the transformation of occipital bones into structures that resemble cervical vertebrae [8].

It is clear from these observations of HOX gene function that abnormalities in temporal or spatial expression patterns may have significant developmental consequences. Identification of HOX target genes will be necessary to complete an understanding of the function of these genes in regulating regional identity. Unfortunately, identification of target genes has remained problematic. It is expected, however, that the identification of target genes in *Drosophila* may then allow candidate target genes to be identified in the mammal.

Finally, HOX genes have been shown to be expressed in normal adult tissues as well as during development [4,40]. Distinct patterns of HOX gene expression have been demonstrated in adult kidney, lung, liver, and colon [40–42]. In addition, HOX genes have been described that are located outside of HOX complexes and appear to be isolated within the genome.

3.3. HOX genes in cancer

Based on their role as important developmental regulatory genes, it has been proposed that HOX genes may be important in oncogenesis [43,44]. Observations supporting a role for HOX genes in malignancy include their ability to transform murine cell lines when constitutively expressed or activated by either proviral insertion or chromosomal rearrangement, differing HOX gene expression patterns in human tumor cells compared with normal cells from a specific organ, and a specific example of altered expression of HOX11 as a result of chromosomal translocation in human T-cell leukemia.

Transfection of CMV promoter-driven expression vectors for HOXA1, A5, A7, B7, and C8 into mouse NIH3T3 cells and rat 208F cells results in cell transformation [45]. Transfected cells grow in foci; grow in soft agar, with the exception of HOXA5; and, again with the exception of HOXA5, form tumors in nude mice. Histologically, the tumors resemble poorly differentiated spindle cell sarcomas. Induction of HOXB8 expression by proviral insertion in bone marrow cells results in a leukemic phenotype. In addition, HOXB8 is constitutively expressed in murine WEHI-3B cells as a result of a chromosomal rearrangement that inserts an intracisternal A particle upstream of HOXB8 [46,47].

Altered HOX gene expression, compared to that of normal tissue, has been observed in renal cell carcinoma and colorectal carcinoma. HOXB5 and HOXB9 are expressed in the normal adult kidney; however, the majority of renal cell carcinomas tested do not show expression of these HOX genes [40,48]. HOXC11 is not expressed in the normal kidney; however, HOXC11 transcripts are present in renal cell carcinomas [40]. Whereas four HOXD4 transcripts are normally found in the adult kidney, only a subset of these transcripts are frequently found in renal cell carcinoma [48]. In the normal colon, HOXA1 through 4 are usually expressed; however, they are often silent in colorectal carcinomas, and HOXD11 transcription is increased in colorectal carcinoma over normal colon [41,48]. HOXB7 and HOXD4, both of which are expressed in the normal colon, demonstrate altered transcript patterns in some colorectal carcinomas [48]. It has additionally been suggested that altered HOX gene expression may be seen in metastatic lesions compared with primary colorectal tumors and normal intestinal mucosa [48].

HOX gene expression has also been described in leukemia, breast cancer, small cell lung carcinoma, Wilms' tumor, and neuroblastoma. Different types of human leukemia are characterized by specific patterns of HOX gene expression, with the most significant variations in HOX gene expression between different types of leukemia occurring in the HOXB cluster. Murine myeloid leukemia and fibrosarcomas have been associated with HOXB8 expression [49]. HOXA1, HOXA10, HOXB6, and HOXC6 are expressed in the human breast cancer cell line MCF7, and further studies may define a role for these genes in the development and progression of human breast cancer [50]. Interestingly, in variant-type small cell lung carcinoma, HOX gene expression has been reported to change in metastatic versus primary tumors [51]. In a case of Wilms' tumor, two abundant HOXC11 transcripts were detected, whereas HOXC11 expression is generally undetectable in the normal kidney [48]. Finally, upregulation of HOXC6, HOXD1, and HOXD8 expression has been shown in human neuroblastoma cells chemically induced to differentiate, suggesting an association of these HOX genes with maturation toward a differentiated neuronal phenotype [52]. In each of these settings, further studies will be necessary to define the role of HOX genes in tissue differentiation and tumor development and progression.

The translocation t(10;14)(q24;q11) is observed in 5%–10% of patients with T-cell acute lymphoblastic leukemia [53]. The genes involved at the translocation breakpoints are the T-cell receptor delta-chain gene at 14q11 and the HOX11 gene at 10q24. HOX11 was initially identified through cloning of the t(10;14) translocation. Although classified as a HOX gene, HOX11 is not a part of the HOX clusters. The result of the translocation is inappropriate expression of HOX11 in T cells that acquire the mutation, which is believed to play a role in cell transformation. The mouse homologue of HOX11, Tlx-1, is a developmental regulatory gene that is expressed in the developing spleen. Tlx-1 knockout mice are asplenic [54,55].

These preliminary studies describe abnormal HOX gene expression patterns in several human malignancies. Clearly, however, further studies need to be carried out to clarify the role of HOX genes in human malignancy. To understand this role, attention must be paid to unifying themes of HOX gene organization and function, such as colinear organization and expression, expression of paralogous HOX gene groups, and dominance of posterior-acting HOX proteins over more anterior-acting HOX proteins. Perhaps only by understanding HOX gene function during normal development will we be able to recognize the disruptions in HOX gene function that contribute to human malignancy. Furthermore, general principles of developmental regulatory control illustrated by the HOX gene family may have application to understanding developmental regulation by other gene families, as well as the dysregulation by other gene families that contributes to human malignancy.

4. Genomic imprinting during mammalian development

Some genetic traits in mammals demonstrate parental dependency. Expression of these traits is based on the genetic material inherited from one parent. Parental dependency may be caused by unequal distribution of genetic information between male and female gametes. While the egg carries the unique mitochondrial and maternal-effect genes and, of course, can only be expressed from maternal inheritance, the sperm carries the unique genes on the Y chromosome that can only be expressed from paternal inheritance. Imprinted hemizygosity or *imprinting*, on the other hand, describes parental-dependent traits in which both the male and female alleles are present but function unequally in the embryo. Through epigenetic modification, an imprinted allele becomes reversibly differentially processed during either male or female gametogenesis. Consequently, during specific developmental periods, either the male or female allele will be exclusively expressed. If the paternal allele is solely expressed, then the gene is maternally imprinted; if the maternal allele alone is expressed, then the gene is paternally imprinted.

Early evidence for parental dependency during development included murine pronuclear experiments, observations of human triploid phenotypes, and observations of trophoblastic diseases demonstrating uniparental disomy. Murine pronuclear experiments showed that neither maternal:maternal 'gynogenetic' nor paternal:paternal 'androgenetic' zygotes could develop to full-term embryos [56,57]. A bipaternal conception formed only a placenta, while a bimaternal conception evolved solely into disorganized embryonal tissues. Biparental status was necessary for the development of a normal placenta and a normal viable fetus. Observations of human triploid phenotypes that resulted in uniparental genomic excess have supported these data and demonstrate retarded embryos accompanied either by hyperplasia of the placenta in cases of paternal excess or hypoplasia of the placenta in cases of maternal excess. Uniparental disomy is demonstrated in naturally occurring complete hydatidiform moles and ovarian teratomas. Complete hydatidiform moles are androgenetic and are made up of highly proliferative extraembryonic membranes, while ovarian teratomas are gynogenetic and are made up of disorganized embryonic tissues. Early observations that cell proliferative rate and growth seemed to be enhanced in situations of paternal uniparental disomy and that growth appeared to be decreased in situations of maternal uniparental disomy led to a hypothesis suggesting that imprinting evolved because of opposing paternal and maternal influences on growth of the embryo [58,59].

Some of the known imprinted genes whose expression is restricted to either the maternal or paternal allele in humans and mice are listed in table 1. The extent of monoallelic expression varies for these genes during development and differentiation. Interestingly, the majority of imprinted genes in the human have been shown to cluster to specific domains on chromosome 11 or 15. This clustering may provide clues to the imprinting mechanism. It has been suggested that groups of genes are imprinted by common cis-acting sequences. One imprinter control gene has been described that maps to the X chromosome [60]. The mechanism of imprinting, however, remains uncertain, and it is not even clear whether each imprinted gene is imprinted by the same mechanism. The mechanism of imprinting must be heritable in somatic tissues during development and must be reversed in the germline. All imprinted genes studied so far contain DNA sequences that have been methylated in a parental-specific manner in the germline, and DNA methylation is currently thought to be the most likely mechanism of imprinting [61,62]. Methylation may be inherited from one gamete or may be acquired during embryonic development. DNA methylation is the enzymatic addition of a methyl group to the 5-position of the cytidine ring in genomic DNA, usually in a CpG dinucleotide by DNA methyltransferase [63]. Mice deficient for DNA methyltransferase die in the early postimplantation period, perhaps due to instability of primary imprints. These mice lose monoallelic expression of several imprinted genes, including H19 and IGF2 [64–66]. Since DNA methyltransferase functions primarily as a maintenance enzyme and demonstrates a preference for hemimethylated sites, it may help maintain methylation stability but probably

Table 1. Mammalian imprinted genes

Gene	Expressed allele	Chromosome	
		Mouse	Human
WT1	M	2	11p
INS	P	7	11p
IGF2	P	7	11p
H19	M	7	11p
p57KIP2	M	7	11p
MASH2	M	7	nd
SNRPN	P	7	15q
ZNF127	P	7	15q
PAR1	P	nd	15q
PAR5	P	nd	15q
IPW	P	nd	15q
IGF2R/MPR300	M	17	6q
MAS	M	17	nd
XIST	P/R	X	X
PEG1/MEST	P	6	nd
SP2	P	11	nd

Mammalian genes that demonstrate parental imprinting are listed. Abbreviations: WT1, Wilms' tumor 1; INS, insulin; IGF2, insulin-like growth factor 2; SNRPN, small nuclear riboprotein particle SmN; IGF2R/MPR300, insulin-like growth factor 2 receptor (also called the mannose 6-phosphate 300-kD receptor); XIST, X chromosome-inactive specific transcript. (Reprinted with permission from Barlow DP 1995. Genomic imprinting in mammals. *Science* 270: 1611. Copyright 1995 American Association for the Advancement of Science.)

does not represent *the* imprinting enzyme. It has been hypothesized that methylation alters chromatin structure and modulates the access of DNA binding proteins that repress or activate transcription of imprinted genes [67]. In addition, it has been observed that imprinted DNA sequences demonstrate regions rich in direct repeats [68,69]. These repeats show a range of size and show no homology to each other in the various imprinted genes studied so far. It is speculated that these regions play a role in the imprinting mechanism.

The expression patterns of several imprinted genes during development have been described. Monoallelic expression of imprinted genes varies during development, during differentiation, and in disease. H19, IGF2, and WT1 are of particular interest for this text. H19 and IGF2 map to 11p15.5, while WT1 maps to 11p13.

The paternally imprinted gene H19 is abundantly expressed during embryogenesis. In the mouse, a methylation imprint appears to repress the paternal H19 allele. Monoallelic maternal expression of H19 has been demonstrated in preimplantation embryonic stages. H19 mRNA transcripts are most abundant in the fetal adrenal gland, skeletal muscle, and kidney [70]. In the fetal kidney, H19 is most strongly expressed in metanephric blastema. Expression decreases dramatically as differentiation into renal tubules occurs [71]. Consistent with this pattern, nephrogenic rests have been shown to have high levels of H19 expression [71]. Prominent H19 expression has also been demonstrated in the urothelium along the urinary collecting system of the fetus but not in the adult. Lower levels of H19 expression have been demonstrated during embryogenesis in the lung, heart, spleen, thymus, and mucosa of the small intestine. Bi-allelic repression of H19 expression has been shown in the developing nervous system. Consistent with these embryonic data, immature ovarian teratomas demonstrate H19 mRNA expression in endodermal and mesodermal derived tissues and not in neuroectodermal elements [71]. Mature tissues in adults and mature tissue elements in mature ovarian teratomas do not show H19 mRNA expression.

The function of the H19 gene is unknown; in fact, there is no evidence that H19 mRNA encodes a protein in the embryo [72]. Maternally expressed H19 appears to inhibit *cis* expression of maternal IGF2, and H19 has been shown to function as a tumor suppressor gene in some tumor cell lines [73,74]. Altered expression of H19, however, is associated with significant pathology. H19 gain-of-function transgenic embryos die at around day 15 of mouse gestation, demonstrating the significant role of H19 during development [75]. H19 reexpression has been observed in malignancies involving tissues that normally demonstrate H19 expression during development, including choriocarcinoma, rhabdomyosarcoma, Wilms' tumor, urothelial carcinoma, and ovarian teratoma [2]. Neuroectodermal tissues do not show H19 expression during development, and tumors of neuroectodermal tissues do not show H19 expression [2].

While H19 is paternally imprinted, insulin-like growth factor 2 (IGF2) is maternally imprinted [76–78]. The maternal IGF2 imprint likely results from methylation and activation of the upstream *cis* H19 gene [73]. The expression patterns of IGF2 and H19 are nearly identical. The few exceptions include the choroid plexus, leptomeninges, and the ciliary anlage of the retina, which do not shown H19 expression [79]. Biallelic expression of IGF2 is seen in the fetal choroid plexus and leptomeninges of the central nervous system and within the adult liver [79]. IGF2 encodes a fetal peptide growth factor that generally mediates its growth-regulating effect through the IGF1 receptor [80]. The gene product is without doubt an important embryonic growth factor for normal development. IGF2 knockout mice show growth retardation at term but have a normal postnatal growth rate and are otherwise fertile and without abnormalities [81]. In addition to the variation in monoallelic expression that occurs in development and differentiation, IGF2 has been shown to switch to biallelic expression in human tumors and in Beckwith–Wiedeman syndrome [82–84].

WT1 is an example of a polymorphic imprinted human gene. It is located at a locus distinct from the IGF2-H19 gene cluster [85]. Its expression is normally biallelic in the kidney, and it plays a crucial role in early urogenital development. Homozygous WT1 knockout mice are embryonic lethal, with failure of kidney and gonadal development [86]. Monoallelic imprinted expression of the WT1 gene has been demonstrated only in the placenta and fetal brain. Paternal imprinting of WT1 is seen in the placenta [87]. Imprinted expression of WT1 appears to be a polymorphic trait, seen in only some individuals in the population [87]. WT1 is generally not subject to transcriptional imprinting in Wilms' tumor or normal fetal kidney [88]. The significance of polymorphic imprinting to normal development and oncogenesis is uncertain.

4.1. Aberrant imprinting in development

Aberrant imprinting could theoretically lead to a double dose of a particular gene product if an 'imprinted' gene is not turned off or could lead to the absence of a gene product if the 'active' allele is not expressed. It is now known that dysregulation of the developmental regulatory process of imprinting may have clinical consequences. Mechanisms that have actually been identified in pathologic human conditions include loss of heterozygosity with uniparental disomy at imprinted loci or loss of imprinting, also referred to as *relaxation* of imprinting. As might be expected, this dysregulation may result in clinical syndromes characterized by multiple birth defects as well as human cancer. Examples of syndromes characterized by altered imprinting include Prader–Willi syndrome, Angelman syndrome, and Beckwith–Wiedeman syndrome.

Prader–Willi syndrome and Angelman syndrome both seem to involve an identical chromosomal segment at 15q11–13. Maternal uniparental disomy for 15q11–12 or a visible cytogenetic deletion of the same region from the paternal chromosome is seen in Prader–Willi syndrome. This syndrome is characterized by a special facies, small hands and feet, hypogonadism, mild to moderate mental retardation, uncontrolled appetite, massive obesity, and infantile hypotonia [89,90]. Paternal uniparental disomy for 15q11–12 or a visible cytogenetic deletion of the same region from the maternal chromosome is seen in Angelman syndrome [91]. Angelman syndrome is characterized by severe mental retardation, hyperactive behavior, happy disposition and outbursts of laughter, red cheeks, a large mouth, seizures, and ataxic movements. Thus, in Prader–Willi syndrome both alleles are maternal, while in Angelman syndrome both alleles are paternal [91]. Gene(s) that contribute to the differential phenotypic presentation of Prader–Willi syndrome and Angelman syndrome must be imprinted and lie within this chromosomal region. Human chromosome 15q11–13 is syntenic with a portion of mouse chromosome 7, where the maternally imprinted mouse Snrpn gene is found [92]. Snrpn is involved in mRNA processing. Human *SNRPN* has been shown to lie in the smallest region of deletion in Prader–Willi syndrome patients, which suggests a role for this gene in the Prader–Willi phenotype [93].

Beckwith–Wiedeman syndrome (BWS) is an overgrowth disorder characterized by gigantism, macroglossia, visceromegaly, abdominal wall defects, exophthalmos, and hypoglycemia. Organs affected by increased growth are the skeletal muscle, tongue, adrenals, kidneys, liver, pancreas, gonads, heart, paraganglia, and placenta [94–96]. Familial cases display a dominant mode of inheritance with a preferential maternal mode of transmission and linkage to 11p15.5 [97,98]. Sporadic cases show paternal uniparental disomy at chromosome 11p15, the region of the human IGF2 and H19 gene cluster [99,100]. Paternal uniparental disomy for the IGF2 locus results in a double dose of expressed IGF2 and may be in part responsible for the overgrowth phenotype. Loss of IGF2 imprinting has been found in normal fibroblasts of some BWS patients [101]. Interestingly, the sites of overgrowth seen in BWS are tissues in which IGF2 is normally abundantly expressed during development [102]. The role of H19 in BWS remains to be defined; however, H19 has been shown to be a tumor suppressor gene in Wilms' tumor cell lines [74,103,104]. These individuals demonstrate an inherited predisposition to cancer, with a 5%–10% incidence of neoplasms including Wilms' tumor, hepatoblastoma, adrenal cortical carcinoma, pancreatoblastoma, neuroblastoma/ganglioneuroma, and rhabdomyosarcoma [98,105–108]. The tumors in patients with BWS have an embryonal histology, show loss of the maternal allele and paternal uniparental disomy for 11p15.5 or relaxation of the IGF2 imprint, and all arise in tissues that normally express relatively high levels of IGF2 and H19 during development [70,109,110].

4.2. Aberrant imprinting in cancer

Several lines of evidence suggest a role for genomic imprinting in human cancer. The earliest observations included the fact that the genome in hydatidiform moles was androgenetic, while the genome in ovarian teratomas was parthenogenetic [111,112]. More recently, preferential loss of a specific parental allele has been demonstrated in several human tumors. Restriction fragment length polymorphisms can be used to distinguish the maternal and paternal alleles. In Wilms' tumor, hepatoblastoma, and embryonal rhabdomyosarcoma, loss of heterozygosity with preferential loss of the maternal allele has been shown at 11p15, while preferential loss of the maternal Rb locus at 13q14 has been shown in sporadic osteosarcoma and bilateral retinoblastoma [113–115].

In Wilms' tumors demonstrating loss of heterozygosity at 11p15, paternal uniparental disomy results in a double dose of paternally transcribed IGF2 [116,117]. In Wilms' tumors without loss of heterozygosity at 11p15, relaxation of the maternal imprint, or loss of imprinting, has been shown to result in a double dose of IGF2 [82,83]. Seventy percent of Wilms' tumors show loss of imprinting of IGF2 and express both the maternal and paternal IGF2 alleles, while 29% of Wilms' tumor show loss of the H19 imprint [82,83]. In Wilms' tumor, loss of imprinting of IGF2 is coupled to downregulation of H19. Abnormal methylation of H19 has been shown in Wilms' tumor and is thought to be the mechanism for the very low or undetectable levels of H19 transcripts [118]. While IGF2 can be considered a potential tumor-promoting gene functioning as an autocrine growth factor in Wilms' tumorigenesis, H19 can be considered a potential tumor suppressor gene in Wilms' tumorigenesis.

It has been hypothesized that loss of imprinting of IGF2 is a general feature of embryonal tumors. In support of this hypothesis, loss of heterozygosity with paternal uniparental disomy has also been reported in embryonal rhabdomyosarcoma [119]. More recently, loss of IGF2 imprinting has been described in the alveolar form of rhabdomyosarcoma as well [110]. In contrast to Wilms' tumor, loss of imprinting of IGF2 is not coupled to downregulation of H19 in embryonal rhabdomyosarcoma [71]. A tumor-promoting role for IGF2 as an autocrine growth factor in rhabdomyosarcoma tumorigenesis has been suggested, and clinical trials taking advantage of this information have been proposed that use suramin to inhibit IGF2 at its receptor. In addition, loss of heterozygosity at 11p15.5 and loss of imprinting have been reported in hepatoblastoma, although perhaps at lower frequency than in Wilms' tumor and rhabdomyosarcoma [120,121]. Similar to rhabdomyosarcoma, loss of imprinting in hepatoblastoma is not associated with downregualtion of H19.

Although neuroblastoma is an embryonal tumor originating from neural crest-derived cells, no evidence for loss of imprinting of H19 or IGF2 has been found [122]. Of interest, however, in cases of neuroblastoma demonstrating *N-myc* amplification, preferential amplification of the paternal allele has been seen, and in cases of neuroblastoma with a single copy of *N-myc*, preferential loss of maternal 1p36 tumor suppressor alleles has been seen [123].

Parental dependency or imprinting may also have relevance to chromosomal translocations in human malignancy. Imprinting has been observed as a mechanism for oncogene activation in the case of the t(9;22) chromosomal translocation in chronic myeloid leukemia [124]. While neither the *bcr* gene nor the *abl* gene are normally imprinted, the translocation is consistently made up of paternal 9 and maternal 22 chromosomal material [124]. It has been suggested that this finding might result from enhanced clonal expansion only of clones containing the translocation that combines material from paternal chromosome 9 and maternal chromosome 22, or that certain chromosomal regions may be more susceptible to rearrangements depending on the parental origin [124]. In either case, preferential participation of paternally derived chromosome 9 and maternally derived chromosome 22 suggests that these chromosomal regions may be imprinted during leukemogenesis. The methylation status of the genes at the translocation breakpoints have been shown to differ from their normal alleles [125,126],

Abnormalities in imprinting clearly relate to pediatric oncogenesis and demonstrate a strong link between developmental regulatory processes and oncogenesis. It is likely that further imprinted genes will be identified and that abnormalities in their expression will be related to childhood cancer. Understanding the mechanisms of imprinting may provide novel strategies for correcting imprinting abnormalities at specific developmental periods and treating embryonal tumors of childhood.

5. The role of specific oncogenes and tumor suppressor genes during development

Genes located at chromosomal translocation breakpoints in childhood tumors include *PAX3* and *FKHR (ALV)* in alveolar rhabdomyosarcoma and *Fli-1* and *EWS* in Ewing's family tumors. Amplified genes in childhood tumors include *N-myc* in neuroblastoma and *GLI* in malignant gliomas. Lost tumor suppressor genes in childhood tumors include *RB* in retinoblastoma and osteosarcoma, and *p53* in rhabdomyosarcoma, osteosarcoma, and brain tumors. It is believed that all these genes play a role during normal embryonic development, based on their restricted temporal and spatial expression patterns during development and on phenotypes produced in gain-of-function transgenic mice or loss-of-function gene knockout mice. In this section, the embryonic function of these genes will be summarized.

5.1. PAX3 and FKHR (ALV)

The paired box domain was first identified as a 128-amino-acid region in the *Drosophila* pair-rule segmentation gene *paired* and in the two-segment polarity genes *gooseberry-proximal* and *gooseberry-distal* [127]. In addition to the paired box domain, these genes contain a conserved region highly related to the homeobox and were called paired-type homeobox genes or *PAX* genes [128]. Like the homeobox, the paired box motif mediates DNA binding. *PAX* genes have subsequently been detected in a variety of organisms, including the mouse, human, chick, and zebra fish [129,130]. The mammalian *PAX* family consists of nine members, called *PAX1–9*, and have been grouped into four classes based on the presence or absence of conserved motifs [129,130]. Class 1 genes include *PAX1* and *PAX9*. Proteins within this class contain the paired DNA binding domain and a conserved region of eight amino acids of unknown function called the *octapeptide*. Class 2 genes include *PAX3* and *PAX7*, and these proteins include the paired domain, the conserved octapeptide, and a paired-type homeodomain. Class 3 genes include *PAX2*, *PAX5*, and *PAX8*, and the proteins contain the paired domain, the octapeptide, and a partial homeodomain. Finally, class 4 genes include *PAX4* and *PAX6*, and these proteins include the paired domain and the homeodomain but lack the octapeptide.

Both class 2 *PAX* genes, namely, *PAX3* and *PAX7*, have been shown to localize to translocation breakpoints in rhabdomyosarcomas and are expressed in restricted temporal and spatial patterns during development. *PAX3* has a transcription-inhibitory domain at its N-terminus and a transcription-activation domain at its C-terminus and has been shown to function as a transcription activator or inhibitor [131]. It is considered a proto-oncogene, since it is able to transform cells, including mouse NIH3T3 cells and rat 208F cells in tissue culture [132]. *PAX3* localizes to human chromosome 2q35 and is found at the breakpoint of the t(2;13)(q35;q14) in alveolar rhabdomyosarcoma. The fusion transcript retains the paired box and the homeodomain DNA binding domains of *PAX3*; however, the putative transcription-activation domain of *PAX3* is replaced by the forkhead DNA binding domain of the *FKHR (ALV)* gene from 13q14 [133]. It has been demonstrated that the PAX3/FKHR chimeric protein binds to the *PAX3* binding sequence [134]. Since it has been demonstrated that *PAX3* can inhibit myogenic differentiation in vitro, it has been suggested that the *PAX3/FKHR* fusion may contribute to the development of rhabdomyosarcoma by preventing terminal differentiation of myoblasts [135].

The *PAX7* gene localizes to human chromosome 1p36 and is found at the breakpoint for the rare t(1;13)(p36;q14) in rhabdomyosarcoma. The forkhead DNA binding domain of *FKHR (ALV)* at 13q14 once again replaces the transcription-activation region of *PAX7* in the fusion transcript [136]. Retention of the DNA binding motifs of *PAX3* and *PAX7* in these fusion transcripts suggests localization to critical target genes involved in the genesis of rhabdomyosarcoma.

Mouse *Pax* genes are expressed during embryonic development in specific spatial and temporal patterns [137]. Class 2, 3, and 4 *Pax* genes are expressed in the developing nervous system of the mouse. Within the developing central nervous system, *Pax3* expression is restricted to mitotically active cells. *Pax3*, *6*, and *7*, which contain a full homeobox, are first expressed in the developing neural tube on embryonic day 8 to 8.5 when the neural folds migrate to form the neural tube. At this stage, the anterior and posterior neuropores remain open. *Pax2*, *5*, and *8*, which contain only a partial homeobox, are not expressed in the developing neural tube until embryonic day 9.5 to 10, after the anterior and posterior neuropores have closed and brain development has started. Restricted localization of *Pax3* expression to the dorsal part of the neural tube and neural crest suggests that *Pax3* may be involved in the establishing dorsoventral polarity of the neural tube. The importance of *Pax3* in neural tube closure and neural crest migration is demonstrated by the fact that most homozygous *Pax3* mutant mice die in utero, with failure of neural tube closure and failure of neural crest cell migration [137]. *Pax3* is also expressed in the developing forebrain, midbrain, and hindbrain [130]. *Pax7* is co-expressed with *Pax3* in the early stages of brain development. As development continues, *Pax7* gene expression localizes to the epithalamus and pretectum. By day 13 of development, *Pax7* expression decreases within the developing brain significantly.

Outside the central nervous system, *Pax3* is expressed in the developing somites, limb buds, and some craniofacial structures such as the tongue, the mandible, and the maxilla [130]. The somites represent bands of mesodermal cells (paraxial mesoderm) running longitudinally along each side of the neural tube. These bands separate into blocks of cells during development, and each block is called a *somite*. *Pax3* is expressed in the developing somites at day 9 to 10 of mouse development. Its expression begins in the dorsal portion of the somite, which eventually gives rise to a dermomyotome. The dermomyotomes give rise to the dermis of the dorsal regions of the body (dermatomes) and the paravertebral musculature (myotomes) and limb musculature. These observations suggest a role for *Pax3* in myogenesis. Similar to the *Pax3* gene, the expression of *Pax7* starts in the dorsal part of the somite, prior to its specification into a dermomyotome. Later, *Pax7* expression is observed in the musculature of the shoulder girdle and of the trunk, suggesting a role for *Pax7* in myogenesis.

Specific phenotypes resulting from mutations in *PAX3* have been reported in the human and in the mouse. In humans, mutations in the *PAX3* gene have been shown to cause the autosomal-dominant disorder Waardenberg syndrome [138]. Waardenberg syndrome is characterized by nerve deafness, heterochromia irides, hypopigmented skin lesions, white forelock, white eyelashes and premature graying, dystopia canthorum, prominent nasal root, bushy eyebrows, high arched palate, cleft lip or palate, occasional spina bifida, Hirschsprung's disease, and contractures or reduction of shoulder and arm muscles. The heterochromia irides, hypopigmented skin lesions, white forelock, white eyelashes, and premature graying suggest failure of melanocyte migration from the neural crest.

Spontaneous *Pax3* deletions or point mutations in the mouse result in loss of *Pax3* function, causing the *splotch (sp)* mutant phenotype. Specific deletions that have been identified occur within the paired box domain or cause frameshift mutations. In addition, substitutions of amino acids in the paired box domain have been observed. The phenotype demonstrates many similarities to the human Waardenburg phenotype. *Splotch* mice demonstrate abnormalities in the brain, neural tube, neural crest derivatives, and muscles [139]. In mice heterozygous for a *Pax3* mutation, white spotting on the belly, limbs, and tail is observed as a result of a neural-crest-associated defect. In mice homozygous for *Pax3* mutations, phenotypic abnormalities include reduction or absence of dorsal root ganglia, Schwann cell deficiency, spina bifida, exencephaly, reduction in axial musculature, and loss of limb musculature.

The *FKHR (ALV)* gene is a member of the Forkhead family of transcription factors, which share a novel DNA binding domain named a *forkhead domain* or a *winged helix domain*. Forkhead was originally identified in *Drosophila* as a nuclear protein expressed in the terminal regions of the embryo [140]. The function of FKHR in mammalian development remains unknown [141].

The *EWS* gene was identified based on its location at the chromosome 22 breakpoint of the t(11;22)(q24;q12) translocation that characterizes the Ewing's sarcoma family of tumors [142]. Based on its homology with the RNA binding protein Cabeza in *Drosophila*, it is believed that human *EWS* encodes an RNA binding protein [143]. Cabeza binds RNA in vitro through a C_2C_2-type zinc finger, and although it is initially widely expressed during fly development, its expression becomes restricted to the central nervous system and gut later in development. Expression of Cabeza within the brain is turned off before the third larval instar, when the juvenile fly larva has undergone its third molt, but Cabeza protein is again expressed within the brain in the adult fly [144]. The role of this protein in development is unknown; however, based on its nuclear localization and its ability to bind RNA, it may be involved in nuclear RNA metabolism such as splicing, polyadenylation, and transport. The expression pattern of *EWS* during mammalian development has not been described.

As a result of the translocation, the N-terminal region of the EWS protein is fused to the DNA binding domain of the *Fli-1* gene. The human *Fli-1* gene codes for a putative transcription activator closely related to the ets family proteins ets, erg, and GABP-a [145]. The expression pattern of the *Fli-1* gene during mammalian development has not been reported. Other ets gene family members, however, regulate embryonic development and the response to growth stimuli [146]. The ets genes are expressed in a number of tissues, and their expression patterns during mouse development are complex. For example, *ets-1* expression is observed in the developing nervous system, including the hindbrain regions, the neural tube, and the neural crest during early gestation [147]. No expression of *ets-1* has been observed after day 8 in the mouse embryo in neuronal tissues. After day 13.5 of mouse gestation, *ets-2* expression is observed in the posterior spinal cord, medulla oblongata, the dentate gyrus, the hippocampus, and the granular layers of the cerebellum. Since human *Fli-1* demonstrates significant sequence homology with ets, it is possible that *Fli-1* may have a similar expression pattern and function during development.

Xl-fli, the *Xenopus* homologue of the *Fli-1* gene, is also expressed during embryogenesis. The Xl-fli protein shows 83% identity to mouse and human Fli-1 proteins. In situ hybridization demonstrates that Xl-fli is expressed in neural crest cells, brain, spleen, kidney, heart, and muscle [148]. The highest level of expression is observed in the spleen. In the adult mouse, *Fli-1* is expressed in the thymus and spleen, suggesting a role in lymphopoiesis.

Fli-1 transgenic mice have been established that overexpress Fli-1 protein in brain, heart, kidney, liver, lung, muscle, thymus, and spleen. By 3 to 6 months of age, a high incidence of immune-mediated tubulointerstitial nephritis and immune-complex glomerulonephritis occurs. The disorders are progressive and ultimately lead to renal failure [149]. The mice also demonstrate hypergammaglobulinemia, B-cell hyperplasia, and splenomegaly, further suggesting an immunologic role for the Fli-1 protein during development.

5.3. N-myc

N-*myc*, a member of the *myc* family of proto-oncogenes, was originally described as an amplified gene in neuroblastoma. It is expressed in restricted temporal and spatial patterns during normal development, primarily in actively proliferating undifferentiated cells. Expression has been described in postmitotic yet undifferentiated cells and generally not in differentiated cells, so it is believed that N-*myc* expression during development may be a marker of an undifferentiated state rather than a marker of proliferation [150]. N-*myc* is expressed in neural crest derivatives within the developing forebrain and hindbrain and within neuroblastic and ganglion cell layers of the developing eye. It is also expressed in the developing epithelium of the lung and bronchioles and in the developing epithelium of the gut.

Genes with sequence homology to N-*myc* have been described in phylogenetically distant organisms, including *Xenopus*, *Drosophila*, and woodchuck [151–153]. In *Drosophila*, the pair-rule segmentation gene *hairy* shows sequence homology with N-*myc* and is expressed during eye imaginal disc development. In the woodchuck, N-*myc2* is expressed during brain development, and in *Xenopus*, N-*myc* is expressed in the central nervous system and the eye during development. These expression patterns suggest an important role for N-*myc* in embryonic neuroectodermal development.

N-*myc* transgenic mice have been produced using the immunoglobulin heavy chain transcriptional enhancer element to drive N-*myc* expression. High levels of N-*myc* expression were observed in lymphoid tissues, and the mice developed early B and B-cell lymphoid malignancies [154]. No developmental defects were observed in these mice. Inactivation of N-*myc* by homologous recombination has resulted in an embryonic lethal phenotype. Mice homozygous for the mutation died between 10.5 and 12.5 days of gestation. These mice demonstrated abnormalities in the central nervous system, lung, heart, kidney, and intestinal tract [155,156]. In the mutant mice, cranial and spinal ganglia were reduced in size, lung branching morphogenesis was blocked, the heart was small and the myocardium was abnormally thin, the genital ridge was hypoplastic, the number of mesonephric tubules was reduced, and defects of the stomach and intestine were present [157].

5.4. GLI

The *GLI* gene was first described as an amplified gene in some cases of malignant glioma and was subsequently found to be amplified in some cases of undifferentiated childhood rhabdomyosarcoma and osteosarcoma [158,159]. *GLI* is a zinc finger containing transcription activator and serves as the prototype for the Gli–Kruppel gene family. Other members of this gene family function as important developmental regulatory genes in *Drosophila, C. elegans*, and mammals. *Cubitus interruptus*, a gene showing significant sequence homology in *Drosophila*, functions as a segment polarity gene and also functions in the hedgehog-patched signaling pathway [160]. A gene showing significant sequence homology in *C. elegans*, *tra-1*, functions as the terminal control gene in the sex determination pathway [161]. The function of *tra-1* is necessary for the development of female sex characteristics. In the mouse and human, the related gene *GLI3* is mutated in the mouse mutant *extra toes* and in the human Grieg syndrome [162,163]. *Extra toes* mice are characterized by extra toes on the preaxial side of the limb, and Grieg syndrome is characterized by craniofacial malformations and mental retardation. In the mouse embryo, *GLI3* is expressed in the developing central nervous system and in primitive mesenchyme [164].

Mouse *gli* is expressed in zones of proliferation within the developing central nervous system, including the ependymal layer of the developing spinal cord and the peri-ventricular region of the brain, in primitive mesenchyme of developing bone, in the mesodermal layer of the developing gastrointestinal tract, and within the genital tubercle [164,165]. In the adult human, *GLI* expression has been described in the testis, ovary, and myometrium. Although downstream targets in development remain unknown, it has been suggested that *GLI* functions in the mammalian Hedgehog–Patched signaling pathway similar to *ci* in *Drosophila* [160].

5.5. RB

The tumor suppressor gene *RB* negatively regulates the cell cycle. The "active" hypophosphorylated Rb protein associates with the transcription factor E2F and arrests cells in the G1 phase of the cell cycle. Phosphorylation of the Rb protein in G1 results in release of E2F and continuation through the cell cycle [166]. *RB* homologues have been found in many vertebrate species that share high sequence homology to the human gene.

The *Rb* gene is normally expressed in a restricted pattern during early embryonic development in the mouse and becomes ubiquitously expressed in adult tissues, including the brain, kidney, spleen, lung, and thymus [167]. During development in the mouse, *Rb* mRNA is first expressed at day 9.5 of gestation and becomes more abundant thereafter. The highest levels of *Rb* mRNA expression are observed in the developing brain, spinal cord, and liver. Rb protein is first detected on day 10.5 of mouse gestation, and the highest level of protein expression is demonstrated in the developing retina, neurons, glia, collecting tubules of the kidney, pancreas, and adrenal cortex [167,168].

When both *Rb* alleles are inactivated by homologous recombination, mouse embryos develop normally until day 12.5, suggesting that the *Rb* gene is not essential for early embryonic development [169–171]. However, these *Rb*-deficient mice die before the 16th day of gestation with multiple abnormalities in the nervous system, including widespread apoptosis of the hindbrain, trigeminal ganglia, spinal cord, and dorsal root ganglia; abnormally high mitotic indices observed in the periventricular region; and abnormal development of the hematopoietic system, including hypoplasia of the liver and abnormal erythrocyte development. Embryos heterozygous for the *Rb* gene appear normal, demonstrating that one copy of the *Rb* is sufficient for normal mouse development.

When extra copies of human *RB* are expressed during mouse development, most of the transgenic mice are smaller than nontransgenic littermates [172]. The size of the mice correlates inversely with the degree of *RB* gene expression [173]. It has been suggested that the small size may result from inhibition of cell cycle progression by Rb protein overexpression during development [174]. It has also been shown that mice with reduced Rb expression are larger than normal mice [175]. These observations collectively demonstrate the importance of *Rb* gene dosage during development.

Surprisingly, there is no correlation between tumors that have been observed in *Rb* loss-of-function mice and humans with familial *RB* mutations. *Rb* loss-of-function mice show no evidence of retinoblastoma development; however, by 10–12 months of age, the majority develop adenocarcinoma of the pituitary. Medullary thyroid carcinoma has been observed in mice with one functional *Rb* gene [176]. There is no explanation for this discrepancy at this time.

5.6. p53

p53 negatively regulates the cell cycle by acting as a "checkpoint" protein that controls progression through the cell cycle and mediates apoptosis during development and following DNA damage [177]. *p53* generally functions as a tumor suppressor gene; however, some mutant forms of *p53* may function as oncogenes [177–179]. Loss of *p53* is very commonly associated with a variety human tumors, including tumors of colon, breast, lung, and brain. In addition, a familial predisposition to breast cancer, leukemia, brain tumors, soft tissue sarcomas, osteosarcoma, and adrenal cortical carcinoma, known as the Li–Fraumeni syndrome, has been associated with germline mutations in *p53* [180].

A role for *p53* during normal development has been suggested, since *p53* is expressed during embryonic development [181]. *p53* is expressed in all cells of the early mouse embryo between days 8.5 and 10.5 of gestation. Later, high levels of expression have been observed in the brain, liver, lung, thymus, intestine, salivary glands, kidney, and during B-cell differentiation [181]. To study the role of *p53* during development, inactivation of *p53* by homologous recombination has been carried out [182,183]. Some *p53* knockout mice appear normal [183]. Developmental abnormalities have been reported in other *p53*-deficient mice [182,183]. In some *p53* null mice, the neural tube fails to close, resulting in exencephaly. This outcome occurs more commonly in female offspring, for unknown reasons. It is believed that neural cell proliferation or apoptosis may be dysregulated in the *p53* null mice, resulting in failure of neural tube closure. In addition, ocular and dental abnormalities have been observed.

p53-deficient mice, however, show an unusually high susceptibility to spontaneous tumor formation. By eight months of age, all the mice develop tumors, predominantly sarcomas and lymphomas.

Transgenic mice have been produced with two different *p53* mutants, each differing from wild-type *p53* by a single amino acid substitution [184]. Mice with the mutant *p53* transgene developed normally; however, they again showed increased susceptibility to spontaneous tumor formation. By 18 months of age, approximately 40% of the transgenic mice developed tumors, mainly adenocarcinomas of the lung, lymphomas, or osteosarcomas.

5.7. Conclusions

In conclusion, a role has been described for each of these genes during normal development. These observations link childhood cancer and embryonic development as related processes at a genetic level and support the idea that a greater understanding of childhood cancer at a genetic level lies within an understanding of the developmental biology of the cell type from which the disease arises. In several instances, these genes seem to demonstrate tissue specificity, i.e., functioning during development and during oncogenesis in the same tissues. This observation is true for *PAX3* in the developing somites and in rhabdomyosarcoma; for *N-myc* in the developing nervous system, and in neuroblastoma, and in gliomas, in the developing lung epithelium, and in small cell lung carcinoma; and for *GLI* in the developing central nervous system, and in glioma, in developing bone, and in osteosarcomas. In addition, it is likely true for *Fli-1* and *EWS*, both of which seem to play a role in central nervous system development and are involved in the Ewing's family of tumors of neuroectodermal origin. Alternatively, these observations suggest that developmental studies may lead to the identification of new developmental regulatory genes in specific tissues that may then be identified as candidate oncogenes/tumor suppressor genes in the corresponding tissue. Comparative biology may be particularly useful for identifying these new developmental regulatory genes and understanding the function of previously identified developmental regulatory genes and oncogenes. Finally, the importance of gene dosage during development and in neoplasia is illustrated by *N-myc* and *RB*. Lack of the oncogene *N-myc* during development results in specific patterns of dysmorphogenesis, while overexpression of *N-myc* during development result in neoplasia. Underexpression of the tumor suppressor gene *RB* during development is associated with neoplasia, dysmorphogenesis, and growth disturbance, while overexpression of *RB* during development results in disturbances of growth.

References

1. Greaves MF. 1988. Speculations on the cause of childhood acute lymphoblastic leukemia. Leukemia 2(2):120–125.
2. Biran H, Ariel I, De Groot N, Hochberg A. 1994. On the oncodevelopmental role of human imprinted genes. Med Hypotheses 43:119–123.
3. Kessel M, Gruss P. 1990. Murine developmental control genes. Science 249:374.
4. Acampora D, D'Esposito M, Faiella A, Pannese M, Migliaccio E, Morelli F, Stornaiuolo A, Nigro V, Simeone A, Boncinelli E. 1989. The human Hox gene family. Nucleic Acids Res 17:10385.
5. Shashikant CS, Utset MF, Violette SM, Wise TL, Einat P, Einat M, Pendleton JW, Schughart KS, Ruddle FH. 1991. Homeobox genes in mouse development. Crit Rev Eukaryot Gene Expresssion 1(3):207.
6. Nusslein-Volhard C, Frohnhofer HG, Lehman R. 1987. Determination of anteroposterior polarity in Drosophila. Science 238:1675.
7. Akam M. 1987. The molecular basis for metameric pattern in the Drosophila embryo. Development 101:1.
8. Gehring WJ, Hiromi Y. 1986. Homeotic genes and the homeobox. Annu Rev Genet 20:147–173.
9. Sheperd JCW, McGinnis W, Carrasco AE, DeRobertis EM, Gehring WJ. 1984. Fly and frog homeodomains show homologies with yeast mating type regulatory proteins. Nature 319:70.
10. Scott MP, Tamkun JW, Hartzell GW. 1989. The structure and function of the homeodomain. Biochem Biophys Acta 989:25.
11. Levine M, Hoey T. 1988. Homeobox proteins as sequence-specific transcription factors. Cell 55:537.
12. Biggin MD, Tijan R. 1989. Transcription factors and the control of Drosophila development. Trends Genet 5:377.
13. Falzon M, Chung SY. 1988. The expression of rat homeobox-containing genes is developmentally regulated and tissue specific. Development 103:601.
14. Regulski M, Harding K, Kostriken R, Karch F, Levine M, McGinnis W. 1985. Homeobox genes of the antennapedia and bithorax gene complexes of Drosophila. Cell 43:71.
15. Karch F, Weiffenbach B, Peifer M, Bender W, Duncan I, Celniker S, Crosby M, Lewis EB. 1985. The abdominal region of the bithorax complex. Cell 43:81.
16. Sanchez-Herreo E, Vernos I, Marco R, Morata G. 1985. Genetic organization of Drosophila bithorax complex. Nature 313:108.
17. Lewis E. 1978. A gene complex controlling segmentation in Drosophila. Nature 276:565–570.
18. Duboule D, Boncinelli E, DeRobertis E, Featherstone M, Lonai P, Oliver G, Ruddle F. 1990. An update of mouse and human Hox gene nomenclature. Genomics 7:458.
19. McAlpine PJ, Shows TB. 1990. Nomenclature for human homeobox genes. Genomics 7:460.
20. Colberg-Poley AM, Voss SD, Chowdhury K, Stewart Cl, Wagner EF, Gruss P. 1985. Clustered homeoboxes are differentially expressed during development. Cell 43:39.
21. Duboule D, Baron A, Mahi P, Galliot B. 1986. A new homeobox is present in overlapping cosmid clones which defines the mouse HOX-1 locus. EMBO J 5:1973.
22. Hart CP, Awgulewitsch A, Fainsod A, McGinnis W, Ruddle FH. 1985. Homeobox gene complex on mouse chromosome 11: molecular cloning, expression in embryogenesis, and homology to a human homeobox locus. Cell 43:9.
23. Brier G, Dressler GR, Gruss P. 1988. Primary structure and developmental expression pattern of Hox 3.1, a member of the murine Hox 3 homeobox gene cluster. EMBO J 7:1329.
24. Featherstone MS, Baron A, Gaunt SJ, Mattei JG, Duboule D. 1988. Hox-5.1 defines a homeobox-containing gene locus on mouse chromosome 2. Proc Natl Acad Sci USA 85:4760.
25. Dolle P, Duboule D. 1989. Two gene members of the murine HOX-5 complex show regional and cell-type specific expression in developing limbs and gonads. EMBO J 8:1507.

30

26. Graham A, Papalopulu N, Krumlauf R. 1989. The murine and Drosophila homeobox gene complexes have common features of organization and expression. Cell 57:367.
27. Krumlauf R. 1994. Hox genes in vertebrate development. Cell 78:191.
28. Simeone A, Acampora D, Nigro V, Faiella A, D'Esposito M, Stornaiuolo A, Mavilio F, Boncinelli E. 1991. Differential regulation by retinoic acid of the homeobox genes of the four HOX loci in human embryonal carcinoma cells. Mech Dev 33:215–228.
29. Akam ME. 1989. Hox and HOM: homologous gene clusters in insects and vertebrates. Cell 57:347.
30. Duboule D, Dolle P. 1989. The structural and functional organization of the murine Hox gene family resembles that of Drosophila homeotic genes. EMBO J 8:1497.
31. Kessel M, Gruss P. 1991. Homeotic transformations of murine vertebrae and concomitant alteration of Hox codes induced by retinoic acid. Cell 67:89–104.
32. Manak JR, Scott MP. 1994. A class act: conservation of homeodomain protein functions. Development (Suppl):61–77. There is no volume number for the supplement.
33. Lufkin T, Dierich A, LeMeur M, Mark M, Chambon P. 1991. Disruption of the Hox-1.6 homeobox gene results in defects in a region corresponding to its rostral domain of expression. Cell 66:1105.
34. Chisaka O, Capecchi MR. 1991. Regionally restricted developmental defects resulting from targeted disruption of the mouse homeobox gene Hox-1.5. Nature 350:473.
35. Gaunt SJ, Krumlauf R, Duboule D. 1989. Mouse homeo-genes within a subfamily, Hox-1.4, -2.6 and -5.1, display similar antero-posterior domains of expression in the embryo, but show stage- and tissue-dependent differences in their regulation. Development 107:131–141.
36. Duboule D. 1994. Temporal colinearity and the phylotypic progression: a basis for the stability of a vertebrate Bauplan and the evolution of morphologies through heterochrony. Development (Suppl):135–142. There is no volume number for the supplement.
37. Izpisua-Belmonte JC, Duboule D. 1992. Homeobox genes and pattern formation in the vertebrate limb. Dev Biol 152:26–36.
38. Duboule D. 1991. Patterning in the vertebrate limb. Curr Opinion Genet Dev 1:211–216.
39. Ramirez-Solis R, Zheng H, Whiting J, Krumlauf R, Bradley A. 1993 Hoxb-4 (Hox-2.6) mutant mice show homeotic transformation of a cervical vertebra and defects in the closure of the sternal rudiments. Cell 73:279–294.
40. Cillo C, Barba P, Bucciarelli G, Magli MC, Boncinelli E. 1992. Hox gene expression in normal and neoplastic kidney. Int J Cancer 51:892–897.
41. De Vita G, Barba P, Odartchenko J, Givel JC, Freschi G, Bucciarelli G, Magli MC, Boncinelli E, Cillo C. 1993. Expression of homeobox-containing genes in primary and metastatic colorectal cancer. Eur J Cancer 29:887–893.
42. Tiberio C, Barba P, Magli MC, Arvelo F, Le Chevalier T, Poupon MF, Cillo C. 1994. HOX gene expression in human small-cell lung cancers xenografted into nude mice. Int J Cancer 58:608–615.
43. Blatt C. 1990. The betrayal of homeo box genes in normal development: the link to cancer. Cancer Cell 6(2):186–198.
44. Castronovo V, Kusaka M, Chariot A, Gielen J, Sobel M. 1994. Homeobox genes: potential candidates for the transcriptional control of the transformed phenotype and invasive phenotype. Biochem Pharmacol 47(1):137–143.
45. Maulbecker CC, Gruss P. 1993. The oncogenic potential of deregulated homeobox genes. Cell Growth Differ 4:431–441.
46. Perkins A, Kongsuwan K, Visvader V, Adams JM, Cory S. 1990. Homeobox gene expression plus autocrine growth factor production elicits myeloid leukemia. Proc Natl Acad Sci USA 87:8398–8402.
47. Blatt CD, Aberdam D, Schwartz R, Sachs L. 1988. DNA rearrangement of a homeobox gene in myeloid leukemic cells. EMBO J 79(13):4283–4290.
48. Barba P, Magli MC, Tiberior Cl, Cillo C. 1993. Hox gene expresssion in human cancers. Adv Exp Med Biol 348:45–57.

49. Aberdam D, Negreanu V, Sachs L, Blatt C. 1991. The oncogenic potential of an activated Hox-2.4 homeobox gene in mouse fibroblasts. Mol Cell Biol 11(1):554–557.

50. Castronovo V, Kusaka M, Chariot A, Gielen J, Sobel M. 1994. Homeobox genes: potential candidates for the transcriptional control of the transformed and invasive phenotype. Biochem Pharmacol 47(1):137–143.

51. Cillo C. 1994. Hox genes in human cancers. Invasion Metastasis 14:38–49.

52. Manohar CF, Salwen HR, Furtado MR, Cohn SL. 1996. Up-regulation of HoxC6, HoxD1, and HoxD8 homeobox gene expression in human neuroblastoma cells following chemical induction of differentiation. Tumor Biol 17:34–47.

53. Lichty BD, Ackland-Snow J, Noble L, Kamel-Reid S, Dube ID. 1995. Dysregulation of Hox11 by chromosome translocations in T-cell acute lymphoblastic leukemia: a paradigm for homeobox gene involvement in human cancer. Leuk Lymphoma 16:209–215.

54. Hatano M, Roberts CWM, Minden M, Crist WM, Korsemeyer SJ. 1991. Deregulation of a homeobox gene, Hox11 by the t(1;14) in T cell leukemia. Science 253:79–82.

55. Zhang N, Gong ZZ, Minden M, Lu M. 1993. The HOX-11 (TCL-3) homeobox proto-oncogene encodes a nuclear protein that undergoes cell cyle-dependent regulation. Oncogene 8:3265–3270.

56. McGrath J, Solter D. 1984. Completion of mouse embryogenesis requires both the maternal and paternal genomes. Cell 37:179.

57. Surani MA, Barton SC, Norris ML. 1984. Development of reconstituted mouse eggs suggests imprinting of the genome during gametogenesis. Nature 308:548.

58. Barton SC, Ferguson-Smith AC, Fundele R, Surani MA. 1991. Influence of paternally imprinted genes on development. Development 113:679–687.

59. Moore T, Haig D. 1991. Genomic imprinting in mammalian development: a parental tug-of-war. Trends Genet 7:45–49.

60. Cattanach B, Beechey C. 1990. Autosomal and X-chromosome imprinting. Development (Suppl):63–72. There is no volume number for the supplement.

61. Razin A, Cedar H. 1994. DNA methylation and genomic imprinting. Cell 77:473–476.

62. Swain JL, Stewart TA, Leder P. 1987. Parental legacy determines methylation and expression of an autosomal transgene: a molecular mechanism for parental imprinting. Cell 50:719–727.

63. Rainier S, Feinberg AP. 1994. Genomic imprinting, DNA methylation, and cancer. J Natl Cancer Inst 86(10):753–759.

64. Tartof KD, Bremer M. 1990. Mechanisms for the construction and developmental control of heterochromatin formation and imprinted chromosome domains. Development (Suppl):35–45. There is no volume number for the supplement.

65. Li E, Beard C, Jaenisch R. 1993. Role for DNA methylation in genomic imprinting. Nature 366:362–365.

66. Beard C, Li E, Jaenisch R. 1995. Loss of methylation activates Xist in somatic but not in embryonic cells. Genes Dev 9:2325.

67. Razin A, Cedar H. 1994. DNA methylation and genomic imprinting. Cell 77:473–476.

68. Neumann B, Kubicka P, Barlow DP. 1995. Characteristics of imprinted genes. Nature Genet 9:12.

69. Pfeifer K, Tilghman SM. 1994. Allele-specific gene expression in mammals: the curious case of the imprinted RNAs. Genes Dev 8:1867.

70. Lustig O, Ariel I, Ilan J, Lev-Lehman E, DeGroot N, Hochberg A. 1994. The expression of the imprinted gene H19 in the human embryo. Mol Reprod Dev 38:239–246.

71. Biran H, Ariel I, DeGroot N, Shani A, Hochberg A. 1994. Human imprinted genes as oncodevelopmental markers. Tumor Biol 15:123–134.

72. Brannan CI, Dees EC, Ingram RS, et al. 1990. The product of the H19 gene may function as an RNA. Mol Cell Biol 10:28–36.

73. Leighton PA, Ingram RS, Eggenschwiler A, Efstratiadis SM, Tilghman SM. 1995. Disruption of imprinting caused by deletion of the H19 gene region in mice. Nature 375:34.

74. Hao Y, Crenshaw T, Moulton T, Newcomb E, Tycko B. 1993. Tumor-suppressor activity of H19 RNA. Nature 365:764–767.
75. Brunkow ME, Tilghman SM. 1991. Ectopic expression of the H19 gene in mice causes prenatal lethality. Genes Dev 5:1092–1101.
76. Giannoukakis N, Deal C, Paquette J, Goodyear CG, Polychronakos C. 1993. Parental genomic imprinting of the human IGF2 gene. Nature Genet 4:98–101.
77. Ohlsson R, Nystrom A, Pfeifer-Ohlsson S, Tohonen V, Hedbourg F, Schofield P, Flam F, Ekstrom TJ. 1993. IGF2 is parentally imprinted during human embryogenesis and in the Beckwith–Wiedemann syndrome. Nature Genet 4:94–97.
78. Zemel S, Bartholomei MS, Tilghman SM. 1992. Physical linkage of the mammalian imprinted genes, H19 and IGF2. Nature Genet 2:61–65.
79. Ohlsson R, Hedborg F, Holmgren L, Walsh C, Ekstrom TJ. 1994. Overlapping patterns of IGF2 and H19 expression during human development. Development 120:361–368.
80. Sara V, Hall K. 1990. Insulin-like growth factors and their binding proteins. Phys Rev 70:591–614.
81. DeChiara TM, Efstratiadis A, Robertson EJ. 1990. A growth deficiency phenotype in heterozygous mice carrying an insulin-like growth factor II gene by disrupted targeting. Nature 345:78–80.
82. Rainier S, Johnson L, Dobry CJ, Ping AJ, Grundy PE, Feinberg AP. 1993. Relaxation of imprinted genes in human cancer. Nature 362:747–749.
83. Ogawa O, Eccles MR, Szeto J, McNoe LA, Yun K, Maw MA, Smith PJ, Reeve AE. 1993. Relaxation of insulin-like growth factor II gene imprinting implicated in Wilms' tumour. Nature 362:749–751.
84. Weksberg R, Shen DR, Fei YL, Song QL, Squire J. 1993. Disruption of insulin-like growth factor 2 imprinting in Beckwith–Wiedemann syndrome. Nature Genet 5:143–150.
85. Junien C, Henry I. 1994. Genetics of Wilms' tumor: a blend of aberrant development and genomic imprinting. Kidney Int 40:1264–1279.
86. Kreidberg JA, Sariola H, Loring JM, Maeda M, Pelletier J, Housman D, Jaenisch R. 1993. WT-1 is required for early kidney development. Cell 74:679–691.
87. Jinno Y, Yun K, Nishiwaki K, Kubota T, Ogawa O, Reeve AE, Nikawa N. 1994. Mosaic and polymorphic imprinting of the WT1 gene in humans. Nature Genet 6:305–309.
88. Little MH, Dunn R, Byrne JA, Seawright A, Smith PJ, Pritchard-Jones K, VanHeyningen V, Hastie JD. 1992. Equivalent expression of paternally and maternally inherited WT1 alleles in normal fetal tissue and Wilms' tumors. Oncogene 7(4):635–641.
89. Nicholls RD, Knoll JHM, Butler MG, Karam S, Lalande M. 1989. Genetic imprinting suggested by maternal heterodisomy in nondeletion Prader–Willi syndrome. Nature 342:281–285.
90. Butler MG, Meaney FJ, Palmer CG. 1986. Clinical and cytogenetic survey of 39 individuals with Prader–Labhart–Willi syndrome. Am J Med Genet 23:783–809.
91. Knoll JHM, Nicholls RD, Magneis RE, Graham JM, Lalande M, Latt SA. 1989. Angelman and Prader–Willi syndromes share a common chromosome deletion but differ in parental orgin of the deletion. Am J Med Genet 32:285–290.
92. Leff SE, Brannan CI, Reed ML, Ozcelik T, Francke U, Copeland NG, Jenkins NA. 1992. Maternal imprinting of the mouse Snrpn gene and conserved linkage homology with the human Prader–Willi syndrome region. Nature Genet 2:259–264.
93. Reed ML, Leff SE. 1994. Maternal imprinting of human SNRPN, a gene deleted in Prader–Willi syndrome. Nature Genet 6:163–167.
94. Beckwith JB. 1969. Macroglossia, omphalocele, adrenal cytomegaly, gigantism, and hyperplastic visceromegaly. Birth Defects 5:188–196.
95. Greenwood RD, Sommer A, Rosenthal A, Craenen J, Nadas AS. 1977. Cardiovascular abnormalities in the Beckwith–Wiedemann syndrome. Am J Dis Child 131:293–294.
96. Shapiro LR, Duncan PA, Davidian MM, Sincer N. 1982. The placenta in familial Beckwith–Wiedemann syndrome. Birth Defects 18:203–206.

97. Ping AJ, Reeve AE, Law D, Young MR, Boehnke M, Feinberg AP. 1989. Genetic linkage of Beckwith–Wiedemann syndrome to 11p15. Am J Hum Genet 44:720–723.

98. Koufos A, Grundy P, Morgan K, Aleck KA, Hadro T, Lampkin BC, Kalbakji A, Cavenee WK. 1989. Familial Wiedemann–Beckwith syndrome and a second Wilms' tumor locus both map to 11p15.5. Am J Hum Genet 44:711–719.

99. Brown KW, Williams JC, Maitland NJ, Mott MG. 1990. Genomic imprinting and the Beckwith–Wiedemann syndrome. Am J Hum Genet 46:1000–1001.

100. Moutou C, Junien C, Henry I, Bonaiti-Pellie C. 1992. Beckwith–Wiedemann syndrome: a demonstration of the mechanisms responsible for the excess of transmitting in females. J Med Genet 29:217.

101. Weksberg R, Shen DR, Fei YL, Song QL, Squire J. 1993. Disruption of insulin-like growth factor 2 imprinting in Beckwith–Wiedemann syndrome. Nature Genet 5:143–150.

102. Hedborg F, Holmgren L, Sandstedt B, Ohlsson R. 1994. The cell type-specific IGF2 expression during early human development correlates to the pattern of overgrowth and neoplasia in the Beckwith-Wiedemann syndrome. Am J Pathol 145(4):802–817.

103. Cohen MM. 1994. Wiedemann–Beckwith syndrome, imprinting, IGF2 and H19: implications for hemihyperplasia, associated neoplasms and overgrowth. Am J Med Genet 52:233–234.

104. Kubota T, Saitoh S, Matsumoto T, Narahara K, Fukushima Y, Jinno Y, Nikawa N. 1994. Excess functional copy of allele at chromosomal region 11p15 may cause Wiedemann–Beckwith (EMG) syndrome. Am J Med Genet 49:378–383.

105. Junien C. 1992. Beckwith–Wiedemann syndrome, tumorigenesis and imprinting. Curr Opinion Genet Dev 2:431–438.

106. Wiedemann HR. 1983. Tumours and hemihypertrophy associated with Wiedemann–Beckwith syndrome. Eur J Pediatr 141:129.

107. Drut R, Jones M. 1988. Congenital pancreatoblastoma in Beckwith–Wiedemann syndrome: an emerging association. Pediatr Pathol 8:331–339.

108. Emery LG, Shields M, Shah NR, Garbes A. 1983. Neuroblastoma associated with Beckwith–Wiedemann syndrome. Cancer 52:176–179.

109. Albrecht S, von Schweinitz D, Waha A, Kraus JA, von Deimling A, Pietsch T. 1994. Loss of maternal alleles on chromosome arm 11p in hepatoblastoma. Cancer Res 54:5041–5044.

110. Pedone PV, Tirabosco R, Cavazzana AO, Ungaro P, Basso G, Luksch R, Carli M, Bruni CB, Frunzio R, Riccio A. 1994. Mono- and bi-allelic expression of insulin-like growth factor II gene in human muscle tumors. Hum Mol Genet 3:1117–1121.

111. Wake N, Fujino T, Hoshi S, Shinkai N, Sakai K, Kato H, Hashimoto M, Yasuda T, Yamada H, Ichinoe K. 1987. The propensity to malignancy of dispermic heterozygous moles. Placenta 8:319–326.

112. Linder D, McCaw B, Hecht F. 1975. Parthenogenetic origin of benign ovarian teratomas. N Engl J Med 292:63–66.

113. Fearon ER, Vogelstein B, Feinberg AP. 1984. Somatic deletion and duplication of genes on chromosome 11 in Wilms' tumours. Nature 309:176–178.

114. Toguchida J, Ishizaki K, Sasaki M, Nakamura Y, Ikenaga M, Kato M, Sugimot M, Kotoura Y, Yamamuro T. 1989. Preferential mutation of paternally derived RB gene as the initial event in sporadic osteosarcoma. Nature 338:156–158.

115. Naumova A, Hansen M, Strong L, Jones PA, Hadjistilianou D, Mastrangelo D, Griegel S, Rajewsky MF, Shields J, Donoso L, Wang M, Sapienza C. 1994. Concordance between parental origin of chromosome 13q loss and chromosome 6p duplication in sporadic retinoblastoma. Am J Hum Genet 54:274–281.

116. Mannens M, Slater RM, Heyting C, Bliek J, deKraker J, Coad N, dePagter-Holthuizen P, Pearson PL. 1988. Molecular nature of genetic changes resulting in loss of heterozygosity of chromosome 11 in Wilms' tumours. Hum Genet 81:41–48.

117. Slater RM, Mannen M. 1992. Cytogenetics and molecular genetics of Wilms' tumor of childhood. Cancer Genet Cytogenet 61:111–121.

34

118. Steenman MJC, Rainier S, Dobry CJ, Grundy P, Horon IL, Feinberg AP. 1994. Loss of imprinting of IGF2 is linked to reduced expression and abnormal methylation of H19 in Wilms' tumour. Nature Genet 7:433–438.

119. Scrable H, Cavenee W, Ghavimi F, Lovell M, Morgan K, Sapienza C. 1989. A model for embryonal rhabdomyosarcoma tumorigenesis that involves genome imprinting. Proc Natl Acad Sci USA 86:7480–7484.

120. Ekstrom TJ. 1994. Parental imprinting and the IGF2 gene. Horm Res 42:176–181.

121. Montagna M, Menin C, Chieco-Bianchi L, D'Andrea E. 1994. Occasional loss of constitutive heterozygosity at 11p15.5 and imprinting relaxation of the IGF II maternal allele in hepatoblastoma. J Cancer Res Clin Oncol 120(12):732–736.

122. Wada M, Seeger RC, Mizoguchi H, Koeffler HP. 1995. Maintenance of normal imprinting of H19 and IGF2 genes in neuroblastoma. Cancer Res 55(125):3386–3388.

123. Caron H, van Sluid P, van Hoeve M, de Kraker J, Bras J, Slater R, Mannens M, Voute PA, Westerveld A, Versteeg R. 1993. Allelic loss of chromosome 1p36 in neuroblastoma is of preferential maternal origin and correlates with N-myc amplification. Nature Genet 4:187–190.

124. Haas OA, Argyriou-Tirita A, Lion T. 1992. Parental origin of chromosomes involved in the translocation t(9;22). Nature 359:414–416.

125. Yamada T, Secker-Walker LM. 1990. Possible evidence for acquired genetic activity at both chromosomal breakpoints of the Philadelphia translocation in chronic myeloid leukemia. Leukemia 4:341–344.

126. Schaefer-Rego KE, Leibowitz D, Mears JG. 1990. Chromatin alterations surrounding the BCR/ABL fusion gene in K562 cells. Oncogene 5:1669–1673.

127. Baumgartner S, Bopp D, Burri M, Noll M. 1987. Structure of the two genes at the gooseberry locus related to the paired gene and their spatial expression during *Drosophila* embryogenesis. Genes Dev 1:1247–1267.

128. Bopp D, Burri M, Baumgartner S, Frigerio G, Noll M. 1986. Conservation of a large protein domain in the segmentation gene paired and in functionally related genes of *Drosophila*. Cell 47:1033–1040.

129. Gruss P, Walther C. 1992. Pax in development. Cell 69:719–722.

130. Strachan T, Read AP. 1994. Pax genes. Curr Opinion Genet Dev 4:427–438.

131. Chalepalas G, Jones FS, Edelman GM, Gruss P. 1994. Pax-3 contains domains for transcription activation and transcription inhibition. Proc Natl Acad Sci USA 91:12745–12749.

132. Maulbecker C, Gruss P. 1993. The oncogenic potential of Pax genes. EMBO J 12:2361–2367.

133. Shapiro DN, Sublett JE, Li B, Downing JR, Naeve CW. 1993. Fusion of PAX 3 to a member of the forkhead family of transcription factors in human alveolar rhabdomyosarcoma. Cancer Res 53:5108–5112.

134. Sublett JE, Jeon IS, Sapiro DN. 1995. The alveolar rhabdomyosarcoma Pax3/FKHR fusion protein is a transcriptional activator. Oncogene 11:545–552.

135. Epstein JA, Lam P, Jepeal L, Maas RL, Sapiro DN. 1995. Pax3 inhibits myogenic differentiation of cultured myoblast cells. J Biol Chem 270:11719–11722.

136. Davis RJ, D'Cruz CM, Lovell MA, Biegel KA, Barr FG. 1994. Fusion of PAX7 to FKHR by the variant t(1;13)(p36;q14) translocation in alveolar rhabdomyosarcoma. Cancer Res 54:2869–2872.

137. Tremblay P, Gruss P. 1994. Pax: genes for mice and men. Pharmacol Therapeut 61:205–226.

138. Baldwin CT, Hoth CF, Macina RA, Milunsky A. 1995. Mutations in PAX3 that cause Waadenburg syndrome type I: ten new mutations and review of the literature. Am J Med Genet 58:115–122.

139. Tremblay P, Kessel M, Gruss P. 1995. A transgenic neuroanatomical marker identifies cranial neural crest deficiencies associated with the Pax3 mutant Splotch. Dev Biol 171:317–329.

140. Wiegel D, Jurgens G, Kuttner F, Seifert E, Jackle H. 1989. The homeotic gene encodes a nuclear protein and is expressed in the terminal regions of the Drosophila embryo. Cell 57:645–658.

141. Hromas R, Costa R. 1995. The hepatocyte nuclear factor-3/forkhead transcription regulatory family in development, inflammation, and neoplasia. Crit Rev Oncol Hematol 20:129–140.

142. Pellin A, Boix J, Blesa JR, Noguera R, Carda C, Llombart-Bosch A. 1994. *EWS/Fli-1* rearrangement in small cell sarcoma of bone and soft tissue detected by reverse transcriptase polymerase chain reaction amplification. Eur J Cancer 30A:827–831.

143. Ohno T, Rao VN, Reddy ES. 1993. EWS/Fli-1 chimeric protein is a transcriptional activator. Oncogene 9:3087–3097.

144. Stolow DT, Haynes SR. 1995. Cabeza, a *Drosophila* gene encoding a novel RNA binding protein, shares homology with EWS and TLS, two genes involved in human sarcoma formation. Nucleic Acid Res 23:835–843.

145. Prasad DD, Rao VN, Reddy ES. 1992. Structure and expression of human *Fli-1* gene. Cancer Res 52:5833–5837.

146. Hromas R, Klemsz M. 1994. The ETS oncogene family in development, proliferation and neoplasia. Int J Hematol 59:257–265.

147. Maroulakou IG, Papas TS, Green JE. 1994. Differential expression of ets-1 and ets-2 proto-oncogenes during murine embryogenesis. Oncogene 9:1551–1565.

148. Meyer D, Wolff CM, Stiegler P, Senan F, Befort N, Befort JJ, Remy P. 1993. Xl-fli, the *Xenopus* homologue of the fli-1 gene, is expressed durig embryogenesis in a restricted pattern evocative of neural crest cell distribution. Mech Dev 44:109–121.

149. Zhang L, Eddy A, Teng Y-T, Fritzler M, Kluppel M, Melet F, Bernstein A. 1995. An immunological renal disease in transgenic mice that overexpress *Fli-1*, a member of the ets family of transcription factor genes. Mol Cell Biol 15:6961–6970.

150. Zimmerman K, Alt FW. 1990. Expression and function of Myc family genes. Crit Rev Oncogenesis 2:75095.

151. Rushlow CA, Hogan A, Pinchin SM, Howe KM, Lardelli M, Ish-Horowicz D. 1989. The *Drosophila* hairy protein acts in both segmentation and bristle patterning and shows homology to N-*myc*. EMBO J 8:3095–3103.

152. Fourel G, Transy C, Tennant BC, Buendia MA. 1992. Expression of the woodchuck N-myc2 retroposon in brain and in liver tumors is driven by a cryptic N-*myc* promoter. Mol Cell Biol 12:5336–5344.

153. Dildrop R, Ma A, Zimmerman K, Hsu E, Tesfaye A, Depinho R, Alt FW. 1989. IgH enhancer-mediated deregulation of N-*myc* gene expression in transgenic mice: generation of lymphoid neoplasias that lack c-*myc* expression. EMBO J 8:1121–1128.

154. Moens CB, Stanton BR, Parada LF, Rossant J. 1993. Defects in heart and lung development in compound heterozygotes for two different targeted mutations at the N-*myc* locus. Development 119:485–499.

155. Davis A, Bradley A. 1993. Mutation of N-*myc* in mice: what does the phenotype tell us? Bioessay 15:273–275.

156. Stanton BR, Perkins AS, Tessarillo L, Sassoon DA, Parada LF. 1992. Loss of N-*myc* function results in embryonic lethality and failure of the epithelial compoment of the embryo to develop. Genes Dev 6:2235–2247.

157. Vize PD, Vaughan A, Krieg P. 1990. Expression of the N-*myc* proto-oncogene during the early development of *Xenopus laevis*. Development 110:885–896.

158. Kinzler KW, Bigner SH, Bigner DD, Trent JM, Law ML, O'Brien SJ, Wong AJ, Vogelstein B. 1987. Identification of an amplified, highly expressed gene in a human glioma. Science 236:70–73.

159. Roberts WM, Douglass EC, Peiper SC, Houghton PJ, Look AT. 1989. Amplification of the *gli* gene in childhood sarcomas. Cancer Res 49:5407–5413.

160. Dominguez M, Brunner M, Hafen E, Basler K. 1996. Sending and receiving the Hedgehog signal: control by the *Drosophila* Gli protein Cubitus interruptus. Science 272:1621–1625.

161. Hodgkin J. 1983. Two types of sex determination in a nematode. Nature 304:267–268.

162. Vortkamp A, Gessler M, Grzeschik KH. 1991. Gli3 zinc-finger gene interrupted by translocation in Greig syndrome families. Nature 352:539–540.

163. Schimmang T, Lemaistre M, Vortkamp A, Ruther U. 1992. Expression of the zinc finger gene Gli3 is affected in the morphogenetic mouse mutant extra-toes (*Xt*). Development 116:799–804.

164. Walterhouse D, Ahmed M, Slusarski D, Kalamaras J, Boucher D, Holmgren R, Iannaccone P. 1993. *gli*, a zinc finger transcription factor and oncogene is expressed during normal mouse development. Dev Dyn 196:91–102.

165. Hui C, Slusarski D, Platt K, Holmgren R, Joyner A. 1994. Expression of three mouse homologs of the *Drosophila* segment polarity gene *cubitus interruptus, Gli, Gli-2, and Gli-3,* in ectoderm- and mesoderm-derived tissues suggests multiple roles during postimplantation development. Dev Biol 162:402–413.

166. Riley DJ, Lee EY-HP, Lee W-H. 1994. The retinoblastoma protein: more than a tumor suppressor. Annu Rev Cell Biol 10:1–29.

167. Bernards R, Schackleford GM, Gerber MR, Horowitz JM, Friend SH, Schartl M, Bogenmann E, Rapaport JM, McGee T, Dryja TP, Weinberg RA. 1989. Structure and expression of the murine retinoblastoma gene and characterization of its encoded protein. Proc Natl Acad Sci USA 86:6474–6478.

168. Szekely L, Jiang QW, Bulic-Jakus F, Rosen A, Ringertz N, Klein G, Wiman KG. 1992. Cell type and differentiation dependent heterogeneity in retinoblastoma protein expression in SCID mouse fetuses. Cell Growth Differ 3:149–156.

169. Clarke AR, Maandag ER, van Roon M, van der Lugt NMT, van der Valk M, Hooper ML, Berns A, te Riele H. 1992. Requirement for a functional Rb-1 gene in murine development. Nature 359:328–330.

170. Jacks T, Fazeli A, Schmitt EM, Bronson RT, Goodell MA, Weinberg RA. 1992. Effects of an Rb mutation in the mouse. Nature 359:295–300.

171. Lee EYH, Chang CY, Hu N, Wang YCJ, Lai CC, Herrup K, Lee WH, Bradley A. 1992. Mice deficient for Rb are nonviable and show defects in neurogenesis and haematopoiesis. Nature 359:288–294.

172. Bignon YJ. 1993. Expression of a retinoblastoma transgene results in dwarf mice. Genes Dev 7:1654–1662.

173. Chang CY, Riley DJ, Lee EY-HP, Lee WH. 1993. Quantitative effects of the retinoblastoma gene on mouse development and tissue-specific tumorigenesis. Cell Growth Differ 4:1057–1064.

174. Goodrich DW, Wang NP, Qian YW, Lee EY, Lee WH. 1991. The retinoblastoma gene product regulates progression throgh the G1 phase of the cell cycle. Cell 67:293–302.

175. Lee WH, Chen PG, Riley D. 1995. Regulatory networks of the retinoblastoma protein. Ann N Y Acad Sci 752:432–445.

176. Clarke AR. 1995. Murine model of neoplasia: functional analysis of the tumor suppressor genes Rb-1 and p53. Cancer Metastasis Rev 14:125–148.

177. Kastan MB, Canman CE, Leonard CJ. 1995. p53, cell cycle, control and apoptosis: implications for cancer. Cancer Metastasis Rev 14:3–15.

178. Clarke AR. 1995. Murine model of neoplasia: functional analysis of the tumor suppressor genes Rb-1 and p53. Cancer Metastasis Rev 14:125–148.

179. Lee JM, Bernstein A. 1995. Apoptosis, cancer and the p53 tumor suppressor gene. Cancer Metastasis Rev 14:149–161.

180. Malkin D. 1993. p53 and the Li–Fraumeni syndrome. Cancer Genet Cytogenet 66:83–92.

181. Rotter V, Aloni-Grinstein R, Schwartz D, Elkind NB, Simons A, Wolkowicz R, Lavigne M, Beserman P, Kapon A, Goldfinger N. 1994. Does wild type p53 play a role in normal cell differentiation? Semin Cancer Biol 5:229–236.

182. Armstrong JF, Kaufman MH, Harrison DJ, Clarke AR. 1995. High-frequency developmental abnormalities in p53-deficient mice. Curr Biol 5:931–936.

183. Sah VP, Attardi LD, Mulligan GJ, Williams BO, Bronson RT, Jacks T. 1995. A subset of p53-deficient embryos exhibit exencephaly. Nature Gen 10:175–180.
184. Lavidueur A, Maltby V, Mock D, Rossant J, Pawson T, Bernstein A. 1989. High incidence of lung, bone, and lymphoid tumors in transgenic mice overexpressing mutant alleles of the p53 oncogene. Mol Cell Biol 9:3982–3991.

2. Immunodeficiency states and related malignancies

Kenneth L. McClain

1. Introduction

The high incidence of malignancies in children with primary immune deficiencies has been well documented over several decades. As increased awareness of the problem drew the interest of experts in lymphoma morphology, it became clear that these were primarily B-lymphoid lymphoproliferations that ranged from benign, but aggressive, to frankly malignant diseases. Some of this understanding came as the result of improved classifications of lymphomas and the realization that a new category diseases — the post-transplant lymphoproliferations — were very similar to many of the neo-plasms of the immune-deficient individuals. These tumors were not the only types found in the transplant patients, however. It was recognized that the renal transplant recipients (mostly adults) had a much higher incidence of skin cancers than expected, as well as some other solid tumors. When the AIDS epidemic began in the 1980s, it soon became clear that HIV-infected children were also having a high incidence of lymphomas and otherwise rare leio-myosarcomas. The obvious reasons behind all these neoplasms were failure of immune surveillance and the opportunity for benign proliferations to achieve independent growth as malignancies. From the initial observations that Epstein–Barr virus DNA is found in many of these tumors to the recent findings of mutations in tumor suppressor genes, there have been significant contributions to our understanding of oncogenesis as a result of studying such cases, although more research is needed. This chapter will summarize informa-tion on the three categories of immune-deficient and cancer-prone patients: primary, posttransplant, and AIDS related (table 1).

2. Malignancies associated with primary immune deficiencies

The majority of comprehensive data available for these patients have come from Immunodeficiency Cancer Registry (ICR) maintained at the University of Minnesota. A detailed summary of ICR data was published in 1990 [1]. At that time, the presence of Epstein–Barr virus (EBV) as cofactor was the most

D.O. Walterhouse and S.L. Cohn (eds), DIAGNOSTIC AND THERAPEUTIC ADVANCES IN PEDIATRIC ONCOLOGY. Copyright © 1997. Kluwer Academic Publishers, Boston. All rights reserved.

Table 1. Cancers of immune-deficient patients

Primary immune deficiencies [1]
Non-Hodgkin's lymphoma >> Leukemias > "Other" >
Hodgkin's disease = Adenocarcinomas
Transplant-related
Lymphoproliferative disease (benign → malignant)
Skin cancers (adults primarily)
AIDS-related
Lymphomas and MALT lesions > Leiomyosarcoma >
Leukemias >> Kaposi's sarcoma

specific etiology recognized. Although it was generally assumed that the underlying immune deficiency was somehow allowing the virus to be more oncogenic, there were no data on cellular genetic defects that could specifically promote a higher incidence of malignancy. It is now understood that in Wiskott–Aldrich syndrome (WAS), patient sialophorin (CD43) is defective [2]. This molecule serves a critical costimulatory role by allowing antigen-presenting cells to bind to the CD43 epitope on T cells. More is known about the genetic defect in ataxia–telengiectasia (A-T) patients since the gene was cloned in 1995 [3]. This gene has extensive homology to known cell cycle checkpoint genes and is critical in signaling other genes when DNA damage occurs. Without the functional A-T gene, cells cannot stop the cell cycle to repair chromosome damage; they do not activate repair enzymes, and they also do not prevent the spontaneous cell death that accompanies DNA damage [4].

2.1. Non-Hodgkin's lymphomas

Fifty percent of all tumors in children with primary immune deficiencies are lymphomas or lymphoproliferations of benign but aggressive nature. In an early report from the ICR, the mortality of various cancer types was compared for the immune-deficient patients versus unselected children [5]. For the unselected children, lymphomas were the cause of 8% mortality, but in the immune-deficient children, 67% died of these neoplasms. Leukemia was the second most common cause of death, with 25% succumbing. Unlike lymphomas of apparently normal individuals, the primary immune-deficient patient often develops the malignancy in multiple sites, including the gastrointestinal tract, brain, lung, or soft tissues of the head and neck. When the different primary immune deficiencies are compared, the relative incidence of lymphomas in each category is as follows: WAS and severe combined immunodeficiency (SCID), 75%; A-T and common variable immunodeficiency (CVI), 46%; hyper IgM syndrome, 56%; hypogammaglobulinemia, 33%; and selective IgA deficiency, 15.8%.

The ICR report summarized clinical and pathological features of 22 WAS patients with lymphoma/lymphoproliferative disorders as to the central review histology versus reported histology, age, survival, and sites of the disease [1]. There were pleomorphic immunocytomas. Two of these had been incorrectly diagnosed as myeloid metaplasia and astrocytoma, and others had been labeled reticulum cell sarcoma — a now archaic term for lymphoma. Only one of these patients survived. Among three patients with immunoblastic sarcoma of B cells or three with lymphoplasmacytoid tumor, some of the tumors were originally called histiocytic lymphomas and one a microglioma. The survival was poor, with one patient living 1.6 years with a central nervous system tumor and the others succumbing quickly to their disease. The other lymphomas included a variety of follicular center cell and polymorphic B-cell lymphomas, although 3 of 22 WAS patients had T-cell lymphoma.

2.2. Hodgkin's disease

Hodgkin's lymphomas were most prevalent in the patients with hyper IgM syndrome (25%) and in patients with hypogammaglobulinemia (14%) [1]. In the other primary immune deficiencies, Hodgkin's disease made up 10% or less of the total malignancies in a given category. The immunodeficient patients exhibit several different clinical characteristics of their Hodgkin's disease when compared to the typical pediatric patient. They are younger (7.8 vs. 11.5 years mean age), are less likely to achieve remission, have poorer survival (five-year survival estimated at 18.5% vs. 84%), and have a predominance of mixed cellularity (42%) and lymphocyte depletion (33%) as compared to 24% and 2%–8% in most pediatric series.

2.3. Other tumors

Other tumors noted by the ICR include adenocarcinomas, which are most common in patients with selective IgA deficiency but make up only 9% of all cancers in immunodeficient patients [1]. Leukemias were not very prevalant except in the hypogammoglobulinemia patients (33%) and the A-T patients (21%). A variety of other tumors account for approximately 20% of the cancers in immunodeficient patients.

2.4. X-linked lymphoproliferative disease

Another interesting group of patients with a primary defective response to EBV infections are those with the X-linked lymphoproliferative (XLP) or Purtillo syndrome [6]. These boys develop benign but aggressive lymphoproliferations, lymphomas, and aplastic anemia. The B-cell lymphoproliferations follow the same pattern of the posttransplant lymphoproliferative diseases described below.

3. Lymphoproliferative diseases in transplant patients

3.1. Organ transplants and lymphoproliferative disease

Besides the patients with congenital immune deficiency, renal transplant patients became an important group with respect to the development of our understanding of EBV and lymphoproliferative disease (LPD). The unusual lymphoproliferative diseases of these patients are related to their immune suppression (prednisone, azathioprine, cyclosporine, anti-OKT3 antibodies, etc.). These cases first became apparent in the late 1960s and early 1970s and have been extensively studied since [7–9]. In recent series, the overall incidence of LPD has decreased but varies with the type of organ transplanted and the type of immunosuppression. LPD in heart transplant patients has typically been the highest, with reported incidences ranging from 1.8% to 9.8% or, with combined heart/lung transplants, 4.6% to 9.4% [8]. Lebland et al. reported an overall 1.7% (24 of 1385) incidence in LPD after solid organ transplantation [9]. Among the 641 kidney graft recipients, the frequency was 1.4%, and lung recipients had the highest (4.5%). Cyclosporine and azathioprine were used in the latter group and only prednisone and azathioprine in the former. Central nervous system (CNS) involvement with the LPD was most frequent after the renal transplants and in those not receiving cyclosporine. The transplanted organ(s) are involved at variable rates: 60% of heart/lung recipients and 15%–30% of the kidney grafts.

Patients with LPD can be segregated into two groups: those with a mean age of 23 years who developed the LPD within nine months after transplantation or after the start of anti-rejection therapy and those with a mean age of 48 years who presented with LPD up to six years after transplant [7]. The younger patients had typical symptoms of infectious mononucleosis: fever, pharyngitis, and lymphadenopathy. The older patients had localized tumor masses. EBV was found in the spectrum of histologic types of LPD from polymorphic diffuse B-cell hyperplasia to monoclonal B-cell lymphoma.

3.2. Bone marrow transplants and LPD

EBV infection is rarely a problem in patients undergoing bone marrow transplants unless the donor marrow is severely depleted of T cells or there is potent posttransplant immunosuppression due to a mismatch situation [10]. The incidence of LPD was 25% among mismatched, T-cell-depleted recipients, 10% in nondepleted marrow/unrelated donor transplants, and only one of 424 among the matched nondepleted transplants in a study from Minnesota [10]. Between 5 and 50 copies of EBV genome/cell were found in the tissues. Most of the LPD occurred in B cells of donor origin, but in 2 of 7 patients the LPD occurred in recipient cells. The onset of LPD was from 30 days to 49 months post bone marrow transplant (BMT). The common presenting features included fever, anorexia, abdominal pain, and hepatitis. Sometimes lethargy, lymphadenopathy, and CNS symptoms were reported. A group of patients who presented in the first two months post BMT with rapidly progressive LPD had received high-dose antithymocyte globulin and prednisone to help engraftment. The other patients developed LPD from three months to three years after the BMT and had slower-paced LPD, but most still died of those processes. Histologically, these LPDs varied from benign polyclonal (as determined by immunochemical staining for immunoglobulins) to monoclonal proliferations that were malignant.

3.3. LPD associated with other immune dysregulatory conditions

Kamel et al. reported EBV-associated, reversible lymphoproliferations in patients receiving methotrexate therapy for rheumatic disease [11]. In reviewing cases at their institutions, they found 18 examples of patients with rheumatoid arthritis or dermatomyositis who developed a variety of LPDs, including lymphoplasmacytic infiltrate, Hodgkin's disease, diffuse large cell lymphoma (immunoblastic and pleomorphic subtypes), large-cell lymphoma, and small-cleaved lymphoma. EBV was found in 6 of 18 cases by in situ hybridization and staining for the EBV latent membrane protein (LMP). Five of these six patients were receiving methotrexate. The authors noted that the 33% incidence of EBV was near the reported 30%–50% in lymphomas of patients with AIDS, but was obviously higher than the 4% incidence of EBV found in lymphomas in general.

3.4. Histologic categories of LPD

The initial response of a B cell infected with EBV is blastogenesis. The cell enlarges and nuclear chromatin changes. Although this change is a radical departure from the morphology of the resting lymphocyte, there is nothing intrinsically "malignant" in appearance about these cells — thus the dilemma in evaluating the early stages of LPD. Frizerra et al. developed a set of guidelines for the different types of LPD based upon morphologic criteria that were correlated with immunophenotypic and cytogenetic data [12]. They stressed that LPDs are different from nonspecific lymphoid hyperplasias, including infectious mononucleosis, because of the location of follicular center cells (FCCs) and other features listed below. The FCCs are large cells with clumped chromatin, multiple prominent nucleoli at the periphery, and a moderate amount of cytoplasm. These large cells are only in the germinal center of lymph nodes with benign hyperplasia, but they invade the involved tissues of LPD patients. Most important, the 'atypical immunoblasts,' invasiveness, and necrosis found in the malignant types of LPD are not found in the benign lymphoid hyperplasias.

The most benign group of LPD was called a polymorphic diffuse B-cell hyperplasia. Lymphoid cells represent a variety of differentiation stages. Many lymphocytes in the lesions had chromatin distributed about the periphery of the nucleus with a central prominent nucleolus and basophilic cytoplasm. These lymphocytes are consistent with plasmacytoid differentiation and were called *B immunoblasts*. There are many large lymphoid cells that invade the lymph nodes or other involved organs.

The LPD qualified as a *lymphoma* only when there were many atypical immunoblasts with invasiveness and necrosis. *Atypia* was defined as very large and irregular nuclei with bilobulation or multilobulation, deep grooves, or contorted margins and giant cell formation. The histologically malignant group was further subdivided into immunoblastic sarcoma of B cells when there were no FCCs and necrosis was present but not prominent.

3.5. Biology of EBV infection in LPD

Epstein–Barr virus (EBV) has been associated with the onset of benign and malignant diseases in a variety of human conditions. In normal individuals, infectious mononucleosis is characterized by a brisk T-lymphocyte response to EBV-infected B lymphocytes. The EBV infection and B-cell growth is limited by the normal immune response. However, in persons with compromised immune function, whether congenital or secondary to immune suppression with a transplant or infection, these B-cell proliferations are often uncontrolled and result in the patient's death.

EBV infection is ordinarily controlled by cytotoxic T lymphocytes that recognize the highly immunogenic coat proteins and nuclear antigens of the virus. EBV infects the oropharyngeal epithelium and B lymphocytes because the complement C3d(CD21) receptor is also the receptor for EBV [13,14]. A productive infection of B lymphocytes occurs when capsid proteins and whole virus are made, causing lysis of the cells. Normally, this process triggers a B-cell response with IgM antibodies to the viral capsid antigen (VCA) followed by the IgG response, which lasts lifelong [15]. Two other early viral antigens (EAs) are distinguished serologically either by their location in the cytoplasm and nucleus [EA(D)] or by their restriction to the cytoplasm [EA(R)]. Both are found in primary EBV infection, but the latter is often a sign of EBV reactivation or of the abnormal serologic responses in lymphoproliferative diseases of children with defective immune systems. A rise in the titers to VCA and EA is often a sign that EBV is in a replicative phase.

Later, the antibodies to the EBV nuclear antigen DNA binding proteins (EBNA) develop. It is thought that these are delayed due to the lag in cytolytic T-cell responses and death of the infected cells [15]. The antibody response to EBNAs provides evidence for a past EBV infection, and the titers are usually quite stable.

Cytolytic T-lymphocyte and natural killer (NK) cell responses to EBV-infected cells provide the ultimate control of infected B cells and thus prevent LPD in normal hosts. T cells are activated by the presence of all the EBNAs (2, 3A, 3B, 3C, 4, and 5) except EBNA-1. The latter antigen is the only one found on chronically infected B cells in normal hosts. Thus, with normal immune surveillance, a nonproductive (latent) viral infection is the rule. Only 1 in 10^7 B cells contains the EBV genome, which is in a limited state of activation [16]. Without the normal immune response, EBV can proliferate and then infect and transform additional B cells. Given multiple replication/infection events without immune control, it is more likely that a permanently cell-transforming event such as the *c-myc* oncogene–immunoglobulin enhancer translocation (t8;14) or other oncogene mutation will occur. However, this event is not necessary to cause a serious life-threatening LPD. The uncontrolled proliferation of apparently normal B lymphocytes in a person with congenital or secondary immune suppression may be fatal.

The EBV infection in patients with posttransplant LPD may be primary, reactivated, or chronic. Although EBV infection may occur in transplant patients without causing an LPD, those with primary EBV infections have the highest risk of LPD. Forty-three percent of LPD patients had primary infections versus 8% of the transplant patients who did not develop LPD. Patients in this latter group are usually less immunosuppressed than those who do develop LPD [17]. A rise in the titers of IgG anti-VCA occurred in 100% of those LPD patients with primary infections and in 57% of those with reactivated infections. About half of each of these groups of patients had increases in the IgM-antiVCA titers. Eighty-three percent of the primary infections and all of the reactivated infections showed elevations of the IgG titers against the restricted early antigen (EA-R). Reactivations occurred between one and seven months after transplantation. The defective immune response to EBV in posttransplant patients is documented by the fact that antibodies to EBNA did not develop in 4 of 6 patients who had primary infections.

Different strains of EBV than are found in other EBV-associated diseases could be involved with LPD. There are two families of EBV (types A and B), as judged by polymorphisms of the EBNA2 gene [18]. Type B is more commonly seen in immunocompromised individuals such as those with Burkitt's lymphoma in Africa and in AIDS patients [19,20]. The type A virus can efficiently immortalize B cells and can infect the oropharyngeal epithelium and peripheral blood lymphocytes. The type B strain is less efficient at immortalizing in vitro and is rarely found in the peripheral blood of normal individuals. In a study of 22 solid organ transplant recipients with LPD, only the type A EBV was found [21]. The authors believed this finding was in concert with the more efficient B cell immortalizing capacity of that strain.

Evaluation of the terminal fragments of EBV DNA for clonality has revealed that 90% of LPD patients have monoclonal or biclonal expansions of virus [22]. These data derive from the variable lengths of the genomic termini of EBV. When multiple clones of EBV are present, probing Southern blots of restriction endonuclease digests of lesional DNA with the terminal EBV fragments can determine whether a polyclonal or monoclonal array of viral genomes is present. The finding of one or two bands suggest monoclonal or biclonal proliferation of the EBV and serves as a surrogate marker of clonal proliferation of the LPD. The size of the terminal fragments also helps show whether the EBV genome is in the closed circular conformation found in the latent phase of virus infection or the linear form seen in the active/replication stage. A homogeneous episomal population in the monoclonal tumors suggests that the EBV infection occurred as an early event in tumorigenesis.

When LPD lesions of solid organ transplant patients were evaluated for EBV gene expression by Western blot studies, the highly immunogenic EBNA2 protein was detected in only 3 of 23 lesions, but the less immunogenic EBNA1 was found in all [23]. The latent membrane protein (LMP) of EBV, a transforming protein [24] with moderate immunogenicity, was found at low levels in all but one of the samples. Serologic data revealed that the patients had appropriate responses to VCA and EA. As had been described earlier in bone marrow transplant recipients with LPD, solid organ transplant patients with LPD had limited (1–3) episomal populations of EBV as determined by terminal repeat analysis. The authors hypothesized that LPDs are like Hodgkin's disease and nasopharyngeal carcinoma in that EBNA2 is absent and LMP, if present, is present at only low levels [25,26]. As with these two latter tumors, LPDs do not usually have rearrangements of an immunoglobulin gene and the *c-myc* oncogene.

In contrast to the results discussed above, Young et al. used immunohistochemical methods to evaluate EBV gene expression in bone marrow transplant patients with LPD [27]. They showed *enhanced* expression of EBNA2 and LMP as well as of the cellular adhesion molecules LFA3 and ICAM 1 and the B-cell activation antigen CD23. The role of EBNA2 as a transforming protein may be a key factor in BMT-LPD, since this viral gene is a key transforming gene of EBV [28]. These investigators found no efficacy for acyclovir in one of their cases. This finding was considered to be consistent with the 'latent' EBV gene pattern found in the patient's tissues. Since the highly immunogenic EBNA2 and adhesion proteins were present on the surface of the LPD cells, it was likely that the normal cytotoxic T-lymphocyte response could clear these cells when immunsuppression was decreased. It is unlikely that the BMT-LPDs are biologically different from the LPDs associated with solid tumors. Therefore, the conflicting data with regard to EBNA2 expression are most likely due to differences in the sensitivity of techniques used by the two groups or to different histologic types of LPD [23,27] (table 2).

Table 2. Associations of lymphoproliferative disease of transplant patients

Profound immune suppression post-organ transplant
T-cell depletion pre-bone marrow transplant
B-cell proliferations
Primary Epstein–Barr virus infection (monoclonal or biclonal)
   ↑ Titers to EBV early antigen-R
   Type A EBV
   EBNA-1, EBNA-2, and latent membrane protein expression
   ↑ Adhesion molecules LFA3 and ICAM 1

The LPDs represent a morphological spectrum from benign but aggressive polymorphic proliferations to obviously malignant lymphomas. Thus, there is interest in correlating the histological variants with EBV gene expression. In a summary of 14 cases of LPD in bone marrow and solid organ transplant recipients, Delecluse et al. showed two distinct groups with regard to expression of EBNA2 and LMP [29]. All the mature B-cell LPDs and the monomorphic large cell lymphomas without plasmacytic differentiation (e.g., immunoblastic) had LMP and/or EBNA2 expression. The number of cells expressing the B-cell markers CD19, 20, and 22 as well as the CD21 EBV receptor antigen were highly variable within each lesion. Lesions in the second group were monomorphic large cell LPD with plasmacytic differentiation. None of these had expression of LMP, EBNA2, or the early B-cell markers. They were, however, positive for the EBV EBER RNA and the mature B cell marker CD38 and an epithelial membrane antigen EMA. The large cell LPD cases were distinct clinically because the LPD developed more than 14 months after transplant. There was no relationship between clonality of the lesions and viral gene expression.

In a comprehensive study of EBV and cellular genes in LPD, Knowles et al. have reported three distinct categories of posttransplantation lymphoproliferative disorders [30]. Since neither morphology or clonality has been a good predictor of clinical outcome in the LPD patients, these authors investigated the LPD tissues for alterations in bcl-1, bcl-2, *c-myc*, the *H-*, *K-*, and *N-ras* proto-oncogenes, and mutations in the p53 tumor suppressor gene. They correlated the findings of those investigations with morphology, immunoglobulin bene clonality, and the presence of EBV as a clonal population or not. In the plasmacytic hyperplasias only 1 of 10 had an immunoglobulin gene rearrangement. Polyclonal EBV was dominant, with only a minor population showing a clonal proliferation. None of these had abnormalities of the cellular oncogenes or a tumor suppressor gene. The LPDs classified as polymorphic B-cell hyperplasia or lymphoma were frequently ones that originated in the lungs or gastrointestinal tract; they had monoclonal immunoglobulin gene rearrangements and distinct clonal proliferations of EBV but lacked any abnormalities of the cellular genes studied. The final group of immunoblastic lymphoma/multiple myeloma LPDs had monoclonal immunoglobulin gene rearrangements, clonal EBV, and a variety of cellular gene mutations. Of the plasmacytoid immunoblastic lymphoma/multiple myeloma cases, one had a mutation in *c-myc*, but all three had the same *N-Ras* mutations of codon 61. There were no *K-* or *H-Ras* mutations in any of the cases. Both the LPD cases classified as pleomorphic immunoblastic lymphoma had mutations of p53. The findings in the most malignant variety of LPD were consistent with findings published previously showing that expression of Ras oncogenes in an EBV cell line caused malignant transformation [31]. In general, the mutations of cellular genes confirmed the clinical nature of these lesions (table 3). If there were no cellular gene abnormalities, the lesions tended to regress when immunosuppressive therapy was minimized. However, the malignant lesions in the third

Table 3. Molecular characteristics of LPD

	Plasmacytic hyperplasia	Polymorphic B-cell hyperplasia	Immunoblastic lymphoma
Immunoglobulin gene rearrangement	Polyclonal	Monoclonal	Monoclonal
EBV infection	Polyclonal	Monoclonal	Monoclonal
c-myc mutations	No	No	Yes
N-Ras mutations	No	No	Yes
p53 mutations	No	No	Yes

LPD group (with the cellular gene mutations) required chemotherapy to treat and most often caused the death of the patients. Overall, the LPDs provide concise examples of the hypotheses relating to malignant transformation of lymphocytes. EBV serves as the 'driver' of the lymphocyte proliferation, which becomes malignant only with mutation of cellular genes. Since these proliferative and mutagenic events may occur independently in an immuno-suppressed patient with LPD, different lesions within the same patient may exhibit any of the three stages of LPD when examined at any specific time in the course of the patient's illness [32].

It is clear that EBV remains the central factor in the development of LPD. Several publications have shown that increasing levels of circulating EBV correlate most highly with the transplant patient developing an LPD [33–35]. An increase in the titer to VCA may be a hint that a patient may develop an LPD. However, the amount of rise is dependent on whether the patient was seropositive before the transplant or not [33]. Preiksaitis et al. showed that quantitation of oropharyngeal EBV shedding by a DNA dot-blot assay could be helpful in following transplant patients at risk for LPD [35]. In their study, serologic responses to EBV underestimated the amount of EBV activity. Subsequently, others have reported that the clearest indication of an incipient LPD is a rise in the amount of EBV DNA amplified by the polymerase chain reaction (PCR) from peripheral blood mononuclear cells. Another indication of profound immune suppression and a fatal outcome was concomitant infection with CMV [34]. In a larger group of patients, Riddler et al. showed dramatically increased levels of EBV in those transplant patients who developed LPD [34]. Of patients who were seropositive before transplant, *all* the LPD patients had over 1000 EBV genomes per 100,000 peripheral blood lymphocytes. The EBV seropositive patients who did *not* develop an LPD had 500 or fewer copies of EBV DNA per 100,000 peripheral blood lymphocytes. Although the amount of EBV in pretransplant seronegative individuals was higher in general after transplant, those with over 50,000 genomes per 100,000 cells were the most likely to have an LPD. In both these patient groups, the absence of or decrease in the serologic titer to EBNA2 was associated with the onset of the LPD. The data show that when EBV infection goes unchecked, there is a higher level of viral replication and thus a greater chance for B cells to develop a malignant change. There was no relationship between the viral load, clonality of EBV, and the morphologic features of the LPD [34]. However, the pretransplant serologic status correlated with outcome. Patients who were seronegative before transplant had the worst outcome in that 3 of 6 patients died of LPD as opposed to 0 of 6 who were seropositive before their transplant.

A correlative means of defining the presence of EBV and the chance of an LPD was found in liver biopsies of liver transplant patients who were being evaluated for hepatitis and graft rejection [36]. Seventy-one percent of the patients with subsequent LPD had EBV detected by in situ hybridization using the EBV EBER RNA probes on a prior liver biopsy. Only 10% of controls who did not develop an LPD had EBV detected. Most (13 of 17) patients with LPD and EBV in a liver biopsy were diagnosed with the LPD within 100 days of the positive biopsy. Ten of the 17 LPDs were in the liver and seven were in other organs. The EBER-positive cells were usually small lymphocytes and larger cells of the blast-transformed morphology. In addition, some bone fide hepatocytes (as determined by double-labeling experiments) were also positive for EBER RNA. Fifteen of the 17 patients had histologic changes indicative of EBV-hepatitis.

3.6. Cytokines in LPD

Interleukin-6 (IL-6), which has a key role in B-cell differentiation, has been implicated in the pathogenesis of multiple myeloma, Castleman's disease, and Kaposi sarcoma [37–39]. IL-6 can work in both autocrine and paracrine pathways to stimulate B-cell growth and secretion of immunoglobulins [40,41]. Likewise, IL-6 is elevated in the serum of LPD patients, and increased levels correlate with a greater chance of developing the LPD [43]. IL-6 is especially relevant to the LPD in transplanted patients because it can be induced by cyclosporine in monocytes and T lymphocytes [43]. Cyclosporine inhibits a variety of T-lymphocyte and natural killer (NK) cell functions including IL-2 production [44]. IL-6 also suppresses NK function and increases the tumorigenicity of B cells [45]. When EBV-infected peripheral blood mononuclear cells are cultured with cyclosporine, the amount of EBV produced in each cell increases by as much as tenfold [42]. These results demonstrate how the combination of EBV, IL-6, and cyclosporine could dramatically increase the chances for LPD in transplant patients.

Although there have been no clinical trials, interleukin-4 (IL-4) could theoretically be used in the therapy of LPD. Schwarz et al. showed IL-4 injections slowed the dissemination of an EBV-infected Burkitt's lymphoma cell line in severe combined immunodeficient (SCID) mice [46]. Mice were injected with 10^6 tumor cells, and 7 to 14 days later, IL-4 injections were begun. The mice without IL-4 therapy rapidly developed diffuse tumor infiltration of all organs. Those with IL-4 had no dissemination of tumor cells. Since IL-4 had no effect on the tumor cells in vitro, it was suggested that the cytokine had recruited NK

Table 4. Role of cytokines in lymphoproliferative diseases

IL-6 promotes	IL-4 controls
By: Enhancing EBV proliferation	Decreasing EBV dissemination
Stimulating B-cell growth and tumorigenicity	Downregulating VCAM-1
Suppressing natural killer cell function	

cells that are present in the SCID mice. Another possible effect of IL-4 could be the downregulation of the vascular adhesion molecule VCAM-1, which would decrease the chance of the tumor cells extravasating via binding of the integrins on the tumor cells [47] (table 4).

3.7. Treatment options for EBV-LPD

Shortly after the problem of LPD in renal transplants began, it was recognized that reduction of immune suppression was the easiest way of controlling the disease [7,48]. This treatment seemed to be effective in many of the diffuse B-cell hyperplasias no matter which drug dose — azathoprine, cyclosporine, or prednisone — was lowered.

Successful anti-EBV therapy with acyclovir or ganciclovir has been reported [7,49]. Both these agents are theoretically effective during times of active EBV replication (lytic infection). Either antiviral agent will clear EBV from throat washings, but there is a rapid rebound after the drug is withdrawn. The latent form of virus in lymphocytes is not affected [35]. It is difficult to judge the role of the antiviral agents because their use often coincides with a decrease in immune suppressive therapy and some patients do not respond to acyclovir [7]. A new antiviral (penciclovir) has effects on replicating virus similar to acyclovir [50].

Anti-B-cell antibodies have also been used to treat patients with LPD [51]. Two children who received mismatched bone marrow transplants for congenital immunodeficiency and were given cyclosporine developed LPD at days 50–60 post BMT. They were treated with a combination of mouse monoclonal antibodies against the CD21 and CD24 antigens of B cells. All symptoms and sign of the LPD resolved after a 10-day treatment, and there were no recurrences.

Alpha-interferon in LPD patients has been a successful therapy for some [52]. In the original group of patients, one lived after receiving high-dose (2 million units/M^2) alpha interferon. Subsequently, 4 of 4 patients were cured of LPD by early institution of the interferon and high-dose intravenous gamma globulin therapy [52].

An alternative method of specific anti-B-cell therapy has been suggested in a mouse model of human EBV-B-cell lymphomas [53]. When human periph-

Table 5. Treatment of lymphoproliferative disease posttransplant

1. Decrease immune suppression
2. Acyclovir treatment of EBV?
3. Anti-B-cell monoclonal antibodies
4. Anti-CD40 monoclonal antibodies
5. Alpha-interferon and IV IgG

eral blood lymphocytes are injected into SCID mice, some of the normally latently EBV-infected cells can proliferate and cause the death of the mice [54]. By using this model, Murphy et al. showed that antibodies to CD40 may inhibit the lymphomagenesis [53]. CD40 stimulation promotes normal B-cell proliferation but inhibits proliferation of human B-cell lymphomas in vitro and in vivo [55]. Although this model system seems very encouraging with regard to LPDs, it should be noted that the authors found no effect of CD40 antibodies on human myeloma cell lines. This fact is discouraging because some of the most malignant LPDs have characteristics of myelomas [30]. Recently, Swinnen et al. showed that aggressive chemotherapy could be curative for LPD patients with malignant lymphomas [56] (table 5).

4. Malignancies of children with HIV infection

A 1994 Center for Disease Control summary of the 6200 cases of AIDS in children noted 42 cases of Burkitt's lymphoma, 32 cases of immunoblastic lymphoma, and 23 primary CNS lymphomas, which gives an overall lymphoma prevalence of 1.6%. (personal communication, Mary Lou Lindegren, M.D., CDC). A European study documented cancer in 8% of children with AIDS [57]. It is believed that this number is low, since only the initial AIDS-defining condition is usually reported and cancer may not be the first condition. In addition, leiomyosarcomas (apparently the second most frequent malignancy of children with AIDS) and several other tumors, including Hodgkin's disease, B-cell leukemias, and other rarer tumors, are not AIDS-defining conditions.

4.1. Non-Hodgkin's lymphoma

As with the congenital immunodeficiencies, a child with AIDS has a markedly increased chance of developing non-Hodgkin's lymphoma (NHL). In hemophiliacs with HIV infection, NHL is 36 times more common than in the HIV-negative children [58]. Most of the NHLs are B-lymphocytic tumors of the small noncleaved cell or immunoblastic histology and have an 8:14 chromosomal translocation. These types of NHL represent approximately 25%–40%

51

of lymphomas in otherwise normal children, so cases may not be recognized as AIDS-associated at first. Thus, all children who develop lymphoma should be tested for HIV infection.

Most pediatric AIDS patients with NHL acquired the HIV infection vertically or from transfusion of blood and clotting factor concentrates. The mean age for discovery of malignancy in the vertically infected group is 35 months, with a range of 6–62 months. [59]. In hemophiliacs, the latency is longer, with cases presenting up to age 18 years [60]. The latency from time of HIV seroconversion to onset of the lymphomas was 22–88 months, and all pediatric patients had CD4 lymphocyte counts less than $50/mm^3$ at diagnosis of the malignancy.

Children with AIDS lymphomas present with fever and weight loss and typically demonstrate extranodal manifestations of hepatomegaly, jaundice, or abdominal distention, evidence of bone marrow involvement, or CNS symptoms. Some of these patients had prior lymphoproliferative diseases such as lymphoid interstitial pneumonitis (LIP) or pulmonary lymphoid hyperplasia (PLH) [57]. Like patients with primary immune deficiency, the AIDS patients often have diffuse (stage III or IV) disease at the time of presentation.

There is a higher than normal incidence of CNS lymphomas in AIDS patients, who may present with developmental delay or loss of developmental milestones, dementia, cranial nerve palsies, seizures, or hemiparesis [61]. The differential diagnosis of infection versus malignancy may be difficult, since CNS symptoms and a mass lesion seen on computed tomography (CT) might be from toxoplasmosis or cryptococcus as well as from lymphoma [62]. Contrast-enhanced CT studies of the brain reveal a rim of enhancement in both neoplastic or infectious etiologies. A sterotactic biopsy can give a definitive diagnosis. Recently, positron emission tomography (PET) has provided help as a noninvasive diagnostic test [63]. A prospective study of AIDS patients using this technique demonstrated that lymphomas were *hyper*metabolic lesions and the toxoplasmosis *hypo*metabolic.

4.2. Treatment of AIDS lymphomas

Effective chemotherapy for NHL in an AIDS patient is possible. Important good prognostic features of the patients include a CD4 lymphocyte count above $100/mm^3$, a near normal serum LDH level, no prior AIDS-defining illnesses, and good Karnofsky score (80%–100%). The number of pediatric AIDS patients treated for lymphoma is low, and no series of patients has been published. There are reports of cyclophosphamide (Cytoxan), vincristine (Oncovin), doxorubicin (adriamycin), methotrexate (amethoperin), cytarabine (cytosine arabinoside), and prednisone plus intrathecal methotrexate and/or cytosine arabinoside providing durable remissions of up to seven years [57,61,64–71]. CNS lymphomas are more difficult because of delay in diagnosis [59]. Intrathecal therapy is indicated even for those without evidence of disease [71]. Radiation therapy may be a helpful adjunct for CNS involvement [67]. In general, HIV-infected children with lymphoma should be treated on standard protocols as recommended by the Pediatric Oncology Group (POG) and the Children's Cancer Group (CCG).

Alpha-interferon is currently under study by the Pediatric Oncology Group (POG) for treatment of AIDS-associated malignancies. This agent was chosen because it has no cross-resistance to chemotherapy, a known anti-HIV activity, and reported responses of some lymphomas [72,73].

Supportive care for patients undergoing chemotherapy should include antiretroviral treatment (as tolerated vis-a-vis cytopenias), pneumocystis carinii prophylaxis, and G-CSF after the completion of chemotherapy.

4.3. Etiology of NHL in AIDS patients

Primary features of HIV infection include lymphadenopathy and atypical lymphoproliferations in many organs [74]. Some of these lymphoproliferative diseases have been associated with EBV infection and include lymphocytic interstitial pneumonitis and CNS lymphoma [64]. Shibata et al. showed the frequency of EBV in benign lymph node biopsies of HIV-infected patients [75]. EBV DNA was present in 13 of 35 biopsies of AIDS patients with persistent generalized adenopathy, but in none of nodes from HIV-negative individuals. Important in this study was the fact that some of these 13 had lymphoma concurrent with the hyperplastic node and others developed lymphoma from 1–22 months later.

Interestingly, not all NHLs of AIDS patients have EBV DNA in the tumor cells. From 35% to 77% of NHLs outside the CNS in adults or in children with AIDS seem to be associated with EBV [76]. For CNS lesions, this rate is 100% as determined by in situ hybridization using probes for the EBER region of the EBV genome [77]. Of the Burkitt-type lymphomas, only 34% had EBV in the tumor cells. This result confirmed findings by others who have documented *c-myc* gene rearrangements rather than evidence of EBV genome in many individuals with AIDS-associated NHLs [78]. HIV has been found only rarely in the lymphoma cells but may be present in surrounding lymphocytes or macrophages [79,80]. It is more likely that any cofactor role of HIV relates to cytokines which are produced as a result of the HIV virus. Interleukins-1, -2, -6, -7, and -10, interferon-gamma, tumor necrosis factor, and B-cell growth factor have all been identified [81–83]. Since EBV cannot always be implicated in the etiology of the NHLs of AIDS patients, some other factors must play an important role.

Mutations or rearrangements in the *c-myc* oncogene are frequent in AIDS NHLs. The classic $t(8:14)$, $t(2;8)$, or $t(8:22)$ that position an immunoglobulin gene enhancer near the *myc* oncogene in Burkitt's lymphoma are well known [84]. The number of HIV-infected patients with NHL and rearrangements in *c-myc* is variable (40%–75%) depending on the methodology, type of patients, and locations of the lymphomas [85,86].

53

Thus, as with most cancers in humans, no one agent or event can be uniformly designated as *the* cause of NHL in AIDS patients. Rather, a multistep pathway to malignancy occurs from immunosuppression, viral infections, enhanced B-cell turnover from growth factors, and finally some genetic change(s).

4.4. AIDS-associated leiomyosarcomas and leiomyomas

Children with HIV infection have a high incidence of benign or malignant smooth muscle tumors [59,87]. Leiomyosarcomas (LSs) and leiomyomas (LMs) occur at a rate of less than 2 cases per 10 million in non-HIV-infected children. More than 16 cases of LS and LM have been reported among the less than 6200 children with AIDS. These tumors originate in the lungs, spleen, and gastrointestinal tract, with symptoms consistent with endobronchial or intestinal obstruction. EBV in situ hybridization studies of the LM and LS demonstrate that EBV, but not HIV, was present in every tumor cell and not in the adjoining normal cells [88]. Quantitative PCR studies corroborated the in situ data by demonstrating high copy numbers of EBV in the tumor and increasing concentrations of EBV DNA in serial studies of patient plasma at times before the tumors were diagnosed. Immunostaining for the EBV receptor (CD21/C3d) on tumor tissue revealed a high concentration, but less on normal smooth muscle or control LN/LS. It is thought that the EBV receptor may be upregulated, allowing EBV to enter the muscle cells in AIDS patients. One of the EBV transforming genes such as EBNA2 may play a key role, since EBNA2 has been identified in a tumor of liver transplant patients that is infected with EBV like the leiomyosarcomas [89].

4.5. Treatment of LM/LS in AIDS patients

There have been no consistent treatments of these patients, but continuous-infusion doxorubicin (adriamycin) or alpha-interferon and/or radiotherapy have provided partial responses. Complete surgical resection is important.

4.6. Other lymphoproliferations of AIDS patients

Reactive and proliferative lymphoid lesions associated with mucosa of the gastrointestinal tract, Waldeyer's ring, salivary glands, respiratory tract and other sites such as the thyroid, thymus, etc. are now known as *mucosa-associated lymphoid tissue* (MALT) [90,91]. Reactive follicles, proliferation of centrocytic cells of the marginal zone, lymphoepithelial lesions, and plasmacytoid differentiation are characteristic. The MALT lesions bridge the continuum of LPD from reactive to neoplastic lesions. Neoplastic lesions are usually of low grade but may progress to high-grade MALT lymphomas [92,93]. The spectrum of other lymphoid lesions of lungs (pulmonary lymphoid hyperplasia/lymphoid interstitial pneumonitis — PLH/LIP — complex) and other organs described previously in children should also be considered as MALT lesions [94,95].

4.7. Leukemias and Hodgkin's disease

Most leukemias of children with AIDS are of B-cell origin, which is consistent with the types of lymphomas [96,97]. They represent the fourth most common malignancy of children with AIDS the first three being NHL, leiomyosarcomas, and various forms of Kaposi's sarcoma. The clinical presentation and biologic features are similar to those found in non-HIV-infected children. Also, these patients have achieved stable remissions with chemotherapy that includes intravenous vincristine, prednisone, cyclophosphamide, doxorubicin, methotrexate, and intrathecal cytosine arabinoside [96,97]. Unlike adults, there is no apparent increase of Hodgkin's disease in children with AIDS [94,98].

4.8. Kaposi's sarcoma

Although Kaposi's sarcoma (KS) occurs in about 25% of adults with AIDS, it is rare in children. A review of 30 cases of KS in children reports that most were HIV-infected children born to mothers in groups at high risk for KS (heterosexual transmission via a bisexual partner) or who acquired HIV infection postnatally via contaminated blood or blood products [99].

There is some controversy about the diagnosis of KS in children, since this lesion may be easily confused with other conditions. For instance, the relative prominence of vascularity in an atrophic lymph node in a child who died of AIDS may be mistaken for KS. Also, there is a nodular spindle-cell vascular transformation of retroperitoneal and other lymph nodes that mimics KS [100]. Infection with *Bartonnela henselae*, which causes bacillary angiomatosis (BA), may create a vasoproliferative lesion. However, BA lacks the spindle cell element and bizarre shapes of the vascular channels seen in KS [101]. The lymphadenopathic form of KS is seen mostly in children born to Haitian parents or in African children and probably represents the epidemic form of KS unrelated to AIDS [102]. Only the cutaneous form is a true indicator of the disease related to AIDS [103]. Thus, it appears that the stated frequency of 6% of HIV-infected children developing KS is a gross overestimate. Visceral involvement (GI tract, lungs, etc.), although clinically suspected in some cases, has not been pathologically documented in children with AIDS.

4.9. Other AIDS-associated malignancies in children

Adolecents are too often forgotten in our consideration of HIV-infected individuals because of the frequency of reports of infants and adults with their various risk factors. Teenagers may exhibit risk-taking behavior that gives them the same problems as adults, and all physicians must be aware of the confluence of these dangers. One example is the human papilloma virus (HPV)-associated condylomatous lesions in children and adolescents with AIDS [94]. There have been reports of cervical condylomata and cervical carcinoma in this age group [104]. The spectrum of cervical dysplasia from minimal to frank intraepithelial neoplasia may progress quickly in patients with AIDS [105]. Physicians caring for adolescent girls with HIV infection should look for the HPV-related genital lesions in their patients, and if found, these lesions should be treated promptly so that their progression to malignancy is prevented.

Only single cases of the following types of tumors have been reported in children with AIDS: hepatoblastoma, embryonal rhabdomyosarcoma of the gall bladder, fibrosarcoma of liver, and papillary carcinoma of thyroid [59,94,106]. These tumors probably represent coincidental occurrences rather than true association with HIV infection.

Since malignancies in children with AIDS are rare, it is important that every one be studied completely with regard to type and incidence, risk factors, and biologic features. The Pediatric Oncology Group (POG) has established a national registry and treatment protocols. Patient information and fresh, frozen, and fixed specimen studies are coordinated through the POG Statistical Office in Gainsesville, Florida (telephone 352–292–5198, FAX 352–392–8162). The collaborative efforts of all physicians treating children with AIDS and malignancies will be needed to advance our knowledge and efficacy in treating these diseases.

Acknowledgments

This work was supported in part by grants CA56296, CA30969, and CA29139 from the National Cancer Institute. Peggy James provided assistance in preparation of the manuscript.

References

1. Filipovich AH, Shapiro R, Robison L, Mertens A, Fizzera G. 1990. Lymphoproliferative disorders associated with immunodeficiency. In McGath IT (ed). The Non-Hodgkin's Lymphomas, London: Edward Arnold, pp 135–154.
2. Park JK, Rosenstein YJ, Rmold-O'Donnell E, Bierer BE, Rosen FS, Burakoff SJ. 1991. Enhancement of T-cell activation by the CD43 molecule whose expression is defective in Wiskott–Aldrich syndrome. Nature 350:706–709.
3. Savitsky K, Bar-Shira A, Gilad S, et al. 1995. A single ataxia telangiectasia gene with a product similar to PI-3 kinase. Science 268:1749–1753.
4. Meyn MS. 1995. Ataxia-teleangiectasia and cellular responses to DNA damage. Cancer Res 55:5991–6001.
5. Kersey JH, Spector BD, Good RA. 1975. Cancer in children with primary immunodeficiency diseases. Pediatrics 84:263–264.
6. Purtilo DT. 1983. Immunopathology of X-linked lymphoproliferative syndrome. Immunol Today 4:291–297.

7. Hanto DW, Gajl-Peczalska KJ, Frizerra G, et al. 1983. Epstein–Barr virus (EBV) induced polyclonal and monoclonal B-cell lymphoproliferative diseases occurring after renal transplantation. Ann Surg 198:356–368.

8. Wilkinson AH, Smith JL, Hunsicker LG, et al. 1989. Increased frequency of posttransplant lymphomas in patients treated with cyclosporine, azathioprine, and prednisone. Transplantation 47:293–303.

9. Leblond V, Sutton L, Dorent R, et al. 1995. Lymphoproliferative disorders after organ transplantation: a report of 24 cases observed in a single center. J Clin Oncol 13:961–968.

10. Shapiro RS, McClain KL, Frizzera G, et al. 1988. Epstein–Barr virus associated B cell lymphoproliferative disorders following bone marrow transplantation. Blood 71:1234–1243.

11. Kamel OW, Rijn Mvd, LeBrun DP, et al. 1994. Lymphoid neoplasms in patients with rheumatoid arthritis and dermatomyositis. Hum Pathol 25:638–643.

12. Frizzera G, Hanto DW, Gajl-Peczalska KJ, et al. 1981. Polymorphic diffuse B-cell hyperplasias and lymphoma transplant recipients. Cancer Res 41:4262–4279.

13. Fingeroth JD, Weiss JJ, Tedder TF, et al. 1994. Epstein–Barr virus receptor of human B lymphocytes is the C3d receptor CR2. Proc Natl Acad Sci USA 4:4510–4514.

14. Sixbey JW, Veterinen EH, Nedrud JG, et al. 1983. Replication of Epstein–Barr virus in human epithelial cells infected in vitro. Nature 306:480–483.

15. Henle W, Henle G, Horowitz CA. 1974. Epstein–Barr virus-specific diagnostic tests in infectious mononucleosis. Hum Pathol 5:551–565.

16. Miyashita EM, Yang B, Lam KMC, et al. 1995. A novel form of Epstein–Barr virus latency in normal B cells in vivo. Cell 80:593–602.

17. Ho M, Miller G, Atchison RW, et al. 1985. Epstein–Barr virus infections and DNA hybridization studies in posttransplant lymphoma and lymphoproliferative lesions: the role of primary infection. J Infect Dis 152:876–886.

18. Zimber U, Aldinger HK, Lenoir GM, et al. 1986. Geographical prevalence of two types of Epstein–Barr virus. Virology 154:56–63.

19. Sculley TB, Apollini A, Hurren L, et al. 1987. Coinfection with A- and B-type Epstein–Barr virus in human immunodeficiency virus-positive subjects. J Infect Dis 162:643–667.

20. Young LS, Yao QY, Rooney CM, et al. 1987. New type B isolate of Epstein–Barr virus from Burkitt's lymphoma and normal individuals in endemic areas. J Gen Virol 68:2853–2859.

21. Frank D, Cesarman E, Liu YF, et al. 1995. Posttransplantation lymphoproliferative disorders frequently contain type A and not type B Epstein–Barr virus. Blood 85:1396–1403.

22. Patton DF, Wilkowski CW, Hanson CA, et al. 1990. Epstein–Barr virus-determined clonality in posttransplant lymphoproliferative disease. Transplantation 49:1080–1084.

23. Cen H, Williams PA, McWilliams HP, et al. 1993. Evidence for restricted Epstein–Barr virus latent gene expression and anti-EBNA antibody response in solid organ transplant recipients with post transplant lymphoproliferative disorders. Blood 81:1393–1404.

24. Wang D, Liebowitz D, Kieff E. 1985. An EBV membrane protein expressed in immortalized lymphocytes transforms established rodent cells. Cell 43:831–840.

25. Li-Fu H, Minarovits J, Shi-Long C, et al. 1991. Variable expression of latent membrane protein in nasophyaryngeal carcinoma can be related to methylation status of the Epstein–Barr virus BNLF-1 5'-flanking region. J Virol 65:1558–1564.

26. Herbst H, Dallenbach F, Hummel M, et al. 1991. Epstein–Barr virus latent membrane protein expression in Hodgkin and Reed–Sternberg cells. Proc Natl Acad Sci USA 88:4766–4771.

27. Young L, Alfieri C, Hennessy K, et al. 1989. Expression of Epstein–Barr virus transformation-associated genes in tissues of patients with EBV lymphoproliferative disease. N Engl J Med 321:1080–1085.

28. Skare J, Farley J, Strominger J, et al. 1985. Transformation by Epstein–Barr virus requires DNA sequences in the region of BamHI fragments Y and H. J Virol 55:286–297.

29. Delecluse H-J, Kremmer E, Roualult J-P, et al. 1995. The expression of Epstein–Barr virus

57

latent proteins is related to the pathological features of post-transplant lymphoproliferative disorders. Am J Pathol 146:1113–1120.

30. Knowles DM, Cesarman E, Chadburn A, et al. 1995. Correlative morphologic and molecular genetic analysis demonstrates three distinct categories of posttransplantation lymphoproliferative disorders. Blood 85:552–565.

31. Seremetis S, Inghirami G, Ferrero D, et al. 1989. RAS oncogenes cause malignant transformation and plasmacytoid differentiation of EBV-infected human B-lymphoblasts. Science 243:660–663.

32. Hanto D. 1995. Classification of Epstein–Barr virus-associated posttransplant lymphoproliferative diseases: implications for understanding their pathogenesis and developing rational treatment strategies. Annu Rev Med 46:381–394.

33. Savoie A, Perpete C, Carpentier L, et al. 1994. Direct correlation between the load of Epstein–Barr virus-infected lymphocytes in the peripheral blood of pediatric transplant patients and risk of lymphoproliferative disease. Blood 83:2715–2722.

34. Riddler SA, Breinig MC, McKnight JLC. 1994. Increased levels of circulating Epstein–Barr virus (EBV)-infected lymphocytes and decreased EBV nuclear antigen antibody responses are associated with the development of posttransplant lymphoproliferative disease in solid-organ transplant recipients. Blood 84:972–984.

35. Preiksaitis JK, Diaz-Mitoma F, Mirzayans F, et al. 1992. Quantitative oropharyngeal Epstein–Barr virus shedding in renal and cardiac transplant recipients: relationship to immunosuppressive therapy, serologic responses, and the risk of posttransplant lymphoproliferative disorder. J Infect Dis 166:988–995.

36. Randhawa PS, Jaffe R, Demetris AJ. 1992. Expression of Epstein–Barr virus-encoded small RNA (by the EBER-1 gene) in liver specimens from transplant recipients with post-transplantation lymphoproliferative disease. N Engl J Med 327:1710–1714.

37. Toshizaki K, Matsuda T, Nishimonto N, et al. 1989. Pathogenic significance of interleukin-6 (IL-6/BSF-2) in Castleman's disease. Blood 74:1360–1363.

38. Miles SA, Rezia AR, Salazar-Golzalez JF, et al. 1990. AIDS Kaposi sarcoma-derived cells produce and respond to interleukin- 6. Proc Natl Acad Sci USA 87:4068–4073.

39. Kawano M, Hirano T, Matusuda T, et al. 1988. Autocrine generation and requirement of BSF-2/IL-6 from human multiple myeloma. Nature 332:83–85.

40. Tanner J, Tosato G. 1992. Regulation of B cell growth and immunoglobulin transcription by interleukin-6. Blood 79:452–457.

41. Tosato G, Tanner JE, Jones KD, et al. 1990. Identification of interleukin-6 as an autocrine growth factor for Epstein–Barr virus-immortalized B cell. J Virol 64:3033–3038.

42. Tosato G, Jones K, Breinig MK, et al. 1993. Interleukin-6 production in post-transplant lymphoproliferative disease. J Clin Invest 91:2806–2810.

43. Tanner JE, Menezes J. 1994. Interleukin-6 and Epstein–Barr virus induction by Cyclosporine A: potential role in lymphoproliferative disease. Blood 84:3956–3964.

44. Sigal NH, Dumont FJ. 1992. Cyclosporine A, FK-506, and ripamycin: pharmacologic probes of lymphocyte signal transduction. Annu Rev Immunol 10:519–533.

45. Tanner JE, Tosato G. 1991. Impairment of natural killer functions by interleukin 6 increases lymphoblastoid cell tumorigenicity in athymic mice. J Clin Invest 88:239–244.

46. Schwarz MA, Tardelli L, Macosko HD, et al. 1995. Interleukin 4 retards dissemination of a human B-cell lymphoma in severe combined immunodeficient mice. Cancer Res 55:3692–3696.

47. Peyron E, Banchereau J. 1994. Interleukin 4. Structure, function and clinical aspects. Eur J Dermatol 4:181–188.

48. Starzl TE, Nalesnik MA, Proter KA, et al. 1984. Reversibility of lymphomas and lymphoproliferative lesions developing under cyclosporin-steroid therapy. Lancet 1:583–587.

49. Pirsch JD, Stratta RJ, Sollinger HW, et al. 1989. Treatment of severe Epstein–Barr virus-induced lymphoproliferative syndrome with ganciclovir: two cases after solid organ transplantation. Am J Med 86:241–244.

50. Bacon TH, Boyd MR. 1995. Activity of penciclovir against Epstein–Barr virus. Antimicrob Agents Chemother 39:1599–1602.

51. Blanche S, LeDeist F, Veber F, et al. 1988. Treatment of severe Epstein–Barr virusinduced polyclonal B-lymphocyte proliferation by anti-B-cell monoclonal antibodies. Ann Intern Med 108:199–203.

52. Shapiro RS, Chauvenet A, McGuire W, et al. 1988. Treatment of B-cell lymphoproliferative disorders with interferon alpha and intravenous gamma globulin. N Engl J Med 318:1334–1335.

53. Murphy WJ, Fuakoshi S, Beckwith M, et al. 1995. Antibodies to CD40 prevent Epstein–Barr virus-mediated human B-cell lymphomagenesis in severe combined immune deficient mice given human peripheral blood lymphocytes. Blood 86:1946–1953.

54. Mosier DE, Gulizia RJ, Baird SM, et al. 1988. Transfer of a functional human immune system to mice with severe combined immunodeficiency. Nature 335:256–259.

55. Funakoshi F, Longo DL, Beckwith M, et al. 1994. Inhibition of human B-cell lymphoma growth by CD40 stimulation. Blood 83:2787–2794.

56. Swinnen LJ, Mullen GM, Carr TJ, et al. 1995. Aggressive treatment for postcardiac transplant lymphoproliferation. Blood 86:3333–3340.

57. Arico M, Caslli D, D'Argenio PD, et al. 1991. Malignancies in children with human immunodeficiency virus Type 1 infection. Cancer 68:2473–2479.

58. Pluda JM, Yarchoan R, Jaffe ES, et al. 1990. Development of non-Hodgkin's lymphoma in a cohort of patients with severe human immunodeficiency virus (HIV) infection on long-term antiretroviral therapy. Ann Intern Med 113:276–280.

59. Mueller BU, Shad AT, Magrath IT, et al. 1994. Malignancies in children with HIV infection. In Pizzo PA, Wilfert CM (eds): Pediatric AIDS, the challenge of HIV infection in infants, children, and adolescents. Baltimore, MD, Williams and Wilkins, pp 603–622.

60. Ragni MV, Belle SH, Jaffe RA, et al. 1993. Acquired immunodeficiency syndrome-associated non-Hodgkin's lymphomas and other malignancies in patients with hemophilia. Blood 81:1889–1894.

61. Epstein LG, DiCarlo FJ, Joshi VV, et al. 1988. Primary lymphoma of the central nervous system in children with acquired immuodeficiency syndrome. Pediatrics 82:355–360.

62. McArthur JC. 1987. Neurologic manifestations of AIDS. Medicine 66:407–416.

63. Pierce MA, Johnson MD, Maciunas RJ, et al. 1995. Evaluating contrast-enhancing brain lesions in patients with AIDS by using positron emission tomography. Ann Intern Med 123:594–598.

64. Andiman WA, Eastman R, Martin K, et al. 1985. Opportunistic lymphoproliferations associated with Epstein–Barr viral DNA in infants and children with AIDS. Lancet 2:1390–1394.

65. Belman AL, Diamond G, Dickson D, et al. 1988. Pediatric acquired immunodeficiency syndrome: neurologic syndromes. Am J Dis Child 142:29–35.

66. Chilcote R, Williams T, Siegel S. 1989. Therapy of Burkitt's lymphoma in children with HIV infection. Pediatr Res 25:149A.

67. Goldstein J, Dickson DW, Rubenstein A, et al. 1990. Primary central nervous system lymphoma in pediatric patient with acquired immmune deficiency syndrome. Cancer 66:2503–2508.

68. Kamani N, Kennedy J, Brandsma J. 1988. Burkitt's lymphoma in a child with human immunodeficiency virus infection. J Pediatr 112:241–247.

69. Nadal D, Caduff R, Frey E, et al. 1994. Non-Hodgkin's lymphoma in four children infected with the human immunodeficiency virus. Cancer 73:224–229.

70. Neumann Y, Toren A, Mandel M, et al. 1993. Favorable response of pediatric AIDS-related Burkitt's lymphoma treated by aggressive chemotherapy. Med Pediatr Oncol 21:661–667.

71. Patton DF, Sixbey JW, Murphy SB. 1988. Epstein–Barr virus in human immunodeficiency virus-related Burkitt lymphoma. J Pediatr 113:951–956.

72. Lane HC, Feinberg J, Davey V, et al. 1988. Anti-retroviral effects of interferon-α in AIDS-associated Kaposi's sarcoma. Lancet 2:1218–1222.

73. Rohatiner AZS. 1991. Interferon alpha in lympoma. Br J Haematol 79 (Suppl 1):26–34.

74. Vellatini C, Horschowski N, Philippon V, et al. 1995. Development of lymphoid hyperplasia in transgenic mice expressing the HIV tat gene. AIDS Res Hum Retrovir 11:21–27.
75. Shibata D, Weiss LM, Nathwani BN. 1991. Epstein–Barr virus in benign lymph node biopsies from individuals infected with the human immunodeficiency virus is associated with concurrent or subsequent development of non-Hodgkin's lymphoma. Blood 77:1527–1533.
76. Hamilton-Dutoit SJ, Raphael M, Audouin J, et al. 1993. In situ demonstration of Epstein–Barr virus small RNAs (EBER 1) in acquired immunodeficiency syndrome-related lymphomas: correlation with tumor morphology and primary site. Blood 82:619–623.
77. MacMahon EME, Glass JD, Hayward SD, et al. 1991. Epstein–Barr virus in AIDS-related primary central nervous system lymphoma. Lancet 338:969–973.
78. Suber M, Neri A, Inghirami G, et al. 1988. Frequent c-*myc* oncogene activation and infrequent presence of Epstein–Barr virus genome in AIDS-associated lymphoma. Blood 72:667–674.
79. Montagnier L, Gruest J, Chamaret S, et al. 1984. Adaption of LAV to replication in EBV transformed B lymphoblastomatoid cell lines. Science 225:63–66.
80. Schittman SM, Lane HC, Higgins SE, et al. 1986. Direct polyclonal activation of B lymphocytes by AIDS virus. Science 233:1084–1095.
81. Jelinek DF, Lipsky PE. 1987. Enhancement of human B cell proliferation and differentiation by tumor necrosis factor-alpha and interleukin 1. J Immunol 139:2970–2974.
82. Paul WE. 1987. Interleukin 4/B cell stimulatory factor 1: one lympholine, many functions. FASEB J 1:456–463.
83. Zlotnik A, Morre KW. 1991. Interleukin 10. Cytokine 3:366–375.
84. Klein G. 1989. Multiple phenotypic consequences of the *Ig/Myc* translocation in B-cell-derived tumors. Genes, Chromosomes Cancer 1:3–9.
85. Ballerini P, Gaidano G, Gong J, et al. 1993. Multiple genetic lesions in acquired immunodeficiency syndrome-related non-Hodgkin's lymphoma. Blood 81:166–170.
86. Meeker TC, Shiramizu B, Kaplan L, et al. 1991. Evidence for molecular subtypes of HIV-associated lymphoma: division into peripheral monoclonal, polyclonal, and central nervous system lymphoma. AIDS 5:669–674.
87. Chadwick EG, Connor EJ, Hanson CG, et al. 1990. Tumors of smooth-muscle origin in HIV-infected children. JAMA 263:3182–3185.
88. McClain KL, Leach CT, Jenson HB, et al. 1995. Association of Epstein–Barr virus with leiomyosarcomas in young people with AIDS. N Engl J Med 332:12–18.
89. Lee ES, Locker J, Nalesnik M, et al. 1995. The association of Epstein–Barr virus with smooth-muscle tumors occurring after organ transplantation. N Engl J Med 332:19–23.
90. Isaacson P, Wright D. 1983. Malignant lymphoma of mucosa associated lymphoid tissue. A distinctive B-cell lymphoma. Cancer 52:1410–1415.
91. Pelstring RJ, Essel JH, Kurtin PJ, et al. 1991. Diversity of organ site involvement among malignant lymphomas of mucosa associated lymphoid tissues. Am J Clin Pathol 96:738–741.
92. Harris NL. 1991. Intranodal lymphoid infiltrates and mucosa associated lymphoid tissue (MALT): a unifying concept. Am J Surg Pathol 15:879–883.
93. Isaacson PG. 1994. Gastrointestinal lymphoma. Hum Pathol 25:1020–1026.
94. Joshi VV. 1993. Pathology of pediatric AIDS: overview, update, and future directions. Ann NY Acad Sci 693:71–82.
95. Joshi VV, Kauffman S, Oleske JM, et al. 1987. Polyclonal polymorphic B-cell lymphoproliferative disorder with prominent pulmonary involvement in children with AIDS. Cancer 59:1455–1459.
96. Montalvo FW, Casanova R, Clavell LA. 1990. Treatment outcome in children with malignancies associated with human immunodeficieny virus infection. J Pediatr 116:735–742.
97. Rechavi G, Ben-Bassat I, Berkowicz M, et al. 1987. Molecular analysis of Burkitt's leukemia in two hemophilic brothers with AIDS. Blood 70:1713–1718.
98. Ames ED, Conjalka MS, Goldberg AF, et al. 1991. Hodgkin's disease and AIDS: twenty-three new cases and a review of the literature. Hematol Oncol Clin North Am 5:343–352.

99. Orlow SJ, Cooper D, Petrea S, et al. 1992. AIDS-associated Kaposi's sarcoma in Romanian children. J Am Acad Dermatol 28:449–455.
100. Cook PD, Czerniak B, Chan JKC, et al. 1995. Nodular spindle-cell vascular transformation of lymph nodes: a benign process occurring predominantly in retroperitoneal lymph nodes draining carcinomas that simulates Kaposi's sarcoma or metastatic tumor. Am J Surg Pathol 19:1010–1014.
101. LeBoit PE. 1995. Bacillary angiomatosis. Mod Pathol 8:218–223.
102. Bouquety JC, Siopathis MR, Ravisse PR, et al. 1989. Lymphadenopathic Kaposi's sarcoma in an African pediatric AIDS case. Am J Trop Med Hyg 40:323–327.
103. Connor E, Boccon-Gibod L, Joshi VV, et al. 1990. Cutaneous AIDS-associated Kaposi's sarcoma in pediatric patients. Arch Dermatol 126:791–795.
104. Maemain M, Fruchter RG, Serur E, et al. 1992. HIV infection and cervical neoplasia. Gynecol Oncol 38:377–381.
105. Matoras R, Ariceta JM, Rementeria A, et al. 1991. HIV induced immunosuppression: a risk factor for human papilloma virus infection. Am J Obstet Gynecol 164:42–46.
106. Diamond FB, Price LJ, Nelson RP. 1994. Papillary carcinoma of thyroid in a 7 year old HIV positive child. Pediatr AIDS HIV Infect Fet Adolesc 5:232–236.

3. Familial cancer syndromes and genetic counseling

Gail E. Tomlinson

1. Introduction

The past several years have witnessed the identification of numerous genes that contribute to cancer development, many of which may be inherited in an altered state so as to predispose to the development of cancer. Collectively, the application of these new gene discoveries will have a significant impact on public health in both pediatric and adult medical practices.

For the oncology specialist, the identification of cancer predisposition genes will provide a new challenge in counseling family members as well as a tremendous power in predicting which patients will be most at risk for second primary cancers. In some cases, identification of a familial form of cancer at diagnosis may have an impact on the course of therapy chosen. A frequent question asked by parents of pediatric cancer patients concerns the possible genetic origins of their child's cancer and the possibility of increased cancer risk to other children in the family. Historically, the cancer specialist has been equipped with little in the way of factual knowledge to address such questions and is left to give the family broad reassurances that most cancers are not hereditary. As data accumulate regarding the genetic epidemiology of childhood cancer, the clinician will soon be able to more accurately assess cancer risks to other family members and, in some cases, to use laboratory data to determine individual risk factors.

As of 1996, over 20 genes had been identified in which heritable constitutional mutations predispose to cancer development [1–20]. These are shown in figure 1 in the order in which they were identified. The identification of multiple genes within a short period of time for the common adult cancers, breast and colon cancer [10–13,15], has attracted much public attention; however, many of the essential concepts of hereditary cancer predisposition derive from the study of genes that predispose to pediatric cancers.

The first cancer predisposition gene to be isolated was *RB1*, the gene for hereditary retinoblastoma [1], which was cloned a decade after cytogenetic studies of retinoblastoma revealed deletions of chromosome 13 in normal and tumor tissues from retinoblastoma patients [21,22]. Similar chromosomal observations in a subset of Wilms' tumor patients demonstrating losses at chro-

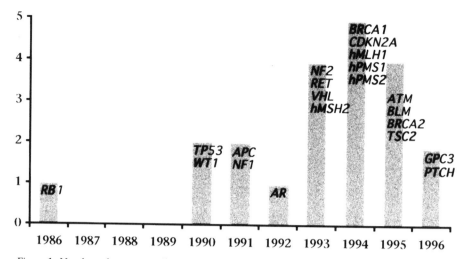

Figure 1. Number of cancer predisposition genes identified to date, shown by year of discovery: *RB1*, hereditary retinoblastoma (1); *WT1*, Wilms' tumor (2); *TP53*, Li–Fraumeni breast sarcoma cancer family syndrome (3); *NF1*, neurofibromatosis type 1 (4); *APC*, adenomatous polyposis coli (5); *AR*, androgen receptor (6); *hMSH2, hMLH1, hPMS1, hPMS2*, nonpolyposis hereditary colon cancer (10–12); *VHL*, von Hippel–Lindau disease (7); *RET*, multiple endocrine neoplasia, type 2, familial medullary thyroid cancer (9); *NF2*, neurofibromatosis, type 2 (8); *CDKN2A*, familial melanoma (14); *BRCA1*, familial breast and ovarian cancer (13); *TSC2*, tuberous sclerosis (18); *BRCA2*, familial breast cancer (15); *BLM*, Bloom's syndrome (16); *ATM*, ataxia telangiectasia (17); *PTCH*, nevoid basal cell carcinoma syndrome (19); *GPC3*, Simpson–Golabi–Behmel syndrome (20).

mosome 11p directed investigators to the isolation of the Wilms' tumor gene *WT1* [23,24]. In the cases of other predisposition genes, such as those for breast and colon cancer, observations of very large pedigrees with multiple affected family members enabled genetic linkage studies to track the inheritance of multiple genetic markers through multiple generations in order to determine the precise chromosomal location harboring the gene of interest [25–27]. It is to be expected that as mapping and sequencing of the human genome proceeds to completion, many more genes that influence the inherited susceptibility to cancer will be identified.

Most of the cancer-predisposing genes discovered to date correspond to a clinically described syndrome. This chapter will highlight some of the known familial cancer syndromes and their corresponding genes with respect to how they may apply to pediatric patients and their families.

Many practicing pediatricians and pediatric oncologists have undoubtedly observed occasional families that do not fit into a recognizable familial cancer syndrome but in which more than one child has been diagnosed with cancer or in which both a child and parent have a cancer diagnosis. It is unclear at this time whether in these situations such familial clustering of childhood cancer is due to chance factors, common environmental exposures, or yet unknown genetic factors. In one large series composed of families in which two children have been diagnosed with a form of cancer, over half of the sibling pairs described did not fall into a recognizable familial cancer syndrome [28]. The most common types of tumor observed to occur in sibling clusters were leukemias or central nervous system (CNS) tumors, which are also the most common types of childhood cancer overall.

As more is learned about the multiple genes known to predispose to cancer, about environmental causes of cancer, and about gene–environmental interactions, it may become easier to ascertain the extent to which genetic predisposition factors, as opposed to environmental factors or chance, play a role in such cases of familial clustering.

2. The two-hit hypothesis: a paradigm for familial cancer

Some of the earliest and most significant advances in understanding basic aspects of familial cancer have come from the study of pediatric cancers. Indeed, the two-hit model predicted over 25 years ago for hereditary retinoblastoma and other pediatric tumors [29–31] has demostrated applicability to many types of cancers, both pediatric and adult.

In 1971, Knudson proposed a model of tumor formation that was based on demographic observations [29]. By analyzing age of onset and tumor laterality, he proposed a mathematical model to explain the pathogenesis of retinoblastoma as occurring in two forms — hereditary and nonhereditary — and suggested that each of these forms requires the same two types of mutations or 'hits.' According to the two-hit model, in cancers of the hereditary form, the initial mutation affects a tumor suppressor locus in the germline. The mutation becomes present in every body cell but does not cause a clinical phenotype — i.e., a tumor — until a second acquired mutation inactivates the other, wild-type allele at the corresponding locus on the other chromosome. However, the same type of tumor may develop in an individual in the absence of a constitutional mutation — i.e., in a nonhereditary form. In this form of the tumor, an individual body cell acquires two separate mutations of the same gene such that both the maternally and paternally derived inherited copies become inactive at times after conception.

The hereditary forms of the tumor occur within a younger age range because in these cases tumor formation only requires one hit postconception, whereas tumors in individuals who do not carry a mutation in the germline develop at a somewhat later age because of the time necessary for two independent mutations to occur in the same cell. In addition, in the hereditary forms of cancer, when an entire organ such as the retina carries a genetic mutation and is thus at risk of developing disease, bilateral or multifocal tumors are seen more frequently.

In this model, the *tendency* to inherit a tumor, the so-called *at-risk* state, is inherited in a dominant fashion, and thus 50% of the offspring of a mutation carrier will be at risk; however, not all such individuals will actually develop cancer. The transformation of 'normal' (although genetically predisposed) cells to tumor depends on the inactivation of the remaining normal copy of the gene — hence the concept of recessiveness in the tumor tissue. Most cancer susceptibility genes are thought to act dominantly, and all the syndromes to be discussed in this chapter involve dominant susceptibility.

Dominant cancer susceptibility genes have the potential of being passed on to 50% of offspring for multiple generations. Mutation of the breast cancer gene *BRCA1* has been estimated to have been transmittable for up to 170 generations [32]. Because of the mortality associated with many types of childhood cancer, however, along with the decreased reproductive capacity associated with cancer treatment, many germline genetic mutations accounting for pediatric cancers have undoubtedly been lost from the population. New mutations occur, however, that compensate for those lost from the population. In fact, most germline mutations for the *RB1* gene are new mutations, as are half of *NF1* mutations [33,34]. As treatment of pediatric cancers and survival rates improve, the potential exists for an increase in the number of carriers of germline mutations in cancer predisposition genes in the population.

3. Retinoblastoma: from genetics to genetic counseling

The detailed understanding of the genetics of retinoblastoma has made possible the counseling of family members and has allowed an estimation of risk to siblings and offspring. The benefit of this ability to recognize at-risk individuals within families permits earlier diagnosis of disease and, in some cases, limits the extent of therapy — benefits that may preserve maximum vision. Therefore, every attempt should be made to identify high-risk individuals.

Approximately 40% of all cases of retinoblastoma are thought to occur in children with a constitutional predisposition, manifested either by the presence of bilateral tumors or a positive family history. In about 10% of cases, the mutation is inherited from an affected parent, while in 30% of cases the mutation is a new germinal mutation [34]. The remaining 60% of cases are unilateral and occur in the absence of a positive family history. These cases are often termed *sporadic*, although in perhaps 10% of them a germline mutation will exist, and this small percentage of cases are the most difficult to identify and counsel as to genetic risk factors [34].

Constitutional mutation of the *RB1* gene is associated with a very high penetrance, i.e., a very high probability of developing the disease. There is no evidence for genetic heterogeneity from family linkage studies, and it is presumed that virtually all cases of bilateral retinoblastoma result from germline mutation of the *RB1* gene. Ninety percent of children born with a germline *RB1* mutation will develop the disease in early childhood, with the mean age of diagnosis being less than one year. A few individuals will appear clinically unaffected, but upon examination of the retina will be found to have a benign retinocytoma. These tumors are thought to be spontaneously regressing benign tumors; however, they may be a manifestation of a constitutional *RB1* mutation [35]. In the absence of an apparent family history, examination of the eyes of parents of every child diagnosed with retinoblastoma is indicated in order to explore the possibility of such sub-clinical lesions, which would then point to an inherited predisposition in the child.

In the absence of molecular studies to determine carrier status, it is estimated that when a positive family history of retinoblastoma is present, siblings of a patient with bilateral retinoblastoma will have a 45% chance of developing disease. This is the observed rate in the large British registry of over 1600 retinoblastoma patients described by Draper et al. [36] and is also consistent with a model of an autosomal-dominant gene with 90% penetrance. Siblings of patients with unilateral disease in a familial setting have a 30% chance of developing retinoblastoma. Interestingly, siblings of bilateral cases also develop bilateral disease, whereas siblings of unilateral cases tend to develop unilateral disease, suggesting that in some families the predisposing mutation may be characterized by a milder phenotype, i.e., lesser number of tumors per individual [36]. The existence of such 'low penetrance' mutations has been confirmed by molecular studies [37,38].

For families in which there is no previous history of retinoblastoma, the risk to siblings is considerably less, even in bilateral cases. In these families, it is thought that approximately 75% of bilateral cases develop due to a new mutation present at conception as a result of a sporadic mutation in a single parental germ cell; however, in a small percentage of cases, there exists a previously unrecognized mutation carried by one of the parents. The observed incidence of retinoblastoma in siblings of bilateral patients in the absence of a family history is 2%; if unilateral, the incidence is 1% [34]. When other siblings in the family are already known to be unaffected, the chance of the parents being carriers is further diminished, and the risk to other siblings decreases to less than 1% [36].

The risk to offspring of survivors of hereditary retinoblastoma is 44%, similar to the risk of retinoblastoma to siblings of children with familial retinoblastoma, and again consistent with the 50% chance of passing the mutant gene to each offspring, coupled with an expected 90% penetrance. For offspring of survivors of sporadic unilateral retinoblastoma, assuming that a small percentage of cases will in fact be carriers of a germline mutation capable of causing retinoblastoma, this risk has been estimated to be 0.7% [36].

Since the cloning and genetic sequence determination of the *RB1* gene [1,39], detection of the disease-causing mutation in a given family has become theoretically possible. The spectrum of molecular abnormalities is wide and includes karyotypic abnormalities, large DNA rearrangements detectable by Southern blotting, point mutations causing amino acid substitutions, and mutations causing DNA splicing alterations [40–45]. Because of the wide range of possible types of mutations, as well as the large size of the *RB1* gene, molecular detection of the precise defect within a given family becomes very labor

67

intensive and costly and has been impractical for routine clinical use. It is considerably easier from a technical standpoint to determine carrier status using polymorphic markers if two affected family members are available for blood sampling [46–48]. The chromosomal origin of the mutant gene can be determined, and it can then be determined if other members of the family also carry the affected allele. Earlier work in this area relied on the technique of restriction fragment length polymorphisms (RFLPs) [46,48]. In recent years, this type of analysis has largely been replaced by the use of polymerase chain reaction- (PCR-) based polymorphic markers, which are more informative [47].

An example of how polymorphic markers can be used to identify mutation carriers within a family is shown in figure 2. The DNA marker used yields highly informative data in 90% of families. DNA fragments generated by PCR vary in size among the normal population from 500 to 600 base pairs [47]. In the family shown in figure 2, the allele common to the mother and affected son is also observed in the daughter (II-3) but not in the unaffected son (II-2). Therefore, the son does not need close surveillance for tumor development. The unaffected daughter (II-3) has inherited the mutant allele and therefore has a 90% chance of developing retinoblastoma in infancy or early childhood. In the absence of molecular diagnostic testing, each child would have a 45% chance of developing the disease and would undergo regular ocular exams under general anesthesia starting in early infancy. Thus, molecular diagnostic testing in informative families can save the risk and expense of frequent eye exams in noncarriers.

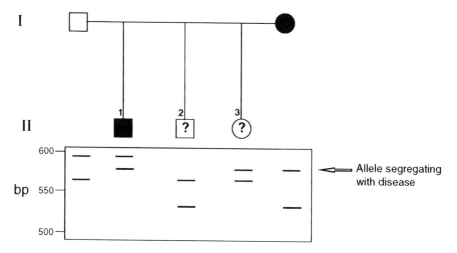

Figure 2. Use of polymorphic markers at the *RB1* locus to genotype members of a nuclear family in which mother and son are affected with the disease retinoblastoma. Squares represent males, circles represent females. Darkened symbols indicate individuals clinically affected with cancer — in this case, retinoblastoma. The arrow designates the allele that the son with retinoblastoma (II-1) has inherited from his mother, who also had retinoblastoma. This same allele is observed in DNA from the daughter (II-3), who is therefore at high risk of developing retinoblastoma.

From follow-up studies, it is apparent that survivors of retinoblastoma have an increased risk of developing a second malignancy. Draper et al. reported the overall second tumor incidence to be 2% at 12 years and 4.2% at 18 years. For patients with retinoblastoma of the hereditary form, the incidence of cancer is 8.4% at 18 years [49]. A population-based study in Denmark analyzed 175 cases of retinoblastoma with an average follow-up of 20 years and found the overall relative risk for a new primary nonocular cancer to be 4.2. For the hereditary form of retinoblastoma, the relative risk was 15.4 [50]. Eng et al. predicted a 26% probability of death from second primary neoplasms at 40 years of age for patients with bilateral retinoblastoma [51].

In all series reported, many of the second tumors occurred within the field of radiation, suggesting that germline mutations of the *RB1* gene and radiation act together. However, a significant number of tumors also occur outside the radiation field, suggesting that *RB1* by itself also predisposes to tumor types other than retinoblastoma. Osteosarcoma is by far the most common second primary tumor type, although other tumors, including other sarcomas, malignant melanomas, and carcinomas, have been observed. In addition, patients with hereditary retinoblastoma develop an excess of benign lipomas [52]. Molecular analyses of the osteosarcomas in retinoblastoma survivors reveal an acquired loss of the wild-type allele, suggesting that the *RB1* gene was involved in the pathogenesis of these tumors and that the *RB1* gene may thus be a pleiotropic cancer predisposition gene [53].

Survivors of hereditary forms of retinoblastoma therefore require both close vigilance for the possible development of second tumors and prompt biopsy and diagnosis of any suspicious mass or lesion. The adult survivor of unilateral retinoblastoma will have a small chance of carrying a germline mutation, and thus the need for surveillance again is an issue; however, specific guidelines as to the type and frequency of screening procedures for these patients as well as their offspring are undetermined.

4. Wilms' tumor: multiple genetic origins

Wilms' tumor occurs in both hereditary and nonhereditary forms and was initially statistically modeled in a fashion similar to retinoblastoma, with bilateral tumors and those occurring in the context of a family history developing at an earlier age than unilateral tumors in the absence of a family history [30]. During the past 25 years, it has become evident, however, that the hereditary forms of Wilms' tumors are more complex than hereditary retinoblastomas in that multiple different genetic syndromes and their associated genes may predispose to Wilms' tumor development.

An early clue to one possible chromosomal location of a gene implicated in Wilms' tumor development was the observation of interstitial deletions at chromosomal band 11p13 in a subset of Wilms' tumor patients with multiple congenital anomalies including aniridia, genitourinary abnormalities, and mental retardation [23,54]. This constellation of physical findings is known as the WAGR (Wilms' tumor, Aniridia, Genitourinary anomalies, and Retardation) syndrome. The karyotypic observations associated with WAGR syndrome prompted molecular biologists to search for a predisposition gene in chromosomal region 11p13 — a search that culminated over a decade later in the isolation of the *WT1* gene [2,55]. This gene is thought to play a critical role in genital development; however, it has been found to be involved in a surprisingly small percentage of Wilms' tumors [56,57]. Even in patients thought to be at high risk of carrying an inborn susceptibility based on the presence of genitourinary anomalies, preliminary analysis demonstrates that only a small percentage carry germline *WT1* mutations [58].

Patients with Denys–Drash syndrome, characterized by nephrotic syndrome and intersex disorders including XX/XY mosaicism and/or ambiguous genitalia, have a predisposition to both Wilms' tumor and gonadoblastoma. This subset of Wilms' tumor patients demonstrates a high frequency of germline mutations in the *WT1* gene. Most of the mutations associated with Denys–Drash syndrome are point mutations causing amino acid substitutions and are concentrated in a narrow region of the gene that encodes zinc finger motifs thought to be important in DNA transcription [59,60].

Wilms' tumor is also seen in the clinical syndrome of Beckwith–Wiedemann (BWS), which is associated with macroglossia, overgrowth of visceral organs resulting in congenital omphalocoele, and the presence of ear lobe pits at birth [61,62]. Like the WAGR syndrome and *WT1*, BWS also maps to the short arm of chromosome 11 but at a distinct locus from *WT1* at 11p15.5 [63,64]. BWS usually is not associated with a family history, although familial forms of BWS have been reported [65–68]. The predisposition to childhood cancer in BWS is not limited to Wilms' tumor, however; it also extends to other embryonal tumors, including hepatoblastoma and adrenocortical carcinoma. Hemihypertrophy also predisposes to the same spectrum of disease, although the genetic etiology and possible relationship of hemihypertrophy to Beckwith–Wiedemann syndrome remain unclear [69,70].

True familial Wilms' tumor — the occurrence of Wilms' tumors in siblings or cousins — is rare, accounting for only 1%–2% of all Wilms' tumors, and has eluded a complete molecular understanding. In these families, the children affected with Wilms' tumor are otherwise phenotypically normal and do not appear to have an increased incidence of genitourinary or other congenital anomalies. In addition, these Wilms' tumor families do not demonstrate a marked increase in the incidence of other tumor types. Although the short arm of chromosome 11 was initially implicated in Wilms' tumors as a likely locus of a cancer predisposition gene, this has not proven to be the predisposition site for familial Wilms' tumor. Genetic linkage studies have shown that in several large families in which multiple members have been affected with Wilms' tumors, there is lack of linkage to either the *WT1* locus on 11p13 or the BWS locus on 11p15 [71,72]. In a separate report, however, a family in which a father and child were both affected with Wilms' tumor demonstrated a heritable mutation in *WT1* [73]. Linkage to familial Wilms' tumor has also been excluded from region 16q, thought to harbor a third Wilms' tumor gene [74]. One recent study demonstrated genetic linkage to chromosomal band 17q12–21 in a large Canadian family with multiple Wilms' tumors [75]. This chromosomal locus also harbors the breast cancer predisposition gene, *BRCA1*; however, due to the lack of breast cancer in Wilms' tumor families and vice versa, it is thought to involve a distinct gene. Future studies will be needed to determine if 17q12–21 is the predisposition locus of other Wilms' tumors families or if a gene at this locus is involved in the pathogenesis of sporadic Wilms' tumors.

A recent study of tumors derived from Wilms' tumor patients who had a family history of Wilms' tumor observed chromosomal deletions of chromosome 4q, 9p, 20p, and 3q. Although these deletions involved tumor DNA and not constitutional DNA, it was inferred that these chromosomal regions could harbor genes important in the pathogenesis of familial Wilms' tumor [76].

Initially, it was predicted that, the familial type of Wilms' tumors, like familial retinoblastoma, would most likely be bilateral. Most analyses of familial Wilms' tumor do not suggest that bilateral tumors predominate. In the combined families for which linkage analysis was performed, 6 out of 22 were observed to be bilateral [71,72,75]. In the population-based study of Draper et al., of six sibling pairs with Wilms' tumor, only one case was bilateral [28]. Although these numbers are small due to the rarity of familial Wilms' tumor, the incidence of bilaterality appears to be only modestly increased over the overall frequency of bilaterality. In addition, the penetrance of Wilms' tumor is thought to be considerably less than complete, e.g., many mutation carriers in high-risk families do not develop Wilms' tumor.

An additional familial syndrome that can be associated with Wilms' tumor is Simpson–Golabi–Behmel (SGB) syndrome, characterized, like BWS, with overgrowth features and a predisposition to Wilms' tumor and other embryonal neoplasms [77,78]. This syndrome is X-linked and localizes the Xq26 [79,80]. The gene responsible for SGB syndrome was recently identified as *GPC3*, an extracellular proteoglycan that forms a complex with insulin-like growth factor-2 (IGF-2) [20]. Since BWS and the sporadic tumors associated with both SGB and BWS are associated with relative overexpression of IGF-2, theses two overgrowth syndromes may share common pathways in tumor development.

Wilms' tumor has been observed to occur in the Li–Fraumeni syndrome, although it is not considered to be a major component tumor of the syndrome [81,82]. The *TP53* gene, mutation of which has been shown to be the underlying defect in many families with Li–Fraumeni syndrome, may be associated with the presence of anaplasia in sporadic Wilms' tumor [83,84]. In one interesting family study, a maternally inherited mutation of *TP53* appears together with a paternally derived apparent predisposition to Wilms' tumor in a child with anaplastic Wilms' tumor [83].

A characteristic feature of Wilms' tumors thought to be associated with a constitutional predisposition, whether the predisposition is due to *WT1* mutation, BWS, or other familial Wilms' gene(s), is the occurrence of nephrogenic rests [85]. The overall median age of patients with Wilms' tumors associated with nephrogenic rests is significantly younger than that of patients with rest-negative tumors. The Denys–Drash syndrome and WAGR, both associated with alteration or loss of *WT1* on chromosome 11p13, are associated with intralobar nephrogenic rests. Kidneys from children with Wilms' and Beckwith–Wiedemann syndrome, associated with chromosome 11p15, are associated with perilobar nephrogenic rests. However, approximately 30%–40% of all Wilms' tumors are associated with nephrogenic rests. Whether or not the presence of nephrogenic rests per se indicates a true constitutional predisposition factor that would signify a risk to offspring will require additional follow-up and study. The presence of nephrogenic rests in association with Wilms' tumor, however, should alert the clinician to the possibility of a genetic predisposition syndrome as well as to the possibility of future development of a subsequent Wilms' tumor in the remaining kidney.

Sporadic unilateral Wilms' tumor (occurring in the absence of a known family history in relatives) appears to be rarely heritable. A series of 179 offspring of 96 long-term survivors studied by Li et al. revealed no Wilms' tumors [86]. Accounting for the limited size of the population studied, this study concluded that the actual risk of Wilms' in the offspring of Wilms' tumor patients is 2% or less. An isolated case of Wilms' tumor in an offspring of a unilateral Wilms' tumor survivor was reported in association with an inherited constitutional mutation of *WT1* [59].

The risk of cancer in offspring of survivors of sporadic bilateral Wilms' tumor is more difficult to evaluate. Bilateral tumors account for only 5%–10% of all Wilms' tumors, and the cure rates of bilateral tumors have historically been generally lower that those of unilateral tumors, accounting for many fewer adult survivors of bilateral Wilms' tumors. The association of nephrogenic rests and the early age of onset of bilateral tumors are suggestive of a constitutional genetic predisposition, and it can be inferred that children with bilateral tumors may carry a mutation of some type that predisposes them to Wilms' tumor development and that would also place their offspring at risk.

The cost-effectiveness of interventional measures in dealing with offspring of Wilms' survivors or siblings of children with familial forms of Wilms' tumor remains to be determined. Factors that need to be considered in any cancer screening program include the prevalence of the type of cancer in the 'at-risk' population, the sensitivity of the screening method empoloyed, the rate of tumor growth in determining the optimal interval between screening exams, and both the clinical benefit and economic impact of cancer screening. Further studies are needed to determine optimal screening methods in high-risk families. At present, it does not appear that screening is indicated in siblings or offspring of survivors of unilateral Wilms' tumors in the absence of genitourinary anomalies or in the absence of an established family history. Although no data confirm the efficacy, children from high-risk families in which two or more individuals have been affected with Wilms' tumor and children with the physical stigmata of Beckwith–Wiedemann syndrome are often followed with abdominal ultrasound performed every 3 to 4 months until they are approximately 6 to 7 years of age.

A small survey study conducted by the National Wilms' Study suggested that there may be a benefit in earlier identification of Wilms' tumors in some genetically predisposed children, thus allowing them to receive less intensive treatment [87]. A recent study by DeBaun projected that screening patients with BWS with abdominal sonogram from birth until age 7 years is possibly a cost-effective approach [88]. There is clearly a need for a multicenter study of screening efficacy in children at increased risk of Wilms' tumor due to genetic predisposition factors.

5. Li–Fraumeni syndrome and the *TP53* gene

The rare syndrome that has come to be known as *Li–Fraumeni syndrome*, also known as the breast sarcoma cancer family syndrome, has received considerable attention in recent years that stems from pioneering work done by the investigators whose name the syndrome now bears [89]. Starting with the clinical observation of a family in which two cousins had developed sarcomas in early childhood, this early investigation was initiated as an epidemiology study of cancers in family members of children with childhood sarcoma; the researchers reviewed charts and searched the cancer mortality record established by Dr. Robert Miller [90]. Out of a total of 641 children with rhabdomyosarcoma, four families were identified in which siblings or cousins had childhood soft-tissue sarcomas. In two of the families, the mother was affected with breast cancer, and in the other two, the fathers of the probands had cancer and other female relatives on the paternal side had early-onset breast cancer. Hence, the possibility of a familial link between childhood rhabdomyosarcoma and early-onset breast cancer was suggested [89].

A follow-up study of these four families over the next 12 years suggested an increased risk of multiple cancer types with a pattern of autosomal dominant transmission, with the most common types of cancers being breast cancer diagnosed before the age of 35 and soft-tissue sarcomas of childhood of young adulthood [81]. A subsequent study of 24 kindreds further defined the clinical syndrome as an autosomal dominantly inherited predisposition to cancers of diverse histologic subtypes that occurred prior to 45 years of age. Characteristic cancers of the breast sarcoma cancer family syndrome include early-onset breast cancer, soft-tissue sarcomas, osteosarcomas, leukemias, brain tumors, and adrenocortical carcinoma. Because of the rarity of childhood adrenocortical carcinoma in the general population (0.3 cases/million), the occurrence of this tumor in multiple families with the syndrome was striking [91].

In addition, multiple primary cancers in the same individual were characteristic. As in hereditary retinoblastoma, second tumors were observed within previously irradiated fields, suggesting that a susceptibility to radiation carcinogenesis was also a feature of the syndrome. A family pedigree characteristic of the Li–Fraumeni syndrome is shown in figure 3, demonstrating tumors of diverse histologies in children and young adults, as well as bilaterality and multiple primary site cancers in an individual.

In 1990, Malkin et al. reported that in five families with Li–Fraumeni syndrome the heritable defect was a mutation of the *TP53* gene, a tumor suppressor gene previously known to be mutated in many different types of cancers [3]. Numerous follow-up studies have documented the occurrence of germline mutations in the *TP53* gene in cancer-prone families [89,92–98]. In addition, germline TP53 mutations have been documented in patients with multiple-site primary tumors regardless of family history [84,99–101]. In some families in which germline *TP53* mutations have been documented, the con-

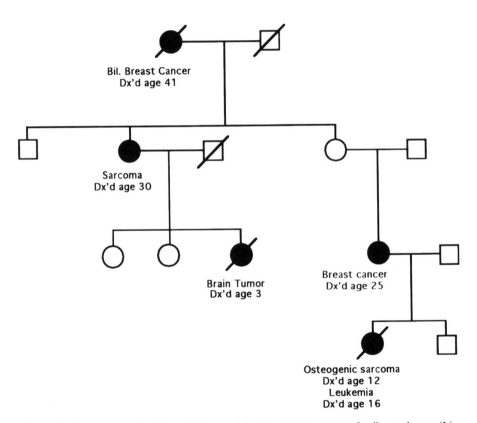

Figure 3. Pedigree typical of the Li–Fraumeni breast sarcoma cancer family syndrome (Li–Fraumeni syndrome), demonstrating autosomal-dominant transmission, bilaterality of tumors, and multiple primary site cancers in same individual. Symbols are as in figure 1.

74

stellation of tumor types that occur are not consistent with the patterns initially described in breast sarcoma families [102]. Thus, germline *TP53* mutations are not strictly synonymous with the clinical description of breast sarcoma cancer family syndrome.

Several site-specific series of patients unselected for family history have demonstrated that *TP53* mutations occur in a small fraction of childhood cancer patients who have the types of tumors that form the syndrome: 3 of 33 (9%) of childhood rhabdomyosarcoma patients; 7 of 235 (3%) of osteosarcomas; and 3 of 6 (50%) of childhood adrenocortical carcinoma [103–105]. Some, but not all, of these cases in which *TP53* germline mutations have been documented were found to have family histories suggestive of Li–Fraumeni syndrome. Felix et al. demonstrated that among acute lymphoblastic leukemia patients, germline mutations are possible although rare even among leukemia patients with a positive family history of leukemia [106,107]. Families with germline *TP53* mutations have been reported that include a wider spectrum of childhood tumors, including Wilms' tumors, hepatoblastoms, and a diverse range of adult cancers [81,108,109]. However, in other families with Li–Fraumeni syndrome, no *TP53* mutation has been documented. It is unclear whether a second gene exists or whether in some families the alteration is simply not detected by the mutation-detection strategies used.

Genetic testing of asymptomatic children in Li–Fraumeni families is thus technically feasible for those families in which a *TP53* mutation has been identified. The test is offered commercially; however, much controversy exists concerning the applicability of *TP53* germline mutation testing. The combination of the highly variable degree of penetrance, the broad spectrum of cancers observed in this syndrome, and the wide variation in age at which cancers occur in predisposed individuals has created difficult issues in the development of predictive testing guidelines [110]. These issues are often somewhat similar to those encountered in genetic testing for Huntington's disease, in which similar social and psychological concerns for mutation carriers exist in the absence of available medical interventions to alter risk of disease [111–113]. At present, routine testing of children, even in high-risk families, is not generally recommended due to the current absence of effective interventional strategies, concerns about adverse psychological outcomes including stigmatization, possible excessive sheltering of the child, the inability of minors to provide adequate consent for testing, and disruption of family relationships.

6. Familial adenomatous polyposis and the pediatric patient

Familial adenomatous polyposis (FAP) is a relatively rare, autosomal dominantly inherited condition affecting approximately 1 in 5000 individuals in the general population. This genetic condition is best known for its associated predisposition to the formation of multiple adenomatous polyps blanketing the colonic mucosa, which place an individual at extremely high risk of colon cancer in early adulthood. Each individual polyp is not any more likely to develop into a colon carcinoma than a polyp from an individual without FAP; however, the number of polyps, often in the hundreds, collectively place an individual at extremely high risk of tumor development. Polyps often develop starting in adolescence, and by age 30 over 90% of genetically affected individuals will show signs of disease. Much of the effort to identify high-risk individuals within polyposis families is geared towards determining optimal methods to prevent colon cancer starting in adolescence. Thus, for many years, an attempt to identify at-risk individuals in polyposis families by means of flexible sigmoidoscopy or colonoscopy has been a standard of medical care. The average age at which adenomatous polyps occur is 10 to 14 years of age, and it is generally recommended that surveillance start at age 8 to 10 and continue yearly. When multiple polyps are noted, total colectomy is the treatment of choice for prevention of cancer. Regular surveillance is recommended in high-risk asymptomatic individuals until at least age 40 [114,115].

Aside from the risk of colon cancer, families with FAP are at risk of both benign and malignant tumors outside the colon, including the upper gastrointestinal track and thyroid [116–125]. Extracolonic manifestations of FAP that are know to occur in children and that may precede the development of colonic polyps are shown in table 1. Of particular interest to health care providers for young children in FAP families is the association of FAP and hepatoblastoma [122–124]. The relative risk of hepatoblastoma is estimated to be over 800-fold in affected children [124].

Benign extracolonic manifestations in association with familial polyposis were originally described by Gardner (125) and include multiple osteomas and epidermoid cysts. This association is sometimes referred to as *Gardner's syndrome*. Osteomas often occur on facial bones, particularly the mandible, but may also occur on long bones. Although benign, osteomas may cause local damage by invasion or destruction of normal tissue. Epidermoid cysts are also considered benign tumors, and in contrast to the general population, in which they occur primarily on the back, in FAP families they occur on the face, scalp, and extremities. These lesions rarely occur in children outside the setting of

Table 1. Extracolonic manifestations of familial adenomatous Polyposis that may occur in childhood

Congenital hypertrophy of the retinal pigmented epithelium
  (CHRPE)
Epidermoid cysts
Abnormal dentition
Desmoid tumors
Malignant tumors
  Hepatoblastoma
  CNS tumors
  Thyroid cancer

familial polyposis. Desmoid tumors, fibromatoid tumors that often occur on the abdominal wall or intraperitoneum, are frequently oberved in polyposis kindreds. Although desmoids do not metastasize, the growth of these tumors can be considerable and may be exacerbated by surgery, hormones, or trauma. An important clinical significance is that these benign manifestations of familial polyposis may precede the appearance of colonic polyps and thus may be an indicator of high-risk status [116].

Another extracolonic finding that has been used diagnostically is the finding of congenital hypertrophy of the retinal pigmented epithelium (CHRPE) [126]. CHRPE is found in some, but not all, FAP families. In families in which CHRPE is observed in affected individuals, eye exams have been used to determine carrier status in children [127].

A clue as to the localization of the gene responsible for FAP arose from the observation of a constitutional deletion of chromosome 5q21 in a patient with FAP [128]. Linkage studies analyzing numerous kindreds with FAP confirmed this as the genetic locus [129–131].

The identification of multiple genetic markers in this region facilitated the identification of gene carriers within an affected family through the use of traditional methods of restriction fragment length polymorphisms later enhanced by the use of highly polymorphic repeat markers [115,132]. As in the case of retinoblastoma, early identification of gene carriers is cost-effective in that it spares nonmutation carriers the need for frequent surveillance procedures.

The gene responsible for FAP was identified in 1991 as the adenomatous polyposis coli (*APC*) gene [5,133–135]. Genetic testing techniques that use surrounding polymorphic markers require typing of at least two known affected family members before another person can be tested for unknown genetic status; therefore, the cloning of the *APC* gene has facilitated the process of genetic testing, since only one affected person is now necessary to document the mutation within the family. The gene is large in size, and mutations have been observed throughout the gene, hampering the feasibility of DNA analysis [136–139].

Over 90% of known mutations in the *APC* gene cause frameshifts that result in a truncated protein product [134–139]. A protein truncation assay for altered *APC* gene product is now available [141,142]. A limitation of this test is that it only detects mutations that terminate protein translation. This test is less labor intensive, however, than direct genetic sequence analysis. A potential advantage of this test is that, in theory, a person from a polyposis family could be tested for altered protein without direct comparison to an affected member; however, a negative test result may not determine with certainty the nonexistence of a disease-causing gene. One must therefore be aware of the possibility of a false negative with the protein truncation assay when it is performed on a single sample from an unaffected individual. Negative lab tests with this assay have been shown to be misinterpreted by nearly a third of physicians utilitizing the commercially available test [143].

No molecular distinction can be made between FAP patients with benign extracolonic manifestations characteristic of Gardner's syndrome. However, some other observed phenotypic variations correlate with the location of the mutation within the gene. Mutations occuring in the 5' region of the gene are characterized by fewer numbers of polyps and a later onset of colon cancer [144]. Germline mutations within a small 200-base-pair region of exon 15 of the *APC* gene are associated with a profuse number of polyps [140]. The presence or absence of CHRPE lesions in FAP families is dependent on the position of the underlying mutation, and CHRPE is absent in families with mutations in the 5' end of the gene [145]. This finding confirms the previously recognized interfamilial variation in the presence or absence of these lesions.

The association of brain tumors and polyps was described in 1959 by Turcot et al. and has since been known as *Turcot's syndrome* [146]. As a clinical syndrome, Turcot's syndrome overlaps considerably with familial polyposis. Analysis of the *APC* gene in cases of polyposis and brain tumors has demonstrated germline mutation and loss of alleles in some but not all cases [147–149]. Although only a few children with CNS tumors have been analyzed, four kindreds analyzed to date with childhood medulloblastoma all have mutations within a narrow region of the gene from codon 1000 to 1114 [147,148]. In a small number of cases, the underlying genetic lesions in patients with polyposis and brain tumors appears not to be *APC*, but rather one of the predisposing genes for non-polyposis hereditary colon cancer [149].

7. Multiple endocrine neoplasia

The multiple endocrine neoplasias (MENs) compose a spectrum of autosomal dominantly inherited cancer predisposition syndromes affecting young adults and children. MEN type 2A and type 2B and familial medullary thyroid cancer (FMTC) are all associated with the development of medullary thyroid cancer at an early age. MEN2A, also known as *Sipple syndrome*, is associated with pheochromocytomas and parathyroid hyperplasia [150]. The penetrance of early signs of thyroid cancer in MEN-2 is over 90% by age 30 [151]. The incidence of pheochromocytoma may vary between families but is considerably lower than that of medullary thyroid cancer. MEN2B is associated with ganglioneuromatosis and mucosal neuromas in addition to the cancers characteristic of MEN-2A. Patients with MEN2B also have a Marfanoid habitus and characteristic facies, whereas patients with MEN2A are phenotypically normal except for the predilection to develop endocrine cancers [152–154]. FMTC consists of thyroid cancer in the absence of the associated tumors or other anomalies characteristic of MEN2A or 2B. The age of onset of thyroid malignancy in FMTC is somewhat older than MEN2A or 2B, and there is some evidence to suggest that the malignancies are more indolent in FMTC [155]. Appoximately 25% of all cases of medullary thyroid cancer will be part of one of these familial syndromes. The medullary thyroid cancers in these familial syndromes occur in the first to fourth decade of life but may occur as early as infancy, particularly in MEN2B [154,156–158], whereas medullary thyroid cancer in the absence of a familial syndrome occurs in the fifth to sixth decade of life.

In linkage studies of large affected kindreds, MEN2 and FMTC were both shown to map to the pericentric region of chromosome 10 [159,160]. The gene for MEN2A was identified in 1993 as the *RET* proto-oncogene [9]. It was soon realized that the germline mutations in MEN2A and FMTC families were localized within a very narrow region of the gene [161], and this finding, together with the predictably observed very high penetrance of disease manifestation and availability of reasonable means of intervention to reduce risk, created an extremely rapid transition from the arena of basic research to clinical diagnostic testing [162,163].

Genotype–phenotype correlation studies have revealed that the mutation at codon 634 is associated with the development of pheochromocytoma in addition to MTC and that a specific CGC mutation at this codon is correlated with the development of parathyroid hyperplasia [164]. Families with MEN2B also have mutations of the *RET* gene; in these families, however, the germline mutations are found at a distinct methionine codon [165,166].

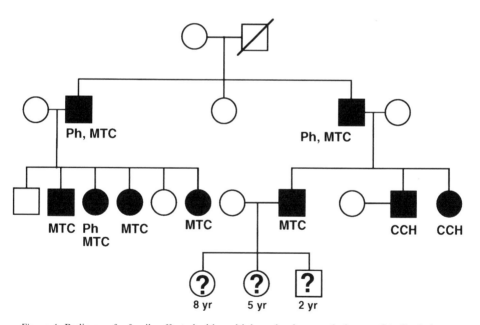

Figure 4. Pedigree of a family affected with multiple endocrine neoplasia, type 2A. Symbols are as in figure 1. MTC, medullary carcinoma of the thyroid; Ph, pheochromocytoma; CCH, clear cell hyperplasia. '?' indicates individuals in whom genetic testing for *RET* mutation was undertaken.

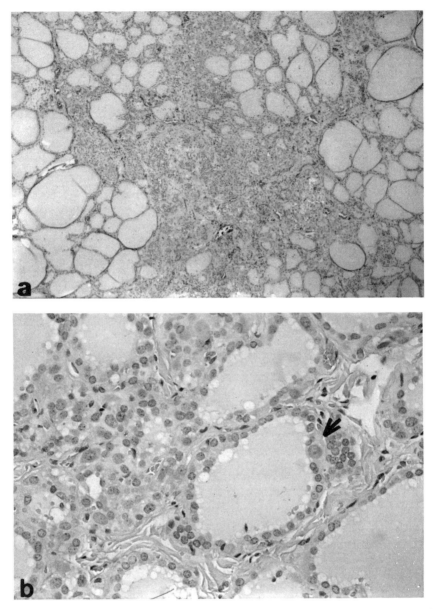

Figure 5. Photomicrograph of resected thyroid glands from 5- and 2-year-old members of the MEN2A kindred shown in figure 4. Both patients tested positive for mutation of the *RET* gene. (**a**) An incipient medullary thyroid carcinoma in resected thyroid gland from the 5-year-old girl who had a borderline positive pentagastrin stimulation test. (**b**) Thyroid follicles with surrounding C-cell hyperplasia taken from the 2-year-old girl who tested genetically positive, but in whom the pentagastrin stimulation test was negative. (**c** and **d**) Calcitonin immunohistochemical staining of the specimens shown in **a** and **b**, respectively.

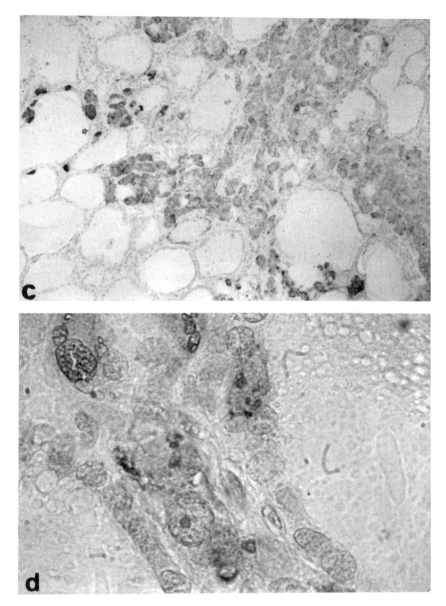

Figure 5 (continued)

Without genetic testing, early detection for thyroid malignancy in MEN families is possible by performing chemical stimulation of parafollicular cells by intravenous infusion of either calcium and pentagastrin, which causes release of calcitonin. Markedly elevated calcitonin levels in response to stimulation are indicative of C-cell hyperplasia or incipient carcinoma. Thyroidectomy has been a standard recommendation for individuals in high-risk families who have positive stimulation tests. Although this biochemical means of screening for occult tumors is sensitive, in some cases the MTC will have spread to lymph nodes, and false positives have been reported [167–169]. This test, however, has unpleasant transient neuropsychological side effects that may cause decreased compliance in high-risk individuals.

With the advent of genetic testing, it has become possible to identify mutation carriers before biochemical evidence of malignancy. Figure 4 demonstrates a pedigree of a family with clinical manifestations of multiple endocrine neoplasia. Three young children had undergone surveillance by pentagastrin stimulation, with equivocal results in the 5-year-old and negative results in the 8- and 2-year-old. After undergoing genetic testing, the younger two children tested positive and underwent thyroidectomy. Histologic examination, as shown in figure 5, revealed incipient medullary thyroid carcinoma in the 5-year-old who had had an equivocal pentagastrin stimulation test and C-cell hyperplasia in the 2-year-old who had been negative for pentagastrin stimulation. These types of observations confirm that the onset of transformation to malignancy occurs at an extremely young age in *RET* mutation carriers and that histologic evidence of malignancy may precede biochemical evidence of malignancy.

Although no long-term studies are yet available, it has been suggested that early thyroidectomy for children who test positive for DNA carrier status may be more likely to be curative than thyroidectomy after biochemical evidence of malignancy [161]. In addition to long-term follow-up studies to determine the benefit of early thyroidectomy in preventing MTC, long-term studies to determine the benefit of surveillance for development of adrenal malignancies are needed.

8. The phakomatoses: neurofibromatosis, types 1 and 2, tuberous sclerosis, and von Hippel–Lindau disease

The phakomatoses (from *phakos,* 'lentil,' 'mole,' or 'freckle') are neurocutaneous disorders that are also, to a varying extent, cancer predisposition syndromes. The clinical expression of these syndromes is variable and can be mild, so signs of disease must be carefully sought in family members of affected individuals. The genes for each of the syndromes to be discussed have been isolated. Genetic testing has become possible but is not routine for any of the phakomatoses.

8.1. Neurofibromatosis (Von Recklinghausen's disease)

The neurofibromatoses are related disorders characterized by café-au-lait spots, neurofibromas, and a predisposition to malignancy. The most common of these disorders is neurofibromatosis type 1 (NF1), which has an estimated frequency of 1 per 2500–3300 births [34]. The diagnosis of NF1 is made by clinical criteria as established by the NIH consensus and listed in table 2 [170]. A study of a large cohort of 212 patients with NF1 in Denmark revealed that the overall relative risk for cancer was 2.5 during a 40-year follow-up period, with a significant excess of brain tumors, primarily gliomas [171]. To assess the risk for malignancy in children with NF1, a review of the Japan Children's Cancer Registry revealed that the incidence of NF1 among cancer patients was 0.21%, 6.45 times that of the general population. The incidence of NF1 was highest in optical nerve glioma (12.5%) and malignant schwannoma (31.4%) but was also increased in rhabdomyosarcoma (1.36%) and myeloid leukemia (0.27%) [172]. A study of children under 6 years of age who had gliomas of the optic pathways and hypothalamus revealed that 33% also carried a diagnosis of NF1; however, tumors were less aggressive in the subset of patients with NF1 [173]. Soft tissue sarcomas of childhood and adulthood are seen and in one family were observed in multiple generations [174]. Myeloproliferative diseases are also seen in NF1, with a predilection for development in boys and a pattern of inheritance favoring maternal inheritance of NF1 [172,175].

The NF1 gene has been identified; like *RB1* and *APC*, it is large, with mutations scattered throughout the gene, making molecular diagnosis costly and laborious [4,176,177]. Testing of asymptomatic relatives of NF1 patients using linkage analysis has been used with some success [178]. Since the diagnosis of NF1 is made by clinical criteria and the possible clinical significance of mutation carriers who do not demonstrate characteristic clinical features is

Table 2. NIH consensus diagnostic criteria for neurofibromatosis [170]

Neurofibromatosis, type 1
    Two or more of the following:
        Six or more café-au-lait macules
            >5 mm in prepubertal persons
            >5 mm in postpubertal persons
        Two or more neurofibromas
        Axillary or inguinal freckling
        Optic glioma
        Two or more iris hamartomas (Lisch nodules)
        Osseous dysplasia
        A first-degree meeting two of the above criteria

Neurofibromatosis, type 2
    Bilateral eighth nerve masses
    or
    A first degree relative with NF2
    or
    Two of the following:
        neurofibroma
        meningioma
        glioma
        schwannoma
        juvenile posterior subcapsular lenticular opacity

unknown, there is no clear indication for molecular testing. Nevertheless, direct mutation detection can help determine definitively whether an affected individual has a new or inherited mutation, which could be of value in counseling parents of an affected child about the likelihood of having a second child with the disorder. Genetic studies may also be helpful in the evaluation of young children in known NF1 families in whom full manifestations of the disease are not yet apparent.

Neurofibromatosis type 2 (NF2), like NF1, is characterized by multiple café-au-lait spots, although the presence of both café-au-lait spots and neurofibromas is less in NF2 than in NF1. The hallmark of NF2 is the development of tumors of the acoustic nerve that are often bilateral. Also characteristic of NF-2 are meningiomas, gliomas, schwannomas, and juvenile posterior subcapsular lenticular opacities [170,179]. The criteria for making a clinical diagnosis of NF2 are given in table 2.

The NF2 gene has been identified [8]. A wide range of mutations have been found, and there is some evidence that the type of mutation correlates with disease severity, with mutations resulting in truncated proteins being associated with a more severe phenotype than mutations causing amino acid substitutions [180,181].

Like NF1, the diagnosis of NF2 is at present usually made on the basis of clinical criteria rather than molecular testing, and it has been recommended that children and young adults at high risk due to a first-degree relative with NF2 be followed with periodic skin and opthalmologic exams as well as audiologic evaluations [179]. As with several of the other syndromes discussed in this chapter, genetic determination of the mutation status of first-degree relatives of affected individuals could possibly lessen the need for periodic screening.

8.2. Tuberous sclerosis (Bourneville's disease)

Tuberous sclerosis (TS) is characteristically associated with white macules (ash leaf spots) that are often present at birth, making affected persons identifiable at an early stage [182]. The mode of inheritance is autosomal dominant, although two distinct genetic loci are involved: *TSC1* at chromosome 9q34 and *TSC2* at chromosome 16p13 [183]. Facial angiofibromas and angiolipomas of the kidney and other organs are common. The incidence of brain tumors in childhood is significant and is estimated to be 5%–14%. The most common histology of CNS tumor is giant cell astrocytoma [184–186].

A distinctive feature of TS is the cardiac rhabdomyoma in infancy [187]. This tumor is considered to be non-malignant; however, it may cause cardiac dysfunction. Over half of cardiac rhabdomyomas are associated with TS; thus, this finding of this tumor in an infant should raise the question of a possible diagnosis of TS and prompt the taking of a careful family history and examination of family members for detection of ash leaf spots.

The *TSC2* gene on chromosome 16p13 has been identified [18], and the search for *TSC1* is still in progress [188]. No genotype–phenotype correlations have yet been determined. Genetic testing is not yet available for most families, and diagnosis of carriers within families is made primarily by clinical features. The yield of routine screening with radiographic or other studies in asymptomatic first-degree relatives of TS patients appears to be low [189].

8.3. Von Hippel–Lindau disease

Von Hippel–Lindau (VHL) disease is an autosomal-dominant inherited disorder characterized by angiomata of the retina and hemangioblastoma of the cerebellum [190]. Renal cell carcinoma and pheochromocytoma have each been observed in approximately 14% of patients with VHL [191]. Renal cell carcinomas constitute a particularly frequent cause of mortality in this disorder, occurring as bilateral and multifocal tumors more frequently than in sporadic, nonfamilial cases, and can develop in children and adolescents.

Because of the frequency of renal cell carcinoma in VHL disease and frequent chromosomal losses on the short arm of chromosome 3 in renal cell carcinoma, investigators were led to examine 3p as a possible genetic locus for VHL (192). The gene was eventually mapped to chromosome 3p25 and isolated by Latif et al. in 1993 [7].

Mutation analysis of the VHL gene reveals mutations corresponding to distinct phenotypes, including renal cell carcinoma without pheochromocytoma, renal cell carcinoma with pheochromocytoma, and pheochromocytoma without renal cell carcinoma [7,193,194]. Such phenotypic correlation could ultimately prove useful in the individual counseling of families.

9. Other counseling issues: weighing the risks and benefits of genetic testing for cancer susceptibility genes in children

The pediatric cancer specialist as well as the general pediatrician will increasingly be asked to play a role in counseling families as to whether and when a child or adolescent should undergo genetic testing for a cancer predisposition gene. Benefits and risks associated with the determination of genetic status should be carefully considered before testing is undertaken. In some cases, the wishes of the parents to know their child's genetic status will need to be weighed against the wishes of the child or adolescent.

Whereas certain benefits regarding early identification of mutations carriers are acknowledged, many concerns have been raised regarding some of the risks that accompany the genetic testing of children. These risks pertain primarily to the psychological and emotional adverse sequelae and may include the risk of creating lowered a feeling of stigmatization on the part of the child that may result in lower self-esteem and an inability to integrate effectively with peers [195,196]. Genetic testing may also tend to divide children within a high-risk family, who were once united by a common feeling of risk, into the 'haves' and 'have-nots' — a situation that may create problems of survivor guilt among noncarriers of germline mutations. Guilt feelings may be also induced among affected parents. Testing of children may be disruptive to parent–child bonding and may disrupt the overall dynamics of the family. Regardless of the degree of medical benefit that a genetic testing opportunity affords, care must be taken to recognize and address these possible problems with appropriate referral and counseling as indicated.

The American Society of Clinical Oncology has classified the priorities for testing for cancer predisposition according to the extent to which medical benefits are available for carriers of germline mutations, given the premise that the greater the benefit, the higher the priority that should be placed on testing [197]. The highest-priority group to consider for testing includes familial retinoblastoma, in which identification of mutation carriers can optimize the cost-effectiveness of screening; familial polyposis, where removal of the colon in adolescence is preventative against development of colon cancer; and MEN2, in which prophylactic removal of the thyroid gland is thought to be preventative against development of medullary carcinoma. In all three of these situations, the likelihood that a mutation carrier will developing disease is in excess of 90%, and therefore the ability to intervene has the potential to reduce both cancer-associated mortality and morbidity. Clearly, among the benefits in this category of genetic testing situations is the benefit to nonmutation carriers, who will not require either frequent screening examinations for early signs of cancer or prophylactic surgeries. In this category of familial syndromes, genetic testing should be incorporated where feasible into standard medical care.

In situations in which medical benefits are less well established, such as testing for mutation of the *TP53* gene, testing should be implemented in the setting of institutional research board approved protocols designed to answer questions about the potential impact of genetic testing. In situations in which there are no known benefits of testing, or in which germline mutations have been reported in only a small number of families, testing should not be undertaken in a clinical setting. It is recommended that, wherever possible, testing within any category be performed in the setting of long-term outcome studies.

The need for informed consent is emphasized, which is to include a thorough discussion as well as written documentation of risks and benefits of testing and medical surveillance options recommended with and without testing. The basic elements of informed consent for genetic testing is given in table 3. These guidelines, however, do not address the unique aspects of genetic testing of children. The extent to which a minor child participates in the process of informed consent for genetic research depends on multiple factors, including the degree of medical benefit and thus the degree of priority placed upon the testing process, as well as the chronological age, state of cognitive

Table 3. Basic elements of informed consent for germline DNA testing [197]

Information on the specific test being performed
Implications of a positive and negative result
Possibility that the test will not be informative
Options for risk estimation without genetic testing
Risk of passing a mutation to subsequent children
Technical accuracy of the test
Fees involved in testing and counseling
Risks of psychological distress
Risks of insurance or employer discrimination
Confidentiality issues
Options and limitations of medical surveillance and screening following testing

development, and maturity of the child. Children 7 years of age and older are generally able to understand the general outline of a medical procedure and in many instances should be asked to assent, e.g., be asked to agree to a parental decision without attaining the necessary autonomy to consent to a procedure on their own. As children reach adolescence, the issue of informed consent often becomes more complex. In polyposis families, it may be particularly difficult in dealing with preadolescents and adolescents to determine when informed consent should be obtained from the young patient in whom prophylactic colectomy has been recommended as an option should a test result be positive. The law has generally regarded 15 years of age as the age at which minors can and should consent to or refuse medical procedures; however, adolescents vary tremendously in their level of emotional maturity and sense of autonomy.

Wertz et al. have defined four categories in which genetic testing of minors may be considered [195]. These include 1) genetic testing that provides a direct benefit to the child; 2) genetic testing that assists the adolescent in making reproductive decisions; 3) genetic testing that provides no direct benefit, but is requested by the child or parent; and 4) genetic testing done solely to provide an estimation of risk to another family member.

The first category includes situations in which immediate benefit is derived for the child, such as the implementation of early detection or prevention strategies that would reduce the risk of developing cancer, dying from cancer, or undergoing extensive treatment. Examples in this category, similar to the high-priority category defined by ASCO, would include MEN2A, FAP, and familial retinoblastoma, in which the benefits or early identification of at-risk children enables early diagnosis and/or prevention of tumor development.

Genetic testing to assist in making reproductive decisions applies primarily to X-linked or autosomal-recessive disorders, but presumably, testing for an autosomal-dominant gene associated with onset of symptoms in adolescence or early adulthood (such as APC) could also influence marital and/or reproductive decisions. This category is also somewhat relevant to clearly adult-onset conditions. The American Society of Human Genetics has strongly felt that in cases in which genetic testing results in no medical benefits nor interventional strategies to be implemented prior to adulthood (as in the case of the breast cancer predisposition genes *BRCA1* or *BRCA2*), testing should be deferred until adulthood [196].

In some cases, genetic testing may be requested by a parent or patient in the absence of any known present or future medical benefit. A survey of mothers of pediatric cancer patients revealed that in hypothetical situations in which genetic factors were defined as causing a child's cancer and the option of genetic testing was available, approximately half the mothers would pursue genetic testing of themselves and 42% would pursue genetic testing of their unaffected children even if no established means of intervention was available [198]. At this time, it is unclear what the true motives are in seeking such testing; however, it is possible that in some cases the desire to test may reflect the strong hope of obtaining a negative test result. However, preliminary observations from a program of predictive testing for germline *TP53* mutations that was offered to adult members of Li–Fraumeni families suggest that when offered a definite testing opportunity, many individuals from high-risk families may actually decline participation [199]. Reasons may include the lack of available interventions for gene carriers, fear of insurance problems, or recent adverse events associated with the diagnosis of cancer in a family member.

Whereas the ASCO statement also endorses the provision of counseling and testing as being within the responsibility of the practicing cancer specialist, in many cases the extent of counseling required to obtain adequate informed consent may exceed the time or resources available to the cancer specialist. In addition, due to the rapid pace of advancements in the field of cancer genetics, many cancer specialists may not be able to provide up-to-date information. Therefore, referral to specialists in the field of genetics or genetic counseling may be indicated. The number and availability of such specialists is limited and may be inadequate to fulfill all the future genetic counseling needs of cancer patients and families. Hence, education of both oncology and primary care specialists is essential. A core curriculum has therefore been designed to serve as a basis for educating health care professionals in the area of genetic counseling and risk assessment, with an acknowledgment of the ongoing need for continuing educational endeavors (200).

References

1. Friend SH, Bernards R, Rogelj S, Weinberg RA, Rapaport JM, Alber DM, Dryja TP. 1986. A human DNA segment with properties of the gene that predisposes to retinoblastoma and osteosarcoma. Nature 323:643.
2. Call KM, Glaser T, Ito CY, Buckler AJ, Pelletier J, Haber DA, Rose EA, Kral A, Yeger H, Lewis WH, Jones C, Housman DE. 1990. Isolation and characterization of a zinc finger polypeptide gene at the human chromosome 11 Wilms' tumor locus. Cell 60:509–520.

3. Malkin K, Li FP, Strong LC, Fraumeni JF, Nelson CE, Kim DH, Kassel J, Gryka MA, Bischoff FZ, Tainsky MA, Friend SH. 1990. Germline p53 mutations in a familial syndrome of breast cancer, sarcomas, and other neoplasms. Science 250:1233–1238.

4. Xu G, O'Connell P, Viskochil D, Cawthon R, Robertson M, Culver M, Dunn D, Stevens J, Gesteland R, White R, Weiss R. 1990. The neurofibromatosis type 1 gene encodes a protein related to GAP. Cell 62:599–608.

5. Groden J, Thliveris A, Samowitz W, et al. 1991. Identification and characterization of the familial adenomatous polyposis coli gene. Cell 66:589–600.

6. Wooster R, Mangion J, Eeles R, Smith S, Dowsett M, Averill D, Barrett-Lee P, Easton DF, Ponder BA, Stratton MR. 1992. A germline mutation in the androgen receptor gene in two brothers with breast cancer and Reifenstein syndrome. Nature Genet 2:132–134.

7. Latif F, Tory K, Gnarra J, et al. 1993. Identification of the von Hippel–Lindau disease tumor suppressor gene. Science 260:1317–1320.

8. Trofatter JA, MacCollin MM, Rutter JL, et al. 1993. A novel moesin-, exrin-, radixin-like gene is a candidate for the neurofibromatosis 2 tumor suppressor. Cell 72:791–800.

9. Mulligan LM, Kwok JBJ, Healey CS, et al. 1993. Germ-line mutations of the RET proto-oncogene in multiple endocrine neoplasia type 2A. Nature 363:458–460.

10. Leach FS, Nicolaides NC, Papadopoullos N, et al. 1993. A mutS homolog in hereditary non-polyposis colorectal cancer. Cell 75:1215–1225.

11. Nicolaides N, Papadopoulos N, Liu B, et al. 1994. Mutations of two PMS homologues in hereditary nonpolyposis colon cancer. Nature 371:75–80.

12. Papadopoulos N, Nicolaides NC, Wei Y-F, et al. 1994. Mutation of a mutL homolog in hereditary colon cancer. Science 263:1625–1631.

13. Miki Y, Swensen J, Shattuck-Eidens D, et al. 1994. A strong candidate for the breast and ovarian cancer susceptibility gene BRCA1. Science 266:66–71.

14. Hussussian CJ, Struewing JP, Goldstein AM, Higgins PAT, Ally DS, Sheahan MD, Clark WH, Tucker MA, Dracopoli MC. 1994. Germline p16 mutations in familial melanoma. Nature Genet 8:15–21.

15. Wooster R, Signold G, Lancaster J, et al. 1995. Identification of the breast cancer suscepti-bility gene BRCA2. Nature 378:789–782.

16. Ellis NA, Groden J, Ye T-Z, Straughen J, Lennon DJ, Ciocci S, Proytcheva M, German J. 1995. The Bloom's syndrome gene product is homologous to recQ helicases. Cell 83:655–666.

17. Savitsky K, Bar-Shira A, Gilad S, et al. 1995. A single ataxia telangiectasia gene with a product similar to PI-3 kinase. Science 268:1749–1753.

18. Wienecke R, Konig A, DeClue JE. 1995. Identification of tuberin, the tuberous sclerosis-2 product. J Biol Chem 270:16409–16414.

19. Johnson R, Rothman A, Xie J, Goodrich L, Bare J, Bonifas J, Quinn E, Myers R, Cox D, Epstein E, Scott M. 1996. Human homolog of patched, a candidate gene for the basal cell nevus syndrome. Science 272:1668–1671.

20. Pilia G, Hughes-Benzie RM, MacKenzie A, Baybayan P, Chen EY, Huber R, Neri G, Cao A, Forabosco A, Schlessinger D. 1996. Mutations in GPC3, a glypican gene, cause the Simpson–Golabi–Behmel overgrowth syndrome. Nature Genet 12:241–247.

21. Francke U, Kung F. 1976. Sporadic bilateral retinoblastoma in 13q-chromosomal deletion. Med Pediatr Oncol 2:379–385.

22. Knudson AG, Meadows AT, Nichols WW, Hill R. 1976. Chromosomal deletion and retinoblastoma. N Eng J Med 295:1120–1123.

23. Riccardi VM, Sujansky E, Smith AC, Francke U. 1978. Chromosome imbalance in the aniridia-Wilms' tumor association: 11p interstitial deletion. Pediatrics 61:604–610.

24. Yunis JJ, Ramsay NKC. 1980. Familial occurrence of the aniridia-Wilms' tumor with dele-tion 11p13-14.1. J Pediatr 96:1027–1030.

25. Wooster R, Neuhausen SL, Mangion J, et al. 1994. Localization of a breast cancer suscepti-bility gene, BRCA2, to chromosome 13q12–13. Science 265:2088–2090.

26. Hall JM, Lee MK, Morrow J, Newman B, Anderson L, Huey B, King MC. 1990. Linkage analysis of early onset familial breast cancer to chromosome 17q21. Science 250:1684–1689.

27. Peltomaki P, Aaltonen LA, Sistonen P, et al. 1993. Genetic mapping of a locus predisposing to human colorectal cancer. Science 260:810–812.

28. Draper GJ, Sanders EL, Lennox EL, Brownhill PA. 1996. Patterns of childhood cancer among siblings. Br J Cancer 74:152–158.

29. Knudson AG. 1971. Mutation and cancer: statistical study of retinoblastoma. Proc Nat Acad Sci USA 68:820–823.

30. Knudson AG, Strong LC. 1972. Mutation and cancer: a model for Wilms' tumor of the kidney. J Natl Cancer Inst 48:313–324.

31. Knudson A, Strong L. 1972. Mutation and cancer: neuroblastoma and pheochromocytoma. Am J Hum Genet 24:514–524.

32. Neuhausen SL, Mazoyer S, Friedman L, et al. 1996. Haplotype and phenotype analysis of six recurrent BRCA1 mutations in 61 families: results of an international study. Am J Hum Genet 58:271–280.

33. The frequency of neurofibromatosis. In Crowe F, Schull W, Neel J (eds.), The Frequency of Neurofibromatosis. Springfield, Illinois: CC Thomas, 1956, pp. 142–146.

34. Vogel F. 1979. Genetics of retinoblastoma. Hum Genet 52:1–54.

35. Gallie BL, Ellsworth RM, Abramson DH, Phillips RA. 1982. Retinoma: spontaneous regression of retinoblastoma or benign manifestation of the mutation? Br J Cancer 45:513–521.

36. Draper GJ, Sanders BM, Brownbill PA, Hawkins MM. 1992. Patterns of risk of hereditary retinoblastoma and applications to genetic counseling. Br J Cancer 66:211–219.

37. Onadim X, Hogg A, Baird P, Cowell J. 1992. Oncogeneic point mutations in exon 20 of the RBI gene in families showing incomplete penetrance and mild expression of the retinoblastoma phenotype. Proc Natl Acad Sci USA 89:6177.

38. Sakai T, Ohtani N, McGee TL, Robbins PD, Dryja TP. 1991. Oncogenic germline mutations in Sp1 and ATF sites in the human retinoblastoma gene. Nature 353:83.

39. Toguchida J, McGee TL, Petersen JC, Eagle JR, Tucker S, Yandell DW, Dryja TP. 1993. Complete genomic sequence of the human retinoblastoma susceptibility gene. Genomics 17:535–543.

40. Dryja T, Rapaport J, Joyce J, Petersen R. 1986. Molecular detection of deletions involving band q14 of chromosome 13 in retinoblastoma. Proc Natl Acad Sci USA 83:7391–7394.

41. Ejima Y, Sasaki MS, Kaneko A, Tamooka H. 1988. Types, rates, origin and expressivity of chromosome mutations involving 13q14 in retinoblastoma patients. Hum Genet 79:118–123.

42. Horsthemke B, Barnert H, Gregor V, Passarge E, Hopping W. 1987. Early diagnosis in hereditary retinoblastoma by detection of molecular deletions at the locus. Lancet 1:511–512.

43. Yandell DW, Campbell TA, Dayton SH, Petersen R, Walton D, Little JB, McConkie-Rosell A, Buckley BG, Dryja TP. 1989. Oncogenic point mutations in the human retinoblastoma gene: their application to genetic counseling. N Engl J Med 321:1689–1695.

44. Dunn JM, Phillips RA, Becker AJ, Gallie BL. 1988. Identification of germline and somatic mutations affecting the retinoblastoma gene. Science 241:1797–1800.

45. Blanquet V, Turleau C, Gross-Morand MS, Senamaud-Beaufort C, Doz F, Besmond C. 1995. Spectrum of germline mutations in the RB1 gene: a study of 232 patients with hereditary and non-hereditary retinoblastoma. Hum Mol Genet 4:383–388.

46. Wiggs J, Nordenskjold M, Yandell D, et al. 1988. Prediction of the risk of hereditary retinoblastoma using DNA polymorphisms within the retinoblastoma gene. N Engl J Med 318:151–157.

47. Yandell DW, Dryja TP. 1989. Detection of DNA sequence polymorphisms by enzymatic amplification and direct genomic sequencing. Am J Hum Genet 45:547–555.

48. Onadim Z, Hungerford J, Cowell JK. 1992. Follow-up of retinoblastoma patients having prenatal and perinatal predictions for mutant gene carrier status using intragenic polymorphic probes from the RB1 gene. Br J Cancer 65:711–716.

49. Draper G, Sanders B, Kingston J. 1986. Second primary neoplasms in patients with retinoblastoma. Br J Cancer 53:661–671.

50. Winther J, Olsen JH, deNully Brown P. 1988. Risk of nonocular cancer among retinoblastoma patients and their parents: a population-based study in Denmark. Cancer 62:1458–1462.

51. Eng C, Li FP, Abramson DH, Ellsworth RM, Wong L, Goldman MB, Seddon J, Tarbell N, Boice JD. 1993. Mortality from second tumors among long-term survivors of retinoblastoma. J Natl Cancer Inst 85:1121–1128.

52. Li FP, Abramson DH, Taron RE, Kleinerman RA, Fraumeni JF, Boice JD. 1997. Hereditary retinoblastoma, lipoma and second primary cancers. J Natl Cancer Inst 89:83–84.

53. Hansen MF, Koufos A, Gallie BL, Phillips RA, Fodstad O, Brogger A, Gedde-Dahl T, Cavenee WK. 1985. Osteosarcoma and retinoblastoma: a shared chromosomal mechanism revealing recessive predisposition. Proc Natl Acad Sci USA 82:6216–6220.

54. Francke U, Holmes LB, Atkins L, Riccardi VM, 1979. Aniridia–Wilms' tumor association: evidence for specific deletion of 11p13. Cytogenet Cell Genet 24:185–192.

55. Gessler M, Poustka A, Cavenee W, Neve RL, Orkin SH, Bruns G. 1990. Homozygous deletion in Wilms' tumours of a zinc-finger gene identified by chromosome jumping. Nature 346:194–197.

56. van Heyningen V, Bickmore WA, Seawright A, Fletcher K, Maule J, Fekete G, Gessler M, Bruns GAP, Huerre-Jeanpierre C, Junien C, Williams BRG, Hastie ND. 1990. Role for the Wilms' tumor gene in genital development? Proc Natl Acad Sci USA 87:5383–5386.

57. Brown K, Wilmore H, Watson J, Mott M, Berry P. 1993. Low frequency of mutations in the *WT1* coding regions in Wilms' tumor. Genes Chromosomes Cancer 8:74–79.

58. Li FP, Breslow N, Morgan JM, Ghahremani M, Miller GA, Grundy PE, Green DM, Diller LR, Pelletier J. 1996. Germline *WT1* mutations in Wilms' tumor patients: preliminary results. Med Pediatr Oncol 27:404–407.

59. Pelletier J, Bruening W, Kashtan CE, et al. 1991. Germline mutations in the Wilms' tumor suppressor gene are associated with abnormal urogenital development in Denys–Drash syndrome. Cell 87:437–447.

60. Coppes MJ, Huff V, Pelletier J. 1993. Denys–Drash syndrome: relating a clinical disorder to genetic alterations in the tumor suppressor gene WT1. J Pediatr 123:673–678.

61. Beckwith JB, 1969. Macroglossia, omphalocoele, adrenal cytomegaly, gigantism and hyperplastic visceromegaly. Birth Defects 5:188–196.

62. Wiedemann H. 1964. Complexe malformatif familial avec hernie ombilicale et macroglossie — 'un syndrome nouveau'? J Genet Hum 13:223–232.

63. Ping AJ, Reeve AE, Law DJ, Young MR, Boehnke M, Feinberg AP. 1989. Genetic linkage of Beckwith–Wiedemann syndrome to 11p15. Am J Hum Genet 44:720–723.

64. Koufos A, Grundy P, Morgan K, Aleck K, Hadro T, Lampkin B, Kalbakju A, Cavenee W. 1989. Familial Wiedemann–Beckwith syndrome and a second Wilms' tumor locus both map to 11p15.5. Am J Hum Genet 44:711–719.

65. Pettenati M, Haines J, Higgins R, Wappner R, Palmer C, Weaver D. 1986. Wiedemann–Beckwith syndrome: presentation of clinical and cytogenetic data on 22 new cases and review of the literature. Hum Genet 74:143–154.

66. Ben-Galim E, Gross-Kieselstein E, Abrahamov A. 1977. Beckwith–Wiedemann syndrome in a mother and her son. Am J Dis Child 131:801–803.

67. Best L, Hoekstra R. 1981. Wiedemann–Beckwith syndome: autosomal-dominant inheritance in a family. Am J Hum Genet 9:291–299.

68. Niikawa N, Ishikiriyama S, Takahashi S, Inagawa A, Tonoki M, Ohta Y, Hase N, Kamel T, Kaju T. 1986. The Wiedemann–Beckwith syndrome: pedigree studies on five families with evidence for autosomal dominant inheritance with variable expressivity. Am J Hum Genet 24:41–55.

69. Fraumeni J, Geiser C, Manning M. 1967. Wilms' tumor and congenital hemihypertrophy: report of five new cases and review of the literature. Pediatrics 40:886–899.

70. Smith P, Sullivan M, Algar E, Shapiro D. 1994. Analysis of paediatric tumour types associated with hemihyperplasia in childhood. J Pediatr Child Health 30:515–517.

91

71. Grundy P, Koufos A, Morgan K, Li F, Meadows A, Cavenee W. 1988. Familial predisposition to Wilms' tumor does not map to the short arm of chromosome 11. Nature 336:374–376.

72. Huff V, Compton D, LY C, LC S, GF S. 1990. Lack of linkage of familial Wilms' tumor to chromosomal band 11p13. Nature 336:6117–6120.

73. Pelletier J, Bruening W, Li F, Haber D, Glaser T, Housman D. 1991. WT1 mutations contribute to abnormal genital system development and hereditary Wilms' tumor. Nature 353:431–434.

74. Huff V, Reeve A, Leppert M, Strong L, Douglass E, Geiser C, Li F, Meadows A, Callen D, Lenoir G, Saunders G. 1992. Nonlinkage of 16q markers to familial predisposition to Wilms' tumor. Cancer Res 52:6117–6120.

75. Rahman N, Arbour L, Tonin P, Renshaw J, Pelletier J, Barchel S, Pritchard-Jones K, Stratton MR, Narod SA. 1996. Evidence for a familial Wilms' tumor gene (FWT1) on chromosome 17q12–21. Nature Genet 13:461–463.

76. Altura RA, Valentine M, Li H, Boyett JM, Shearer P, Grundy P, Shapiro DN, Look AT. 1996. Identification of novel regions of deletion in familial Wilms' tumor by comparative genomic hybridization. Cancer Res 56:3837–3841.

77. Hughes-Benzie RM, Hunter AGW, Allanson JE, MacKenzie AE. 1992. Simpson–Golabi–Behmel Syndrome associated with renal dysplasia and embryonal tumor: localization of the gene to Xqcen-q21. Am J Med Genet 43:428–435.

78. Verloes A, Massart B, Dehalleux I, Langhendries J-P, Koulischer L. 1995. Clinical overlap of Beckwith–Wiedemann, Perlman and Simpson–Golabi–Behmel syndromes: a diagnostic pitfall. Clin Genet 47:257–262.

79. Xuan J, Besner A, Ireland M, Hughes-Benzie R, MacKenzie A. 1994. Mapping of Simpson–Golabi–Behmel syndrome to Xq25–27. Hum Mol Genet 3:133–137.

80. Orth U, Gurrieri F, Behmel A, Genuardi Cremer M, Gal A, Neri G. 1994. Gene for Simpson–Golabi–Behmel syndrome is linked to HPRT in Xq26 in two European families. Am J Med Genet 50:388–390.

81. Li FP, Fraumeni JF. 1982. Prospective study of a family cancer syndrome. JAMA 247:2692–2694.

82. Hartley AL, Birch JM, Tricker K, Wallace SA, Kelsey AM, Harris M, Morris Jones PH. 1993. Wilms' tumor in a Li–Fraumeni cancer family syndrome. Cancer Genet Cytogenet 67:133–135.

83. Bardeesy N, Falkoff D, Petruzzi M-J, Norma N, Zable B, Adam M, Aguiar M, Grundy P, Shows T, Pelletier J. 1994. Anaplastic Wilms' tumor, a subtype displaying poor prognosis, harbours p53 gene mutations. Nature Genet 7:91–97.

84. Malkin D, Sexsmith E, Yeger H, Williams BR, Coppes M. 1994. Mutations of the p53 tumor suppressor gene occur infrequently in Wilms' tumor. Cancer Res 54:2077–2079.

85. Beckwith JB. 1993. Precursor lesions of Wilms tumor: clinical and biological implications. J Pediatr 21:158–168.

86. Li FP, Williams WR, Gimbrere BA, Flamant F, Green DM, Meadows AT. 1988. Heritable fraction of unilateral Wilms' tumor. Pediatrics 81:147–149.

87. Green D, Breslow N, Beckwith J, Norkool P. 1993. Screening of children with hemihypertrophy, aniridia, and Beckwith–Wiedemann syndrome in patients with Wilms' tumor: a report from the National Wilms' Tumor Study. Med Pediatr Oncol 21:188–192.

88. DeBaun M, Brown M, Kessler L. 1996. Screening for cancer in children with Beckwith Wiedemann syndrome (BWS): a cost-effective analysis. Am J Hum Genet 57:A57.

89. Li FP, Fraumeni JF. 1969. Soft-tissue sarcomas, breast cancer and other neoplasms. Ann Intern Med 71:747–752.

90. Miller R. 1968. Deaths from childhood cancer in sibs. N Eng J Med 279:122.

91. Li F, Fraumeni J, Mulvihill J, Blattner WA, Dreyfus MG, Tucker MA, Miller RW. 1988. A cancer family syndrome in twenty-four kindreds. Cancer Res 48:5358–5362.

92. Srivastava S, Zou Z, Pirollo K, Blattner W, Chang E. 1990. Germ-line transmission of a mutated p53 gene in a cancer-prone family with Li–Fraumeni syndrome. Nature 348:747–749.

93. Warneford S, Witton L, Townsend M, Rowe P, Reddel R, Dalla-Possa L, Symonds G. 1992. Germ-line splicing mutation of the p53 gene in a cancer-prone family. Cell Growth Differ 3:839–846.

94. Law J, Strong L, Chidambara A, Ferrell R. 1991. A germline mutation in exon 5 of the p53 gene in an extended cancer family. Cancer Res 51:6385–6387.

95. Santibanez-Koref M, Birch J, Harley A, Morris Jones P, Craft A, Eden T, Crowther D, Kelsey A, Harris C. 1991. p53 germline mutation in Li–Fraumeni syndrome. Lancet 338:1490–1491.

96. Brugieres L, Gardes M, Moutou C, Chompret A, Meresse V, Martin N, Poisson F, Flamant F, Bonaiti-Pellie C, Lemerle J, Feunteun J. 1993. Screening for germ-line p53 mutations in children with malignant tumors and a family history of cancer. Cancer Res 53:452–455.

97. Stolzenberg M-C, Brugieres L, Garders M, Dessarps-Freichey F, Chompret A, Bressac B, Lenoir G, Bonaiti-Pellie C, Lemerle J, Feunteun J. 1994. Germ-line exclusion of a single p53 allele by premature termination of translation in a Li–Fraumeni syndrome family. Oncogene 9:2799–2804.

98. Frebourg T, Barbier N, Yan Y-X, Garber J, Dreyfus M, Fraumeni J, Li F, Friend S. 1995. Germ-line p53 mutations in 15 families with Li–Fraumeni Syndrome. Am J Hum Genet 56:608–615.

99. Gutierrez MI, Bahatia KG, Barreiro C, Spangler G, Schvartzmann E, Sackmann F, Magrath M, Magrath IT. 1994. A de novo p53 germline mutation affecting codon 151 in a six year old child with multiple tumors. Hum Mol Genet 3:2247–2248.

100. Eeles R, Warren W, Knee G, Bartek J, Averill D, Stratton M, Blake P, Tait D, Lane D, Easton D, Yarnold J, Cooper C, Sloane J. 1993. Constitutional mutation in exon 7 of the p53 gene in a patient with multiple primary tumors: molecular and immunohistochemical findings. Oncogene 8:1269–1276.

101. Felix CA, Strauss EA, D'Amico D, et al. 1993. A novel germline p53 splicing mutation in a pediatric patient with a second malignant neoplasm. Oncogene 8:1203–1210.

102. Horio Y, Suzuki H, Uedo R, Koshikawa T, Sugiura T, Ariyoshi Y, Shimokata K, Takahashi T. 1994. Predominantly tumor-limited expression of a mutant allele in a Japanese family carrying a germline p53 mutation. Oncogene 9:1231–1235.

103. Diller L, Sexsmith E, Gottlieb A, Li F, Malkin D. 1995. Germline p53 mutations are frequently detected in young children with rhabdomyosarcoma. J Clin Invest 95:••.

104. McIntyre JF, Smith-Sorensen B, Friend SH, et al. 1994. Germline mutations of the p53 tumor suppressor gene in children with osteosarcoma. J Clin Oncol 12:925–930.

105. Wagner J, Portwine C, Rabin K, Jean-Marie L, Narod S, Malkin D. ••. High frequency of germline p53 mutations in childhood adrenocortical cancer. J Natl Cancer Inst 86:1707–1710.

106. Felix C, Nau M, Takahashi T, Mitsudomi T, Chiba I, Poplack D, Reaman G, Cole D, Letterio J, Whang-Peng J, Knutsen T, Minna J. 1992. Hereditary and acquired p53 gene mutations in childhood acute lymphoblastic leukemia. J Clin Invest 89:640–647.

107. Felix C, D-Amico D, Mitsudomi T. 1992. Absence of hereditary p53 mutations in 10 familial leukemia pedigrees. J Clin Invest 90:653–••.

108. Toguchida J, Yamaguchi T, Dayton S, et al. 1992. Prevalence and spectrum of germline mutations of the p53 gene among patients with sarcoma. N Engl J Med 326:1301–1308.

109. Sameshima Y, Tsunematsu Y, Watanabe S, Tsukamoto T, Kawa-ha K, Hirata Y, Mizoguchi H, Sugimura T, Terada M, Yokota J. 1992. Detection of novel germline p53 mutations in diverse cancer-prone families identified by selecting patients with childhood adrenocortical carcinoma. J Natl Cancer Inst 89:703–707.

110. Li FP, Garber JE, Friend SH, Strong LC, Patenaude AF, Juengst ET, Reilly PR, Correa P, Fraumeni JF. 1992. Recommendations on predictive testing for germ line p53 mutations among cancer-prone individuals. J Natl Cancer Inst 84:1156.

111. Huggins M, Bloch M, Kanani S, Quarrell O, Theilman J, Hedrick A, Dickens B, Lynch A, Hayden M. 1990. Ethical and legal dilemmas arising during predictive testing for adult-onset disease: the experience of Huntington disease. Am J Hum Genet 47:4–12.

112. Turner DR, Willoughby JO. 1990. Ethical issues in Huntington disease presymptomatic testing. Aust NZ J Med 20:545–547.

113. Wiggins S, Whyte P, Huggins M, Adam S, Theilmann J, Bloch M, Sheps S, Schechter M, Hayden M. 1992. The psychological consequences of predictive testing for Huntington's disease. N Eng J Med 327:1401–1405.

114. Berk T, Cohen Z, McLeod R, Cullen J. 1987. Surveillance in relatives of patients with adenomatous polyposis. Semin Surg Oncol 3:105–108.

115. Petersen GM, Slack J, Nakamura Y. 1991. Screening guidelines and premorbid diagnosis of familial adenomatous polyposis using linkage. Gastroenterology 100:1658–1664.

116. Bulow S. 1987. Incidence of associated diseases in familial polyposis coli. Semin Surg Oncol 3:84–87.

117. McAdam WAF, Goligher JC. 1970. The occurrence of desmoids in patients with familial polyposis coli. Br J Surg 57:618–631.

118. Smith W, Kern B. 1973. The nature of the mutation in familial multiple polyposis: papillary carcinoma of the thyroid, brain tumors and familial multiple polyposis. Dis Colon Rectum 16:264–271.

119. Jagelman DG. 1987. Extracolonic manifestations of familial polyposis coli. Cancer Genet Cytogenet 27:319–325.

120. Giardiello FM, OG, Lee DH, et al. 1993. Increased risk of thyroid and pancreatic carcinoma in familial adenomatous polyposis. Gut 34:1394–1396.

121. Plail R, Glazer G, Thompson J, Bussey H. 1995. Adenomatous polyposis: an association with carcinoma of the thyroid? Br J Surg (Suppl) 72:138.

122. Kingston J, Herbert A, Draper G, Mann J. 1983. Association between hepatoblastoma and polyposis coli. Arch Dis Children 58:959–962.

123. Garber J. ••. Hepatoblastoma and familial adenomatous polyposis. J Natl Cancer Inst 80:1626–1628.

124. Giardiello F. 1991. Risk of hepatoblastoma in familial adenomatous polyposis. J Pediatr 119:766–768.

125. Gardner E, Richards R. 1953. Multiple cutaneous and subcutaneous lesions occuring simultaneously with hereditary polyposis and osteomationsis. Am J Hum Genet 5:139–148.

126. Blair N, Trempe C. 1980. Hypertrophy of the retinal pigment eipithelium associated with Gardner's syndrome. Am J Opthalmol 90:661–667.

127. Lewis RA, Crowder WE, Eierman LA, Nussbaum RL, Ferrell RE. 1984. The Gardner syndrome: significance of ocular features. Opthalmology 91:916–925.

128. Herrera L, Kakati S, Gibas L, Pietrzak E, Sandbery A. 1986. Brief clinical report: Gardner Syndrome in a man with an interstitial deletion of 5q. Am J Med Genet 25:473–476.

129. Bodmer W, Bailey C, Bodmer J, et al. 1987. Localization of the gene for familial adenomatous polyposis on chromosome 5. Nature 328: 614–616.

130. Leppert M, Dobbs M, Scambler P, et al. 1987. The gene for familial polyposis coli maps to the long arm of chromosome 5. Science 238:1411–1413.

131. Khan PM, Tops CMJ, Broek MV, et al. 1988. Close linkage of a highly polymorphic marker (D5S37) to familial adenomatous polyposis (FAP) and confirmation of FAP localization on chromosome 5q21–q22. Hum Genet 79:183–185.

132. Spirio L, Nelson L, Jolyn G, Leppert M, White R. 1991. A CA Repeat 30–70 KB downstream from the adenomatous polyposis coli (APC) locus. Nucleic Acid Res 19:6348.

133. Kinzler KW, Nilbet MC, Su L-K, et al. 1991. Identification of FAP locus genes from chromosome 5q21. Science 253:661–664.

134. Joslyn G, Carlson M, Thliveris A, et al. 1991. Identification of deletion mutations and three new genes at the familial ploypopsis locus. Cell 66:601–613.

135. Nishisho I, Nakamura Y, Miyoshi Y, et al. 1991. Mutations of chromosome 5q21 genes in FAP and colorectal cancer patients. Science 253:665–669.

136. Miyoshi YAH, Nagase H, Nishisho I, et al. 1992. Germ-line mutations of the APC gene in 53 familial adenomatous polyposis patients. Proc Natl Acad Sci USA 89:4452–4456.

137. Cottrell S, Bickness D, Kaklamanis L, Bodmer WF. 1992. Molecular analysis of APC mutations in familial adenomatous polyposis and sporadic colon carcinomas. Lancet 340:626–630.
138. Varesco L, Gismondi V, James R, et al. 1993. Identification of APC gene mutations in Italian adenomatous polyposis coli patients by PCR-SSCP analysis. Am J Hum Genet 52:280–285.
139. Olschwang S, Laurent-Puig P, Groden J, White R, Thomas G. 1993. Germ-line mutations in the first 14 exons of the adenomatous polyposis colin (APC) gene. Am J Hum Genet 52:273–279.
140. Nagase HMY, Horii A, Aoki T, Ogawa M, Utsunomiya J, Baba S, Sasazuki T, Nakamura Y. 1992. Correlation between the location of germ-line mutations in the APC gene and the number of colorectal polyps in familial adenomatosis ployposis patients. Cancer Res 52:4055–4057.
141. Luijt RVD, Khan M, Vasen H, van Leeuwen CV, Tops C, Roest P, den Dunnen J, Fodde R. 1994. Rapid detection of translation-terminating mutations at the adenomatous polyposis coli (APC) gene by direct protein truncation test. Genomics 20:1–4.
142. Powell SM, Krush AJ, Booker S, Jen J, Giardiello FM, Hamilton SR, Vogelstein B, Kinzler KW. 1993. Molecular diagnosis of familial adenomatous polyposis. N Engl J Med 329:1982–1987.
143. Giardiello FM, Brensinger JD, Petersen GM, Luce MC, Hylind LM, Bacon JA, Booker SV, Parker RD, Hamilton SR. 1997. The use and interpretation of commercial APC gene testing for familial adenomatous polyposis. N Engl J Med 336:823–827.
144. Spirio L, Olschwang S, Groden J, et al. 1993. Alleles of the APC gene: an attenuated form of familial polyposis. Cell 75:951–957.
145. Olschwang S, Tiret A, Laurent-Puig P, Muleris M, Parc R, Thomas G. 1993. Restriction of ocular fundus lesions to a specific subgroup of APC mutations in adenomatous polyposis coli patients. Cell 75:959–968.
146. Turcot J, Despres J, St Pierre F. 1959. Malignant tumors of the central nervous system associated with familial polyposis of the colon: report of two cases. Dis Colon Rectum 2:465–468.
147. Mori T, Nagase H, Horii A, et al. 1994. Germ-line and somatic mutations of the APC gene in patients with Turcot syndrome and analysis of APC mutations in brain tumors. Genes Chromosomes Cancer 9:168–172.
148. Tomlinson G, Chao L, Stastny V, Ater J, Saunders G, Strong L. 1995. Involvement of the APC gene in medulloblastoma in two familial polyposis kindreds. Med Pediatr Oncol 25:255.
149. Hamilton SR, Liu B, Parsons R, et al. 1995. The molecular basis of Turcot's syndrome. N Engl J Med 332:839–847.
150. Sipple J. 1961. The association of pheochromocytoma with carcinoma of the thyroid gland. Am J Med 31:163–166.
151. Easton DF, Ponder MA, Cummings T, Gagel RF, Hansen HH, Reichlin S, Tashjian AH, Telenius-Berg M, Ponder B. 1989. The clinical and screening age-at-onset distribution for the MEN-2 syndrome. Am J Hum Genet 44:208–215.
152. Carney J, Sizemore G, Lovestedt S. 1976. Mucosal ganglioneuromatosis, medullary thyroid carcinoma, and pheochromocytoma: multiple endocrine neoplasia, type 2b. Oral Surg Oral Med Pathol 41:739–752.
153. Schimke R, Hartmann W, Prout T, Rimoin D. 1968. Syndrome of bilateral pheochromocytoma, medullary thyroid carcinoma and multiple neuromas: a possible regulatory defect in the differentiation of chromaffin tissue. N Engl J Med 279:1–7.
154. Brown RS, Colle E, Tashjian AH. 1975. The syndrome of multiple mucosal neuromas and medullary thyroid carcinoma in childhood: importance of recognition of the phenotype for the early detection of malignancy. J Pediatr 86:77–83.
155. Farndon JR, Leight GS, Dilley WG, Baylin SB, Smallridge RC, Wells SA. 1986. Familial medullary thyroid carcinoma without associated endocrinopathies: a distinct clinical entity. Br J Surg 73:278–281.

156. Samaan N, Draznin M, Halpin R, Bloss R, Hawkins E, Lewis R. 1991. Multiple endocrine syndrome type IIb in early childhood. Cancer 68:1832–1834.

157. Stjernholm MR, Freudenbourg JC, Mooney HS, Kinney FJ, Deftos LJ. 1980. Medullary carcinoma of the thyroid before age 2 years. J Clin Endocrinol Metab 51:252–253.

158. Telander RL, Zimmerman D, Sizemore GW, van Heerden JA, Grant CS. 1989. Medullary carcinoma in children. Arch Surg 124:841–843.

159. Lairmore TC, Howe JR, Korte JA, Dilley WG, Aine L, Aine E, Wells SA, Donis-Keller H. 1991. Familial medullary thyroid carcinoma and multiple endocrine neoplasia type 2B map to the same region of chromosome 10 as multiple endocrine neoplasia, type 2A. Genomics 9:181–192.

160. Norum RA, Lafreniere RG, O'Neal LW, et al. 1990. Linkage of the multiple endocrine neoplasia Type 2B gene (MEN2B) to chromosome 10 markers linked to MEN2A. Genomics 8:313–317.

161. Donis-Keller H, Dou S, Chi D, Carlson KM, Toshima K, Lairmore TC, Howe JR, Moley JF, Goodfellow P, Wells SA. 1993. Mutations in the RET proto-oncogene are associated with MEN 2A and FMTC. Hum Mol Genet 2:851–856.

162. Lips CJM, Landsvater RM, Hoppener JWM, et al. 1994. Clinical screening as compared with DNA analysis in families with multiple endocrine neoplasis type 2A. N Engl J Med 331:828–834.

163. Skinner MA, DeBenedetti MK, Moley JF, Norton JA, Wells SA. 1996. Medullary thyroid carcinoma in children with multiple endocrine neoplasia, type 2A and 2B. J Pediatr Sur 31:177–182.

164. Mulligan LM, Eng C, Healey CS, et al. 1994. Specific mutations of the RET proto-oncogene are related to disease phenotype in MEN 2A and FMTC. Nature Genet 6:70–74.

165. Carlson KM, Dou S, Chi D, Scavarda N, Toshima K, Jackson CE, Wells SA, Goodfellow PJ, Donis-Keller H. 1994. Single missense mutation in the tyrosine kinase catalytic domain of RET proto-oncogene is associated with multiple endocrine neoplasia, type 2B. Proc Natl Acad Sci USA 91:1579–1583.

166. Hofstra RMW, Landsvater RM, Ceccherini I, et al. 1994. A mutation in the RET proto-oncogene associated with multiple endocrine neoplasia type 2B and sporadic medullary thyroid carcinoma. Nature 367:375–376.

167. Melvin KEW, Miller HH, Tashjian AH. 1971. Early diagnosis of medullary carcinoma of the thyroid gland by means of calcitonin assay. N Engl J Med 285:1115–1120.

168. Graze K, Spiler IJ, Tashjian AH, et al. 1978. Natural history of familial medullary thyroid carcinoma. N Engl J Med 299:980–985.

169. Gagel RF, Tashjian AH, Cummings T, Papathanasopoulos N, Kaplan MM, DeLellis RA, Wolfe HJ, Reichlin S. 1988. The clinical outcome of prospective screening for multiple endocrine neoplasia type 2a: an 18-year experience. N Engl J Med 318:478–484.

170. NIH Consensus Development Conference. 1988. Neurofibromatosis: conference statement. Arch Neurol 45:575–578.

171. Sorensen SA, Mulvihill JJ, Nielsen A. 1986. Long-term follow-up of von Recklinghausen neurofibromatosis. N Engl J Med 314:1010–1015.

172. Matsui I, Tanimura M, Kobayashi N, Sawada T, Nagahara N, Akatsuka J-I. 1993. Neurofibromatosis type 1 and childhood cancer. Cancer 72:2746–2754.

173. Janss AJ, Grundy R, Cnaan A, et al. 1995. Optic pathway and hypothalamic/chiasmatic gliomas in children younger than age 5 years with a 6-year follow-up. Cancer 75:1051–1059.

174. Hartley AL, Birch JM, Kelsey AM, Harris M, Morris Jones PH. 1990. Sarcomas in three generations of a family with neurofibromatosis. Cancer Genet Cytogenet 45:245–248.

175. Shannon K, Watterson J, Johnson P, O'Connell P, Lange B, Shah N. 1992. Monosomy 7 myeloproliferative disease in children with neurofibromatosis, type 1: epidemiology and molecular analysis. Blood 79:1311–1318.

176. Heim RA, Kam-Morgan LNW, Binnie CG, Corns DD, Cayouette MC, Farber RA, Aylsworth AS, Silverman LM, Luce MC. 1995. Distribution of 13 truncating mutations in the neurofibromatosis 1 gene. Hum Mol Genet 4:975–981.

177. Shen MH, Harper PS, Upadhyaya M. 1996. Molecular genetic of neurofibromatosis type 1 (NF1). J Med Genet 33:2–17.
178. Hofman KJ, Boehm CD. 1992. Familial neurofibromatosis type 1: clinical experience with DNA testing. J Pediatr 120:394–398.
179. Evans DGR, Huson SM, Donnai D, Neary W, Blair V, Newton V, Strachan T, Harris R. 1992. A genetic study of type 2 neurofibromatosis in the United Kingdom. II. Guidelines for genetic counselling. J Med Genet 29:847–852.
180. MacCollin M, Ramesh V, Jacoby LB, et al. 1994. Mutational analysis of patients with neurofibromatosis 2. Am J Hum Genet 55:314–320.
181. Bourn D, Carter SA, Mason S, Evans DGR, Strachan T. 1994. Germline mutations in the neurofibromatosis type 2 tumour suppressor gene. Hum Mol Genet 3:813–816.
182. Gomez MR. 1979. Tuberous Sclerosis. New York: Raven Press.
183. Povey S, Burley MW, Attwood J, et al. 1994. Two loci for tuberous sclerosis: one on 9q34 and one on 16p13. Ann Hum Genet 58:107–127.
184. Marshall D, Saul GB, Sachs E. 1995. Tuberous sclerosis: a report of 16 cases in two family trees revealing genetic dominance. N Engl J Med 261:1102–1105.
185. Pascual-Castroviejo I, Patron M, Gutierrez M, Carceller F, Pascual-Pascual SI. 1995. Tuberous sclerosis associated with histologically confirmed ocular and cerebral tumors. Pediatr Neurol 13:172–174.
186. Boesel CP, Paulson GW, Kosnik EJ, Earle KM. 1979. Brain hamartomas and tumors associated with tuberous sclerosis. Neurosurgery 4:410–417.
187. Harding CO, Pagon RA. 1990. Incidence of tuberous sclerosis in patients with cardiac rhabdomyoma. Am J Med Genet 37:443–446.
188. Au KS, Murrell J, Buckler A, Blanton SH, Northrup H. 1996. Report of a critical recombination further narrowing the TSC1 region. J Med Genet 33:559–561.
189. Fryer AE, Chalmers AH, Osborne JP. 1990. The value of investigation for genetic counselling in tuberous sclerosis. J Med Genet 27:217–223.
190. Melmon KL, Rosen SW. 1964. Lindau's disease: review of the literature and study of a large kindred. Am J Med 36:595–617.
191. Maddock IR, Moran A, Maher ER, et al. 1996. A genetic register for von Hippel–Lindau disease. J Med Genet 33:120–127.
192. Seizinger BR, Rouleau GA, Ozelius LJ, et al. 1988. Von Hippel–Lindau disease maps to the region of chromosome 3 associated with renal cell carcinoma. ••.
193. Crossey PA, Richards FM, Foster K, et al. 1994. Identification of intragenic mutations in the von Hippel–Lindau disease tumour suppressor gene and correlation with disease phenotype. Hum Mol Genet 3:1303–1308.
194. Zbar B, Kishida T, Chen F, et al. 1996. Germline mutations in the von Hippel–Lindau Disease (VHL) gene in families from North America, Europe, and Japan. Hum Mutat 8:348–357.
195. Wertz D, Fanos J, Reilly R. 1994. Genetic testing for children and adolescents. JAMA 272:875–881.
196. American Society of Human Genetics Board of Directors and The American College of Medical Genetics Board of Directors. 1995. Points to consider: ethical, legal, and psychosocial implications of genetic testing in children and adolescents. Am J Hum Genet 57:1233–1241.
197. American Society of Clinical Oncology. 1996. Statement of the American Society of Clinical Oncology: genetic testing for cancer susceptibility. J Clin Oncol 14:1730–1736.
198. Patenaude AF, Basili L, Fairclough DL, Li FP. 1996. Attitudes of 47 mothers of pediatric oncology patients towards genetic testing for cancer predisposition. J Clin Oncol 14:415–421.
199. Schneider K, Patenaude A, Garber J. 1995. Testing for cancer genes; decisions, decisions. Nature Med 1:302–303.
200. American Society of Clinical Oncology, 1997. Resource document for curriculum development in cancer genetics education. J Clin Oncol. 15:2157–2169

II

Embryonal Tumors

4. Molecular basis of Wilms' tumor

Paul Grundy

1. Introduction

Wilms' tumor, the most common primary malignant renal tumor of childhood, has been a model for the multimodal treatment of pediatric malignant solid tumors. The generally favorable outcome for Wilms' tumor patients can be partly attributed to medical advances, including refinement in surgical technique, the sensitivity of Wilms' tumor to irradiation, and the availability of several active chemotherapeutic agents. The successful application of these treatment modalities to Wilms' tumor has been largely facilitated by the National Wilms Tumor Study Group (NWTSG) which has studied the majority of Wilms' tumor patients in North America on randomized clinical trials since 1969. In conjunction with these therapeutic trials, data on numerous clinical features and from central pathological review have been collected and analyzed. Such systematic study of a large proportion of the Wilms' tumor population has contributed not only to the clinical management of affected children but also to our understanding of the etiology and pathogenesis of Wilms' tumor.

Refinement of the prognostic classification of Wilms' tumor patients by features such as the histological pattern of the tumor, presence of lymph node metastases, and degree of local invasion has allowed the progressive individualization of therapy for subsets of patients. Thus, reductions in therapy for patients with favorable factors while preserving excellent outcome have been possible, while reserving more intensive therapies for patients at higher risk of relapse who, as a result, now have almost as good an eventual outcome. For example, patients with stage I favorable histology tumors can now be treated with only two drugs, namely, vincristine and dactinomycin, for 11 weeks without abdominal irradiation with an expected four-year relapse-free survival percentage of 89% [1]. In contrast, patients with more advanced-stage disease require chemotherapy with the addition of a third drug, doxorubicin, as well as abdominal irradiation with 1000 cGy — although when so treated, they have a similar four-year survival percentage of 90.9% [1]. Further progress in improving the cure rate or in decreasing therapy to minimize late effects, however, is now limited. With overall survival percentages in the 90% range, it becomes

D.O. Walterhouse and S.L. Cohn (eds), DIAGNOSTIC AND THERAPEUTIC ADVANCES IN PEDIATRIC ONCOLOGY. Copyright © 1997. Kluwer Academic Publishers, Boston. All rights reserved.

impractical to conduct randomized trials unless novel prognostic factors can be identified to further stratify patient groups.

Abundant progress has been made in understanding the molecular basis of Wilms' tumorigenesis since Knudson's proposal of the *two-hit* hypothesis in 1971 [2]. The study of children with specific congenital abnormalities, including aniridia, mental retardation, and abnormal genitourinary development ranging from hypospadias and undescended testes to pseudohermaphrodism, led to the localization and subsequent cloning of the first Wilms' tumor gene at chromosome 11p13 [3–5]. This gene, *WT1*, was found to encode a transcription factor that is critical to normal kidney and gonadal development. The study of another congenital Wilms' tumor predisposition sydrome, Beckwith–Wiedemann syndrome, uncovered evidence of genomic imprinting [6] and other unusual chromosomal inheritance patterns, implicating a second genetic locus, *WT2*, at chromosome 11p15. The existence of large pedigrees with familial transmission of susceptibility to Wilms' tumor implicates at least a third genetic locus. Histological analysis has strengthened the link between Wilms' tumor and normal kidney development, as illustrated by its association with nephrogenic rests, the foci of primitive renal cells [7], whose characteristics may vary with involvement of different Wilms' tumor-associated genetic loci.

Study of the molecular basis of Wilms' tumor in the last decade has thus contributed to our understanding of the pathogenesis of embryonal tumors, to the identification of previously unrecognized mechanisms of genetic aberration, and to the possible identification of novel prognostic factors necessary to make further progress in the clinical treatment of this disease.

This chapter will examine the genetic concepts and evidence for involvement of various loci, which have arisen from the molecular analyses of Wilms' tumors, and their implications for understanding the diverse clinical features associated with this tumor.

2. The two-event hypothesis

In 1971, Knudson proposed a model to explain the earlier age of onset and the bilateral presentation of eye tumors in children with a family history of retinoblastoma, compared with sporadic cases [8]. A similar model for Wilms' tumor was proposed a year later [2], although it should be noted that fewer familial and bilateral cases were available for analysis due to the lower incidence of familial Wilms' tumor and the poor disease survival at that time. The Knudson model predicted that tumor formation depends on two *rate-limiting* genetic events. Children with genetic susceptibility would have a constitutional lesion, either inherited from a parent or resulting from a de novo mutation. Thus, since all cells would harbor the first lesion, only one new genetic event would be needed for tumorigenesis, greatly increasing the likelihood of tumor formation. This model was postulated to explain the average younger age at diagnosis and the occurrence of multiple tumors compared with sporadic cases in which two rare, independent somatic mutations in the same cell would be required. Subsequent genetic studies of a number of tumors have confirmed the concept of the two-event hypothesis, demonstrating that the two postulated genetic events consist of inactivation of both alleles of a tumor-suppressor gene [9]. In many cases, the first allele is inactivated by a mutation within the gene itself. Although the second allele might incur a similar, although independent intragenic mutation, it is often inactivated by a loss of chromosomal material. This loss of chromosomal material may result from simple deletion, either of the whole or of part of the chromosome, or by somatic recombination.

Somatic recombination involving a chromosome harboring a mutant allele would result in one of the daughter cells containing two copies of the mutant allele. Although cytogenetic analysis can detect deletions, if large enough, somatic recombination cannot be detected, since two copies of the chromosome, not distinguishable by cytogenetic criteria, are present. Molecular genetic analysis, on the other hand, is capable of identifying loss of chromosomal material whether due to deletion or somatic recombination by detection of the phenomenon known as loss of heterozygosity (LOH). Thousands of polymorphic DNA segments, i.e., DNA segments that vary in sequence within the population, have been identified and mapped throughout the genome. If an individual is constitutionally heterozygous for a particular locus (usually assayed using DNA from peripheral blood lymphocytes), each member of the chromosome pair can be distinguished. If a tumor from such a heterozygous individual contains only one of the two patterns seen constitutionally, it is said to have undergone loss of heterozygosity. In turn, this finding implies that the tumor has lost chromosomal material, whether through deletion or recombination, involving the chromosomal region to which the polymorphic locus has been mapped. Further, if DNA from the individual's parents is available, it can be determined whether the allele lost from the tumor was derived from the mother or father. The detection of these chromosomal changes, whether by cytogenetic or molecular analyses, has inferred the existence and chromosomal localization of many tumor-associated genes.

3. Chromosome 11p13 and *WT1*

In 1964, Miller and coworkers reported an association between aniridia, a rare congenital abnormality of the iris, and Wilms' tumor [10]. Subsequently, a complex of developmental anomalies, including aniridia, genitourinary malformations, and mental retardation, was found to be associated with a high probability (>30%) of developing Wilms' tumor (the WAGR [*W*ilms' tumor with *a*niridia, *g*enitourinary malformations, and mental *r*etardation] syndrome) [11]. Constitutional karyotypes from children with the WAGR syndrome demonstrated variably sized deletions within the short arm of one copy of chromosome 11, which overlapped at band p13 [12]. This constitutional deletion was thought to represent the 'first' hit in these children and provided the initial clue to the location of a gene involved in the development of Wilms' tumor. It is now known that the WAGR deletion encompasses a number of contiguous genes, including the aniridia gene *PAX6* and Wilms' tumor suppressor gene *WT1*, so the WAGR syndrome constitutes a contiguous gene syndrome. Germline absence of one allele of the *PAX6* gene is responsible for aniridia [13], whereas germline deletion or mutation of one *WT1* allele results in the genitourinary defects [14,15], in addition to constituting the first event required for the development of Wilms' tumor [16]. The basis of the mental retardation remains unclear. Although mutation of *WT1* appears to be the initiating event in Wilms' tumors arising in the context of WAGR syndrome, the role of *WT1* is more limited in sporadic Wilms' tumor. In two large studies, mutations in the *WT1* gene were found in only 10% of 175 tumors analyzed [17,18]. Thus, in contrast with retinoblastoma, where inactivation of the *RB1* gene underlies the development of most, if not, all tumors, Wilms' tumor is clearly more heterogeneous at the genetic level. However, the close link between *WT1's* role in normal kidney development and its inactivation in Wilms' tumors provides a model for other Wilms' tumor suppressor genes that have not yet been isolated.

3.1. WT1 *structure and function*

The 10 exons of the *WT1* gene encode four different messenger RNAs resulting from a complex pattern of alternative splicing [19]. *WT1* protein is 45 to 49 kDa in size and contains functional domains indicating that it is a transcription factor, a protein that regulates the expression of other genes. Specifically, the carboxy terminus of *WT1* contains four *zinc finger* domains that confer the ability to bind DNA in a sequence-specific manner. The amino terminus contributes a functional domain that appears responsible for the regulation of transcription of potential target genes.

The identity of the genes targeted by *WT1* during normal kidney development is unknown, but through in vitro reconstitution experiments, several DNA sequences that bind *WT1* have been identified. *WT1* appears to bind promoters with guanine-cytosine (GC)-rich DNA sequences, as does a family of genes that are induced shortly after cellular exposure to a mitogen. In general, these growth-promoting genes tend to promote transcription upon binding to the so-called EGR1 (for *early growth response*) consensus sequences, while *WT1* tends to suppress transcription [20]. A number of growth-inducing genes such as insulin-like growth factor II (*IGF2*) and platelet-derived growth factor A chain (*PDGFA*) contain this DNA consensus sequence and hence have been postulated to be potential targets of *WT1* [20]. However, *WT1* also binds to other DNA sequences within the *PDGFA* promoter and can function either as a suppressor or activator of transcription, depending on the target promoter [21,22].

WT1 was recently found to form a physical complex with the p53 protein [23]. This association appears to depend on the integrity of both the WT1 and p53 proteins and has implications for the function of both genes. In the absence of functional p53 protein, WT1 appears to acquire potent transcriptional activating activity [23]. WT1, on the other hand, appears to exert a cooperative effect on p53, enhancing its transcriptional activating ability. The functional significance of this interaction and its role in tumorigenesis remains to be defined.

The roles of the four different mRNA transcripts also remain unclear. The relative levels of expression of the different transcripts appears to be the same in different tissues and at different stages of development. The most abundant transcript contains a small insertion that results in three additional amino acids inserted between zinc fingers 3 and 4 [19] and that prevents the protein from binding to the originally defined *EGR1*-like consensus sequence [24]. It is not known whether this isoform of the WT1 protein, which cannot regulate transcription due to its lack of DNA binding activity, has other functions.

The normal function of *WT1* and its in vivo target genes remains a very complex area of investigation, given the existence of multiple transcripts with differing DNA-binding specificity, the inherent ability to activate or suppress transcription, and the interactions with other transcription factors. Whether the ability to suppress the expression of growth-associated genes such as *IGF2* or *PDGFA* contributes to the function of *WT1* as a tumor suppressor gene also remains to be conclusively proven. The lack of good Wilms' tumor cell lines, in which one would to be able to manipulate some of these factors, has hindered the ability to obtain clear answers to some of these questions.

3.2. WT1 *expression patterns*

Unlike other tumor suppressor genes such as *RB1* or *p53*, which are expressed in all tissues, *WT1* is expressed only in specific types of cells [3,14,25]. As might be expected, the genetic consequences of *WT1* inactivation appear to be restricted to organs that normally express the gene. The pattern of normal *WT1* expression has provided important clues to the function of *WT1* during differentiation. In the kidney, *WT1* is expressed only in condensing blastemal cells, renal vesicles, and glomerular epithelium [25], all thought to be the sites of origin of Wilms' tumor. Normal expression of *WT1* may be necessary for the differentiation of renal blastemal cells to mature epithelial components, and its disruption may result in cells with the inappropriate potential for further proliferation either as nephrogenic rests or tumors. Classical triphasic Wilms' tumors contain variable histological components, including blastemal, epithelial and stromal cell types. Two studies have demonstrated an association between stromal predominance and reduced *WT1* expression. It remains a matter of debate whether the reduced *WT1* expression results in stromal differentiation or whether the reduced *WT1* expression simply reflects the fact that stromal cells do not normally express *WT1* [14,26].

Renal *WT1* expression peaks around the time of birth and then rapidly declines as the organ matures [25,27]. In contrast to its transient expression in the developing kidney, *WT1* is expressed continuously in mesothelial cells, Sertoli cells of the testis, and granulosa cells of the ovary [28]. *WT1* mutations have been found occasionally in gonadoblastomas and mesothelial tumors [29,30] but not in the common tumors derived from testes or ovaries [31]. Nevertheless, the critical developmental role of *WT1* is evident in the severe genitourinary and mesothelial abnormalities of mice whose *WT1* alleles have been deleted [32].

3.3. WT1 *mutations*

Prior to the cloning of *WT1*, it was expected that the gene would represent a so-called tumor suppressor gene, since it was loss of the gene that appeared to be critical, as exemplified by the constitutional deletions in WAGR patients and by loss of heterozygosity in Wilms' tumors. Many of the mutations identified to date have involved large deletions of part or all of the *WT1* gene. Smaller mutations such as small deletions or insertions also tend to result in premature truncation of the RNA transcript and therefore a predicted non-functional protein [33]. Although a large number of localized mutations have not yet been characterized, there is a potential mutational hot spot involving repetitive CCTG sequences in exon 1 [33].

Very few examples of *WT1* mutation transmitted from one generation to the next have been identified. This may possibly be attributed to the genitourinary and other anomalies affecting such individuals. The few examples documented do illustrate, however, that there is not a strict genotype–phenotype correlation. For example, in one case in which both a father and child had a one-base-pair mutation in exon 6, the father had Wilms' tumor but no congenital anomalies whereas the child had hypospadias and cryptorchidism in addition to bilateral Wilms' tumor [15].

3.4. Denys–Drash syndrome

In addition to inactivating deletions, specific alterations may convert a tumor suppressor gene into a dominant negative oncogene [34]. Proteins altered in this way may disrupt the function of normal gene products (including that of the remaining normal allele) through the formation of protein complexes or through abnormal interactions with DNA targets. Thus, loss of normal function of both alleles may result from a dysfunctional mutation in only one allele (a dominant effect).

The existence of dominant negative mutations of *WT1* is supported by the observation of specific constitutional mutations of *WT1* in children with the Denys–Drash syndrome [29,35], a congenital syndrome with predisposition to Wilms' tumor consisting of intersex disorders and mesangial sclerosis [36]. The phenotypic effects of constitutional *WT1* mutations found in Denys–Drash syndrome are far more severe than those resulting from complete deletion of *WT1*, seen in patients with WAGR syndrome. This finding suggests that the altered *WT1* protein in patients with the Denys–Drash syndrome is dysfunctional rather than nonfunctional. Potential dominant negative *WT1* mutations are also seen in sporadic Wilms' tumor specimens containing only one mutated *WT1* allele [37–39]. In contrast with the previously described inactivating mutations, which generally result in loss of WT1 protein, the mutations in Denys–Drash syndrome patients are single-base-pair mutations with a mutational hot spot in exon 9 [35]. Exon 9 encodes the third zinc finger, and most such mutations are predicted to alter the specificity of the target DNA sequence. Although a striking genotype–phenotype correlation therefore exists for Denys–Drash syndrome, the correlation is not absolute, as exemplified by the report of a normal father and child with Denys–Drash syndrome who both had identical constitutional exon 9 mutations [40]. Even more so than for *WT1* deletions, Denys–Drash mutations would not be expected to be frequently transmitted because of the severe genitourinary defects in affected individuals.

With the characteristics discussed above, *WT1* clearly fulfills the criteria one would expect for a tumor suppressor gene. The unexpectedly low frequency of *WT1* mutations, however, suggests that other genetic alterations account for the majority of cases. Such alterations might include additional tumor-associated loci as discussed below. On the other hand, given the complex pattern of *WT1* transcription, DNA binding specificity, and transcriptional regulating capacity, it remains possible that *WT1* may be involved in more cases than is immediately obvious or that a further Wilms' tumor suppressor locus may reside in the 11p13 region.

4. Chromosome 11p15 and *WT2*

The existence of a putative second Wilms' tumor locus was first appreciated due to the fact that a subset of Wilms' tumors undergo loss of heterozygosity restricted to markers located at chromosome 11p15, not affecting the neighboring 11p13 loci including *WT1* [41–44]. Although this second putative gene has not been isolated, it has been designated *WT2*. The chromosome 11p15 region is also associated with a congenital syndrome, Beckwith–Wiedemann syndrome (BWS). BWS is characterized by overgrowth, ranging from gigantism to regional hypertrophy (hemihypertrophy) and/or visceromegaly and macroglossia. It is also characterized by hyperinsulinemic hypoglycemia and a predisposition to embryonal tumor formation in about 5%–15% patients, predominantly Wilms' tumor [45,46]. BWS is usually sporadic, but 15% of cases are familial, and genetic analysis has demonstrated linkage to 11p15.5 markers [42,47]. Whether one genetic locus is responsible for both BWS and Wilms' tumor or adjacent loci are involved as in the contiguous gene syndrome WAGR is not known.

A striking feature of the 11p15 Wilms' tumor locus is the apparent distinction between the maternal and paternal alleles. The 11p15 allele lost in Wilms' tumors is invariably that derived from the mother [41,48], a result not predicted by a model involving somatic inactivation of both alleles of an auto-

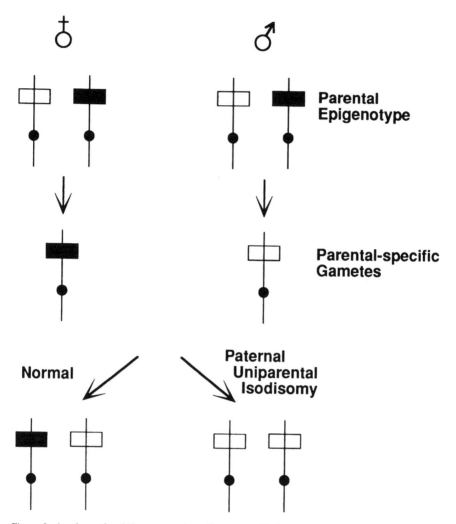

Figure 1. A schematic of the segregation of a maternally imprinted locus such as *IGF2*. Both parents carry two alleles of the *IGF2* locus, with one imprinted allele (darkened symbol). The gametes produced are different, however — dependent on the sex of the transmitting parent. The mother produces only gametes with an imprint at the *IGF2* locus, while the father produces only gametes without the imprint. Normally, offspring would have the same epigenotype as their parents, with one imprinted allele. In the case of uniparental paternal isodisomy, however, since the child has inherited both *IGF2* alleles from the father, neither is imprinted and hence both are active.

somal locus, in which no bias would be expected. In addition, karyotype analysis of BWS children revealed that some had a constitutional duplication of chromosome 11p15, always paternal [49]. In some BWS cases with grossly normal karyotypes, both copies of chromosome 11 are identical and in fact represent two copies of the same chromosome inherited from the father and none from the mother, a condition termed *uniparental isodisomy* [50,51] (figure 1). Taken together, these findings have suggested that the BWS/*WT2* gene represents an imprinted locus. In general terms, the term *imprint* implies a functional difference between the two alleles of a locus that is dependent on the parent of origin. The imprint is not based on the DNA sequence but on a reversible modification that must take place during gametogenesis. Thus, if the BWS/*WT2* gene is normally expressed solely from the paternal allele, the inheritance of two copies of the paternal BWS gene in the form of either trisomy or paternal isodisomy would be expected to double the level of expression. It is noteworthy, then, that the loss of heterozygosity that occurs in some Wilms' tumors is usually the result of somatic recombination, as opposed to deletion, resulting in two copies of paternal 11p15. Thus the tumor is rendered isodisomic for paternal 11p15, similarly to the constitutional genotype of some BWS patients (figure 1).

Uniparental disomy for chromosome 11p15 has been shown to be an uncommon occurrence in Wilms' tumor patients without concomitant manifestations of BWS [52]. However, one instance of a Wilms' tumor patient with isolated hemihypertrophy and uniparental isodisomy for chromosome 11 has been reported [50]. Additionally, several Wilms' tumor patients have been described with mosaicism for uniparental isodisomy [53]. These finding would infer that although alteration of 11p15 loci may be necessary for tumorigenesis, such alterations cannot be the penultimate tumorigenic event since these children had normal kidney tissue in addition to the Wilms' tumor.

4.1. Candidate 11p15 loci

Several genes that map to chromosome 11p15 have been evaluated as candidate loci for either *WT2* or BWS or both. The study of these genes has advanced our understanding of imprinting as a genetic phenomena, but to date, proof of their involvement in Wilms' tumor pathogenesis remains to be found.

The insulin-like growth factor II (IGF2) gene encodes an embryonal growth factor that is highly expressed in fetal kidney and Wilms' tumors [54]. *IGF2* is the first gene shown to be imprinted in humans, with expression only of the paternally derived allele [55–57]. This pattern of imprinting is found in the kidney but is both developmentally regulated and tissue specific [58,59]. Since *IGF2* induces cell growth, an increased dosage of this imprinted gene could conceivably contribute to both BWS and Wilms' tumorigenesis. If this were the case, tumor-specific loss of heterozygosity for 11p15 may represent duplication of the active *IGE2* allele rather than loss of a tumor suppressor allele.

Among Wilms' tumors that have not lost heterozygosity at 11p15, some demonstrate loss or relaxation of the imprint at the *IGF2* locus so that both alleles are expressed, resulting in increased expression [55,56]. Likewise, a constitutional loss of the imprint has been associated with some cases of BWS [60]. Analysis of *IGF2* expression by Northern blot has confirmed that both tumors with loss of heterozygosity or loss of the imprint have an average twofold increase in mRNA levels relative to tumors with no such alteration, but the increase in individual tumors ranges from minimal to very large [61], leaving the functional consequences of the altered levels open to speculation. Although one might have hypothesized that BWS patients with regional overgrowth might be somatically mosaic for loss of the imprint, with the abnormality restricted to the hypertrophied tissue, this has been shown not to be the case [60,62].

Although *IGF2* might be the BWS gene and contribute to predisposition to Wilms' tumor, there is also evidence to support an adjacent tumor suppressor locus. Another 11p15 gene, *H19*, is adjacent to *IGF2* and imprinted in a reciprocal manner with expression restricted to the maternal allele [63]. The *H19* gene is transcribed into mRNA, but it has no open reading frame, suggesting that it functions as regulatory RNA molecule [64]. Transfection of an H19 expression construct into Wilms' and rhabdomyosarcoma cell lines suppressed both growth and tumorigenicity, suggesting that loss of this imprinted gene may also contribute to Wilms' tumorigenesis [65]. Since *H19* is only transcribed from the maternal allele, loss of DNA heterozygosity would be expected to result in complete loss of expression as a result of this single genetic event, and indeed this has been shown to be the case [61,66].

Most Wilms' tumors, however, do not show evidence of loss of heterozygosity. It is striking then, that Wilms' tumors that have lost the imprint at the *IGE2* locus and that have increased expression of *IGF2* have a complete loss of *H19* expression [61,66].

The mechanism underlying imprinting is unknown. However, DNA methylation may play a role in the regulation of imprinted genes (for reviews, see [6,67]). The *H19* locus has been shown to be differentially methylated on the maternal versus paternal allele. It is intriguing to note that concomitantly with the loss of *H19* expression, a switch of the *H19* promoter methylation pattern from the maternal (active) to paternal (inactive) pattern occurs [61,66]. Thus, three different genetic aberrations — constitutional paternal isodisomy, LOH involving the maternal allele, and loss of the maternal imprint — all result in two copies of the paternally imprinted chromosome 11p15 (figure 2).

It is speculated that *IGF2* and *H19* may be only two examples of imprinted loci within this region. An additional example, p57^{KIP2} mapping 500 kb centromeric to *IGF2*, has recently been studied [68]. This locus also shows evidence for imprinting, with preferential maternal expression in normal tissues. In this case the imprint is not absolute in that slight paternal expression is also observed in most tissues. In 2 of 10 informative Wilms' tumors, however, equal expression from both alleles was observed, implicating the possible

110

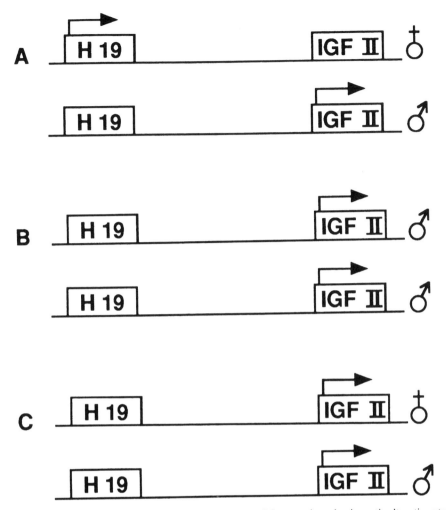

Figure 2. A schematic of the functional consequences of the genetic and epigenetic alterations to chromosome 11p15 known to occur in Wilms' tumors. (**A**) Normally, only the maternal copy of *H19* and the paternal copy of *IGF2* are transcriptionally active. (**B**) In the case of uniparental paternal isodisomy, the child has inherited two identical copies of 11p15, both with the paternal pattern of the imprint. (**C**) In tumors with loss of the imprint at *IGF2*, and a switch to the maternal imprint at *H19*, the functional consequences to transcription are the same as for uniparental isodisomy.

involvement of this cyclin-dependent kinase inhibitor in the genesis of some tumors.

Finally, it has been shown that transfection of a subchromosomal fragment of 11p15, not including *IGFII* or *H19*, into a rhabdomyosarcoma cell line resulted in growth suppression [69]. This suggests that an additional tumor-suppressor locus may also be located at 11p15. In fact, the high proportion of tumors exhibiting either loss of heterozygosity or loss of imprint, as opposed to more localized deletions, may imply that the tumor-suppressor activity at 11p15 can not be ascribed to a single locus but may involve multiple loci. The same phenomena could apply to Beckwith Wiedemann Syndrome and could conceivably account for the variability in phenotype. If this is the case, it will make assignment of relative importance of the different loci much more difficult.

In summary, there is strong evidence that alterations at one or more imprinted loci on chromosome 11p15.5 underlie the development of BWS and predisposition to the development of Wilms tumor. Whether the syndrome and the tumor result from alterations of the same gene/s or whether multiple loci are affected by a single genetic mechanism remains uncertain. It is possible in some cases that the epigenetic changes are secondary to a primary genetic event affecting the locus responsible for regulating the imprint, a locus which could be on chromosome 11 or elsewhere.

5. Familial Wilms' tumor

Familial Wilms' tumor is rare, composing only 1.5% of all Wilms' tumors [70]. Curiously, only half the familial cases registered with the National Wilms' Tumor Study have had affected siblings, parents, or children, while the remainder have involved more distant relatives including aunts, uncles, nieces, nephews, cousins, or more distant relatives [70]. Three families with an inherited susceptibility to Wilms' tumor, large enough to allow genetic linkage analysis, have been reported. These families appear to manifest an autosomal-dominant mode of inheritance but with incomplete penetrance. Linkage analyses of these families have excluded both the chromosome 11p13 and 11p15 regions and chromosome 16q as the genomic locations of the genes responsible for inherited predisposition [71–73]. These findings have therefore inferred the existence of at least a third Wilms' tumor gene responsible for conferring familial predisposition to Wilms' tumor.

Linkage analysis of a large Canadian family with seven known cases of Wilms' tumor has recently been reported [74]. No congenital anomalies or other cancers were observed in the pedigree. Significant evidence for linkage was obtained for an interval mapping to chromosome 17q12–q21, an interval bounded by D17S933 and D17S787. Tumor-specific loss of heterozygosity at these loci was not seen by these authors in a series of 13 sporadic Wilms' tumors and was seen in only one of 22 tumors in another series [75]. It is not yet known whether this chromosome 17q locus, *FWT1*, is involved in other Wilms' tumor families or whether this locus is involved in sporadic tumors.

Wilms' tumor also occurs with increased frequency in the sometimes familial Simpson–Golabi–Behmel syndrome (SGBS) [76]. This overgrowth syndrome has many phenotypic similarities with Beckwith–Wiedemann syndrome, although SGBS may also include congenital heart defects, cryptorchidism, vertebral and rib anomalies, and postaxial hexadactyly [77]. Familial SGBS is an X-linked condition that has been mapped to Xq25–q27 [78]. Through the study of two female SGBS patients with chromosome X autosome translocations, the responsible gene, GPC3, was recently cloned [79]. GPC3 encodes an extracellular proteoglycan, glypican 3, that may play an important role in the growth and differentiation of mesodermal tissues.

It had been previously hypothesized by some that a locus controlling parental allele-specific imprinting might be expected to reside on the X chromosome. Although the SGBS locus might have been a candidate for this imprintor gene, the apparent biochemical function of glypican 3 does not seem to support such a role. Intriguingly, however, glypican 3 may form a complex with IGF2, thereby modulating its action [79]. This might then explain the phenotypic similarities between SGBS and BWS.

Wilms' tumor has also been occasionally reported in association with a number of other familial disorders, including Perlman syndrome, another overgrowth syndrome [80]; the Li–Fraumeni syndrome, a subset of which is attributable to mutations in the p53 gene at chromosome 17p13 [81]; neurofibromatosis type 1, which is attributable to mutations in the NF1 gene at 17q11 [82]; the hereditary hyperparathyroid jaw tumor syndrome, mapping to chromosome 1q21–q31 [83]; and the breast–ovarian cancer syndrome caused by mutations in *BRCA1* at chromosome 17q21 in many families [84]. These varied clinical associations would suggest that alterations to numerous loci may confer predisposition to Wilms' tumor in selected cases. How often mutations at these specific loci may be involved in the greater proportion of familial tumors, and how often these loci might be involved somatically in sporadic tumors, remains to be defined.

Familial Wilms' tumors have also recently been analyzed by comparative genomic hybridization on the assumption that detection of somatic amplification or deletion might point to the location of the inherited defect. Briefly, this technique involves hybridizing flurochrome-labeled tumor DNA to normal DNA that has been labeled with a different flurochrome and then hybridizing the mixture to a normal metaphase spread. Regions of the chromosomes represented equally in the tumor and normal DNA appear as one color, while sequences overrepresented or underrepresented in the tumor show up as different colors. Using this methodology, analysis of eight tumors from patients with a documented family history revealed deletion of 4q21–ter in 4 of the 8 cases, including tumors from two siblings. Chromosome 9p21–ter was deleted in a similar proportion, while 3 of the 8 cases had lost the short arm of chromosome 20 [85]. Studies such as these may provide important clues to help focus linkage analyses.

6. Other potential Wilms' tumor loci

Two published studies have attempted to identify additional Wilms' tumor loci by screening other chromosomal arms for loss of heterozygosity [75,86]. From these and other ongoing studies, there is evidence that several additional chromosomal arms may harbor tumor suppressor genes involved in Wilms' tumorigenesis.

6.1. Chromosome 16q

Approximately 20% of Wilms' tumors have undergone allelic loss for the long arm of chromosome 16, suggesting that this is the location of Wilms' tumor-associated gene [75,87]. Although the proportion of cases with LOH at this site is small, this rate of loss is significantly greater than the 'background' rates for other chromosomes (see [75] and unpublished data). The smallest region of deletion common to all tumors maps between the HP locus at 16q22 and the CTRB locus at 16q23 [87]. Loss of each parentally derived allele appears to occur equally frequently, in contrast to the bias to loss of the maternal copy of chromosome 11p, so there is no evidence to suggest that this putative Wilms' tumor gene is subject to imprinting [75].

There are also differences in the pattern of allele loss when 11p and 16q probes are hybridized to Southern blots of Wilms' tumors. Loss of heterozygosity detected by chromosome 11p probes usually results in complete loss of one band, whereas with chromosome 16q probes, we have often observed a significant reduction but not complete loss of one band (P. Grundy, unpublished data). This finding has been consistent even in tumors with loss at both chromosomal regions, excluding the possibility of contamination of the tumor by normal kidney tissue. This finding would suggest, then, that loss of the 16q locus takes place within an already established tumor and more likely reflects an event related to tumor progression rather than an etiologic event. Consistent with this hypothesis, the 16q locus has been excluded as the familial Wilms' tumor locus [88].

Also consistent with a role as a tumor progression event, tumor-specific loss of 16q appears to be an adverse prognostic factor. In an analysis of 232 Wilms' tumor patients registered on the National Wilms' Tumor Study, including those with tumors of all stages and both favorable and anaplastic histology, tumor-specific loss of 16q was associated with a statistically significantly poorer two-year relapse-free survival and overall survival [87]. Allelic loss at 16q occurred at equivalent frequency in tumors of each stage, and in tumors of favorable or anaplastic histology, indicating that this event was independent of these previously known clinical prognostic factors. One of the main objectives of the 5th National Wilms' Tumor Study is to confirm the prognostic significance of 16q loss and to ascertain the potential clinical significance within each tumor stage.

Tumor-specific 16q deletions have also been noted in hepatocellular carcinoma [89], breast carcinoma [90], and prostate cancer [91], among others. It remains possible that this putative Wilms' tumor locus may also be involved in determining the malignant phenotype of other more common tumors.

6.2. Chromosome 1p

Loss of heterozygosity also occurs at chromosome 1p in approximately 11% of Wilms' tumors [87]. Almost all cases with loss of markers mapping to the most telomeric band, 1p36.3, reveal loss at markers mapping to 1p32, suggesting that the deletion is very large, spanning half of 1p (P. Grundy, unpublished data). Analysis of 50 tumors at multiple 1p loci revealed only two cases with an interstitial deletion, with the minimal region of deletion flanked by locus D1S8 at 1p32 and locus D1Z2 at 1p36.3. Again, as for chromosome 16q, analysis of the parental origin of the child's alleles revealed that loss of each parental allele occurs approximately equally (P. Grundy, unpublished data).

With reference to the 232 patients referred to above, there was no apparent association between loss of chromosome 1p and either stage or histological classification. Analysis of outcome with cases classified by loss of 1p revealed a threefold increase in relapse and mortality rates for cases with loss of 1p, but these results did not quite reach statistical significance [87]. Because the low incidence of both the marker frequency and adverse outcome may have limited the statistical power of this study, the fifth National Wilms' Tumor Study will also determine whether loss of 1p is an independent adverse prognostic factor.

Loss of 1p also occurs in other tumors, most notably in another pediatric tumor, neuroblastoma, in which it has also been associated with worse outcome [92,93]. The consensus region of deletion in neuroblastoma, at 1p36, lies well within the much larger consensus region of deletion in Wilms' tumor [94]. A more proximal second region of deletion has been postulated in neuroblastoma, at 1p32, which may be involved in a separate subset of neuroblastoma tumors [94]. Too few Wilms' tumor deletions have been characterized to determine whether more than one Wilms' tumor suppressor locus might reside on 1p, although the deletion in most Wilms' tumors encompasses both of the putative neuroblastoma loci. Loss of 1p is also frequently observed in many tumor types (reviewed in [94]), but it is premature to speculate whether the putative Wilms' 1p locus might be involved in such a spectrum of tumors.

6.3. Chromosome 7p

Cytogenetic analyses of both the constitutional karyotypes of Wilms' tumor patients and of Wilms' tumors have identified recurrent deletions and translocations involving chromosome 7p (reviewed in [95]). One case of a Wilms' tumor patient with a constitutional balanced translocation between chromosomes 1 and 7, t(1;7)(q42;p15), has been described in which the child's tumor had loss of the remaining short arm of chromosome 7. Four additional independent Wilms' tumor-specific deletions have been described with a consensus region of deletion of 7p15–p11 [96,97]. Our laboratory has also observed chromosome 7p loss of heterozygosity in 5 of 35 tumors (P. Grundy, unpublished data). The combination of constitutional alterations to 7p15 in Wilms' tumor patients and somatic LOH at a rate apparently above background would suggest that chromosome 7p may harbor yet another gene associated with the development of Wilms' tumor. It is not yet known whether tumor-specific 7p LOH is associated with any particular subset of Wilms' tumors nor whether it could be the site of a putative familial locus.

6.4. p53

Mutations of the p53 tumor suppressor gene, located at chromosome 17p13, have been identified as the most frequent specific alteration in human cancer. They occur in a variety of adult-onset tumors but have been infrequently identified in childhood cancers. p53 mutation analysis has been reported for one large series of Wilms' tumors, and only five tumors (4%) were found to harbor a mutant p53 allele [98]. However, all the p53 mutations occurred in tumors with anaplastic histology, either focal or diffuse, while none were found in the 92 tumors known to be of favorable histology. The apparent association between p53 mutation and anaplastic histology suggests that p53 mutation may be the primary alteration underlying the development of this histologic variant of Wilms' tumor, which is associated with a poor prognosis. However, a p53 mutation has also been identified in a Wilms' tumor with favorable histologic features [99], the most common histopathological phenotype. The association of p53 mutation with the anaplastic histology is strengthened, though, by the finding that in tumors where both anaplastic and non-anaplastic cells can be identified, the p53 mutation is generally confined to the anaplastic cells [100]. The anaplastic cells appeared to have a decreased rate of apoptosis, suggesting a p53-mediated mechanism for a selective growth advantage that might account for the poor outcome of such cases [100]. As mentioned previously, there is also evidence to suggest that p53 and WT1 may interact [23], although the functional significance of this interaction and its role in Wilms' tumorigenesis remains to be defined.

It also remains to be determined whether the presence of a p53 mutation in a tumor histologically classified as favorable might confer a worse prognosis despite the absence of classical features of anaplasia.

7. Nephrogenic rests

The presence of Wilms' tumor within a kidney is often associated with renal developmental abnormalities. The most common of these, nephrogenic rests, are small foci of persistent primitive blastemal cells that are occasionally found in neonatal kidneys [7]. The kidneys of virtually all children with inherited susceptibility to Wilms' tumor contain nephrogenic rests, suggesting that these are markers for a constitutional or early somatic defect in kidney development. However, 25% to 40% of children with sporadic Wilms' tumor also have nephrogenic rests within otherwise normal kidney tissue [7]. In two such children, from whom DNA was extracted from both the microdissected rests and the tumor, the same somatic mutation of *WT1* was present in both tissues, indicating a common cell of origin for both lesions [101]. Thus, nephrogenic rests may represent clonal precursor lesions, which are at least one step along the pathway to tumor formation. The natural history of these reste is variable: some regress spontaneously, whereas other degenerate into Wilms' tumor [102].

The association between nephrogenic rests and the genetic loci implicated in Wilms' tumor may also be reflected in the anatomical location of the premalignant lesions [102]. Nephrogenic rests developing at the periphery of the renal lobe (perilobar nephrogenic rests) are usually found in children with the Beckman–Wiedemann syndrome, which is linked to the 11p15 Wilms' tumor locus. In contrast, intralobar nephrogenic rests, which may arise anywhere within the renal lobe (as well as in the renal sinus and the wall of the pelvicaliceal system), are typically found in children with aniridia or other features associated with the *WT1* locus at 11p13. These observations suggest that the different Wilms' tumor genes may be involved in distinct developmental pathways within the kidney and that their inactivation may interrupt normal kidney development at specific times.

8. Conclusions

The past few years have provided breakthroughs in understanding some of the genetic factors involved in Wilms' tumor and their relation to normal kidney development as well as uncovering novel mechanisms of tumorigenesis. Preventing the delineation of a clear model of etiology, however, is the overwhelming evidence for genetic heterogeneity among Wilms' tumors and the increasing evidence for involvement of numerous loci. Although clearly not all the putative loci herein described are involved in each case of Wilms' tumor, it is currently difficult to predict how many and what combinations of loci might be involved in each individual case. Given the frequency of loss of heterozygosity for chromosome 11p and the apparent frequency of altered imprinting in the remaining proportion of cases, it would seem likely that a locus or loci on 11p are involved in the early development of most tumors. At the same time, given the fact that patients with constitutional uniparental paternal isodisomy for chromosome 11p or with a constitutional alteration of the 11p15 imprint have normal kidney in addition to their Wilms' tumor; and given the evidence that some nephrogenic rests already harbor homozygous inactivation of the *WT1* locus, the inference is that chromosome 11p15 alterations may only be an early and predisposing event in the Wilms' tumorigenesis pathway. It may be that most or at least many tumors require alterations of one or more additional loci and that the involvement of these additional loci is associated with specific characteristics of the tumor that have not yet been defined.

Clinical use of some of these findings can already be entertained. For example, the identification of *WT1* allows more precise genetic counseling for the subset of children with aniridia or other WAGR syndrome-associated anomalies and may be used for their clinical management. Children who present with sporadic aniridia have a greatly increased risk of Wilms' tumor, and frequent renal ultrasound examinations have usually been recommended for them. Molecular analysis of germline DNA in such children should distinguish those with a mutation restricted to the *PAX6* gene, who have no increased risk for Wilms' tumor, from those with a chromosomal deletion encompassing the neighboring *WT1* gene. Similarly, identification of the Wilms' tumor gene at chromosome 11p15 and its relation with the Beckwith–Wiedemann syndrome gene will hopefully allow genetic counseling and appropriate screening for children with hemihypertrophy, whose increased risk of embryonal tumors is now poorly defined.

The clinical care of children with Wilms' tumor may also improve with a better understanding of underlying genetic factors. The efforts of the National Wilms' Tumor Study have been aimed at intensifying treatment for patients with the poor clinical prognostic features, high tumor stage, or anaplastic histology, while reducing interventions for those without such risk factors. As a result, over 80% of patients with Wilms' tumor can be cured with modern multimodality therapy, some with minimal chemotherapy and without radiation therapy. To continue this process so as to maximize the number of children cured of their disease, while attempting to reduce the number of children exposed to anthracyclines or radiation, will require the identification of additional prognostic markers. It is likely that further dissection of the molecular pathogenesis of the disease will yield such factors. Of course, the ultimate goal is to understand the biochemical abnormalities that occur as a result of the genetic alterations so that more specific therapy can be designed.

References

1. D'Angio GJ, Breslow N, Beckwith B, Evans A, Baum E, DeLorimier A, Fernbach D, Hrabovsky E, Jones B, Kelalis P, Othersen B, Tefft M, Thomas PRM. 1989. Treatment of Wilms's tumor. Results of the Third National Wilms' Tumor Study. Cancer 64:349–360.
2. Knudson AG, Strong LC. 1972. Mutations and cancer: a model for Wilms' tumor of the kidney. J Nat Cancer Inst 48:313–324.
3. Call KM, Glaser T, Ito CY, Buckler AJ, Pelletier J, Haber DA, Rose EA, Kral A, Yeger H, Lewis WH, Jones C, Housman DE. 1990. Isolation and characterization of a zinc finger polypeptide gene at the human chromosome 11 Wilms' tumor locus. Cell 60:509–520.
4. Gessler M, Poustka A, Cavenee W, Neve RL, Orkin SH, Bruns GAP. 1990. Homozygous deletion in Wilms tumours of a zinc-finger gene identified by chromosome jumping. Nature 343:774–778.

5. Bonetta L, Kuehn SE, Huang A, Law DJ, Kalikin LM, Koi M, Reeve AE, Brownstein BH, Yeger H, Williams BRG, Feinberg AP. 1990. Wilms tumor locus on 11p13 defined by multiple CpG island-associated transcripts. Science 250:994–997.

6. Hall JG. 1990. Genomic imprinting: review and relevance to human diseases. Am J Hum Genet 46: 857–873.

7. Beckwith JB, Kiviat NB, Bonadio JF. 1990. Nephrogenic rests, nephroblastomatosis, and the pathogenesis of Wilms' tumor. Perspect Pediatr Pathol 10:1–36.

8. Knudson AG. 1971. Mutation and cancer: a statistical study of retinoblastoma. Proc Natl Acad Sci USA 68:820–823.

9. Comings DE. 1973. A general theory of carcinogenesis. Proc Natl Acad Sci USA 70:3324–3328.

10. Miller RW, Fraumeni JF, Manning MD. 1964. Association of Wilms' tumor with aniridia, hemihypertrophy and other congenital anomalies. N Engl J Med 270:922–927.

11. Narahara K, Kikkawa K, Kimira S, Ogata M, Kasai R, Hamawaki M, Matsuoka K. 1984. Regional mapping of catalase and Wilms' tumor — aniridia, genitourinary abnormalities, and mental retardation triad loci to the chromosome segment 11p1305→p1306. Hum Genet 66:181–185.

12. Riccardi VM, Sujansky E, Smith AC, Francke U. 1978. Chromosomal imbalance in the aniridia–Wilms' tumor association: 11p interstitial deletion. Pediatrics 61:604–610.

13. Ton CCT, Hirvonen H, Miwa H. 1991. Positional cloning and characterization of a paired box- and homeobox-containing gene from the aniridia region. Cell 67:1059–1074.

14. Huang A, Campbell CE, Bonetta L, McAndrews-Hill M, Chilton-MacNeill S, Coppes MJ, Law DJ, Feinberg AP, Yeger H, Williams BRG. 1990. Tissue, developmental, and tumor-specific expression of divergent transcripts in Wilms tumor. Science 250:991–994.

15. Pelletier J, Bruening W, Li FP, Haber DA, Glaser T, Housman DE. 1991. WT1 mutations contribute to abnormal genital system development and hereditary Wilms' tumor. Nature 353:431–434.

16. Coppes MJ, Campbell CE, Williams BRG. 1993. The role of WT1 in Wilms tumorigenesis. FASEB J 7:886–895.

17. Varanasi R, Bardeesy N, Ghahremani M, Petruzzi M-J, Nowak N, Adam MA, Grundy P, Shows TB, Pelletier J. 1994. Fine structure analysis of the *WT1* gene in sporadic Wilms tumor. Proc Natl Acad Sci USA 91:3554–3558.

18. Gessler M, Konig A, Arden K, Grundy P, Orkin S, Sallan S, Peters C, Ruyle S, Mandell J, Li F, Cavenee W, Bruns G. 1994. Infrequent mutation of the *WT1* gene in 77 Wilms' tumors. Hum Mutat 3:212–222.

19. Haber DA, Sohn RL, Buckler AJ, Pelletier J, Call KM, Housman DE. 1991. Alternative splicing and genomic structure of the Wilms tumor gene *WT1*. Proc Natl Acad Sci USA 88:9618–9622.

20. Rauscher FJ III. 1993. The WT1 Wilms tumor gene product: a developmentally regulated transcription factor in the kidney that functions as a tumor suppressor. FASEB J 7:896–903.

21. Wang Z-Y, Qui Q-Q, Deuel TF. 1993. The Wilms' tumor gene product WT1 activates or suppresses transcription through separate functional domains. J Biol Chem 268:9172–9175.

22. Wang Z-Y, Qiu Q-Q, Enger KT, Deuel TF. 1993. A second transcriptionally active DNA-binding site for the Wilms tumor gene product, WT1. Proc Natl Acad Sci USA 90:8896–9000.

23. Maheswaran S, Park S, Bernard A, Morris JF, Rauscher FJ III, Hill DE, Haber DA. 1993. Physical and functional interaction between WT1 and p53 proteins. Proc Natl Acad Sci USA 90:5100–5104.

24. Rauscher FJ, Morris JF, Tournay OE, Cook DM, Curran T. 1990. Binding of the Wilms' tumor locus zinc finger protein to the EGR-1 consensus sequence. Science 250:1259–1262.

25. Pritchard-Jones K, Fleming S, Davidson D, Bickmore W, Porteous D, Gosden C, Bard J, Buckler A, Pelletier J, Housman D, Van Heyningen V, Hastie N. 1990. The candidate Wilms' tumour gene is involved in genitourinary development. Nature 346:194–197.

26. Miwa H, Tomlinson GE, Timmons CF, Huff V, Cohn SL. 1992. RNA expression of the WT1 gene in Wilms tumors in relation to histology. J Natl Cancer Inst 84:181–186.

27. Buckler AJ, Pelletier J, Haber DA, Glaser T, Housman DE. 1991. Isolation, characterization, and expression of the murine Wilms' tumor gene (WT1) during kidney development. Mol Cell Biol 11:1707–1712.

28. Pelletier J, Schalling M, Buckler AJ, Rogers A, Haber DA, Housman D. 1991. Expression of the Wilms' tumor gene WT1 in the murine urogenital system. Genes Dev 5:1345–1356.

29. Pelletier J, Bruening W, Cashtan CE, Mauer SM, Manivel JC, Striegel JE, Houghton DC, Junien C, Habib R, Fouser L, Fine RN, Silverman BL, Haber DA, Housman D. 1991. Germline mutations in the Wilms' tumor suppressor gene are associated with abnormal urogenital development in Denys–Drash syndrome. Cell 67:437–447.

30. Park S, Schalling M, Bernard A, Maheswaran S, Shipley GC, Roberts D, Fletcher J, Shipman R, Rheinwald J, Demetri G, Griffin J, Minden M, Housman DE, Haber DA. 1993. The Wilms tumour gene WT1 is expressed in murine mesoderm-derived tissues and mutated in a human mesothelioma. Nature Genet 4:415–420.

31. Coppes MJ, Ye Y, Rackley R, Zhao Z-L, Liefers GJ, Casey G, Williams BRG. 1993. Analysis of *WT1* in granulosa cell and other sex cord-stromal tumors. Cancer Res 53:2712–2714.

32. Kreidberg JA, Sariola H, Loring JM, Maeda M, Pelletier J, Housman D, Jaenisch R. 1993. WT-1 is required for early kidney development. Cell 74:679–691.

33. Huff V, Jaffe N, Saunders GF, Strong LC, Villalba F, Ruteshouser EC. 1995. WT1 exon 1 deletion/insertion mutations in Wilms tumor patients, associated with di- and trinucleotide repeats and deletion hotspot consensus sequences. Am J Hum Genet 56:84–90.

34. Herskowitz I. 1987. Functional inactivation of genes by dominant negative mutations. Nature 329:219–222.

35. Coppes MJ, Huff V, Pelletier J. 1993. Denys–Drash syndrome: relating a clinical disorder to genetic alterations in the tumor suppressor gene WT1. J Pediatr 123:673–678.

36. Jadresic L, Leake J, Gordon I, Dillon MJ, Grant DB, Pritchard J, Risdon RA, Barratt TM. 1990. Clinicopathologic review of twelve children with nephropathy, Wilms tumor, and genital abnormalities (Drash syndrome). J Pediatr 117:717–725.

37. Haber DA, Buckler AJ, Glaser T, Call KM, Pelletier J, Sohn RL, Douglass EC, Housman DE. 1990. An internal deletion within an 11p13 zinc finger gene contributes to the development of Wilms' tumor. Cell 61:1257–1269.

38. Little MH, Prosser J, Condie A, Smith PJ, Van heyningen V, Hastie ND. 1992. Zinc finger point mutations within the WT1 gene in Wilms tumor patients. Proc Natl Acad Sci USA 89:4791–4795.

39. Haber DA, Timmers HT, Pelletier J, Sharp PA, Housman DE. 1992. A dominant mutation in the Wilms tumor gene WT1 cooperates with the viral oncogene E1A in transformation of primary kidney cells. Proc Natl Acad Sci USA 89:6010–6014.

40. Coppes MJ, Liefers GJ, Higuchi M, Zinn AB, Balfe JW, Williams BR. 1992. Inherited WT1 mutation in Denys-Drash syndrome. Cancer Res 52:6125–6128.

41. Mannens M, Slater RM, Heyting C, Blick J, De Kraker J, Coad N, De Pagter-Holthuizen P, Pearson PL. 1988. Molecular nature of genetic changes resulting in loss of heterozygosity of chromosome 11 in Wilms' tumors. Hum Genet 81:41–48.

42. Koufos A, Grundy P, Morgan K, Aleck KA, Hadro T, Lampkin BC, Kalbakji A, Cavenee WK. 1989. Familial Weidemann-Beckwith syndrome and a second Wilms' tumor locus both map to 11p15.5. Am J Hum Genet 44:711-719.

43. Wadey RB, Pal N, Buckle B, Yeomans E, Pritchard J, Cowell JK. 1990. Loss of heterozygosity in Wilms' tumour involves two distinct regions of chromosome 11. Oncogene 5:901–907.

44. Coppes MJ, Bonetta L, Huang A, Hoban P, Chilton-MacNeill S, Campbell CE, Weksberg R, Yeger H, Reeve AE, Williams BRG. 1992. Loss of heterozygosity mapping in Wilms tumor indicates the involvement of three distinct regions and a limited role for nondisjunction or mitotic recombination. Genes Chromosomes Cancer 5:326–334.

45. Wiedemann HR. 1964. Complexe malformatif familial avec hernie ombilicale et macroglossie — un syndrome nouveau? J Genet Hum 13:223–232.

46. Beckwith JB. 1969. Macroglossia, omphalocele, adrenal cytomegaly, gigantism, and hyperplastic visceromegaly. Birth Defects: Original Article Series 5:188–190.
47. Ping AJ, Reeve AE, Law DJ, Young MR, Boehnke M, Feinberg AP. 1989. Genetic linkage of Beckwith–Weidmann syndrome to 11p15. Am J Hum Genet 44:720–723.
48. Schroeder WT, Chao L, Dao DD, Strong LC, Pathak S, Riccardi V, Lewis WH, Saunders GF. 1987. Nonrandom loss of maternal chromosome 11 alleles in Wilms' tumors. Am J Hum Genet 40:413–420.
49. Waziri M, Patil SR, Hanson JW, Bartley JA. 1983. Abnormality of chromosome 11 in patients with features of Beckwith–Wiedemann syndrome. J Pediatr 102:873–876.
50. Grundy P, Telzerow P, Haber D, Berman B, Li F, Paterson MC, Garber J. 1991. Chromosome 11 uniparental isodisomy predisposing to embryonal neoplasms. Lancet 338:1079–1080.
51. Henry I, Bonaiti-Pellie C, Chehensse V, Beldjord C, Schwartz C, Utermann G, Junien C. 1991. Uniparental paternal disomy in a genetic cancer-predisposing syndrome. Nature 351:665–667.
52. Grundy P, Wilson B, Telzerow P, Zhou W, Paterson MC. 1994. Uniparental disomy occurs infrequently in Wilms tumor patients. Am J Hum Genet 54:282–289.
53. Chao LY, Huff V, Tomlinson G, Riccardi VM, Strong LC, Saunders GF. 1993. Genetic mosaicism in normal tissues of Wilms' tumour patients. Nature Genet 3:127–131.
54. Scott J, Cowell J, Robertson ME, Priestley LM, Wadey R, Hopkins B, Pritchard J, Bell GI, Rall LB, Graham CF, Knott TJ. 1985. Insulin-like growth factor II gene expression in Wilms' tumour and embryonic tissues. Nature 317:260–262.
55. Rainier S, Johnson LA, Dobry CJ, Ping AJ, Grundy PE, Feinberg AP. 1993. Relaxation of imprinted genes in human cancer. Nature 362:747–749.
56. Ogawa O, Eccles MR, Szeto J, McNoe LA, Yun K, Maw MA, Smith PJ, Reeve AE. 1993. Relaxation of insulin-like growth factor II gene imprinting implicated in Wilms tumour. Nature 362:749–751.
57. Giannoukakis N, Deal C, Paquette J, Goodyer CG, Polychronakos C. 1993. Parental genomic imprinting of the human IGF2 gene. Nature Genet 4:98–100.
58. Davies SM. 1994. Developmental regulation of genomic imprinting of the IGF2 gene in human liver. Cancer Res 54:2560–2562.
59. Pedone PV, Tirabosco R, Cavazzana AO, Ungaro P, Basso G, Luksch R, Carli M, Bruni CB, Frunzio R, Riccio A. 1994. Mono- and bi-allelic expression of insulin-like growth factor II gene in human muscle tumors. Hum Mol Genet 7:1117—1122.
60. Weksberg R, Shen DR, Fei Y-L, Song Q-L, Squire J. 1993. Disruption of insulin-like growth factor 2 imprinting in Beckwith–Wiedemann syndrome. Am J Hum Genet 53:17.
61. Steenman MJC, Rainier S, Dobry CJ, Grundy P, Horon IL, Feinberg AP. 1994. Loss of imprinting of IGF2 is linked to reduced expression and abnormal methylation of H19 in Wilms tumour. Nature Genet 7:433–439.
62. Reik W, Brown KW, Schneid H, Ie Bouc Y, Bickmore W, Maher ER. 1995. Imprinting mutations in the Beckwith–Wiedemann syndrome suggested by an altered imprinting pattern in the IGF2-H19 domain. Hum Mol Genet 4:2379–2385.
63. Zhang Y, Tycko B. 1993. Monoallelic expression of the human H19 gene. Nature Genet 1:40–44.
64. Bartolomei MS, Zemel S, Tilghman SM. 1991. Parental imprinting of the mouse H19 region. Nature 351:153–155.
65. Hao Y, Crenshaw T, Moulton T, Newcomb E, Tycko B. 1993. Tumour-suppressor activity of H19 RNA. Nature 365:764–767.
66. Moulton T, Crenshaw T, Hao Y, Moosikasuwan J, Lin N, Dembitzer F, Hensle T, Weiss L, McMorrow L, Loew T, Kraus W, Gerald W, Tycko B. 1994. Epigenetic lesions at the H19 locus in Wilms tumour patients. Nature Genet 7:440–447.
67. Nicholls RD. 1994. New insights reveal complex mechanisms involved in genomic imprinting. Am J Hum Genet 54:733–740.
68. Matsuoka S, Thompson JS, Edwards MC, Barletta JM, Grundy P, Kalikin LM, Harper JW,

121

Elledge SJ, Feinberg AP. 1996. Imprinting of the gene encoding a human cyclin-dependent kinase inhibitor, p57^{KIP2}, on chromosome 11p15. Proc Natl Acad Sci USA 93:3026–3030.

69. Koi M, Johnson LA, Kalikin LM, Little PFR, Nakamura Y, Feinberg AP. 1993. Tumor cell growth arrest caused by subchromosomal transferable DNA fragments from chromosome 11. Science 260:361–364.

70. Breslow N, Olsen J, Moksness J, Beckwith J, Grundy P. 1996. Familial Wilms tumors: a descriptive study. Med Pediatr Oncol. 27:398–403.

71. Grundy P, Koufos A, Morgan K, Li FP, Meadows AT, Cavenee WK. 1988. Familial predisposition to Wilms' tumour does not map to the short arm of chromosome 11. Nature 336:374–376.

72. Huff V, Compton DA, Chao L, Strong LC, Geiser CF, Saunders GF. 1988. Lack of linkage of familial Wilms' tumour to chromosomal band 11p13. Nature 336:377–378.

73. Schwartz CE, Haber DA, Stanton VP, Strong LC, Skolnick MH, Housman DE. 1991. Familial predisposition to Wilms tumor does not segregate with the WT1 gene. Cenomics 10:927–930.

74. Rahman N, Arbour L, Tonin P, Renshaw J, Pelletier J, Baruchel S, Pritchard-Jones K, Stratton MR, Narod SA. 1996. Evidence for a familial Wilms' tumour gene (*FWT1*) on chromosome 17q12–q21. Nature Genet 13:461–463.

75. Maw MA, Grundy PE, Millow LJ, Eccles MR, Dunn RS, Smith PJ, Feinberg AP, Law DJ, Paterson MC, Telzerow PE, Callen DF, Thompson AD, Richards RI, Reeve AE. 1992. A third Wilms' tumor locus on chromosome 16q. Cancer Res 52:3094–3098.

76. Hughes-Benzie RM, Hunter AG, Allanson JE, MacKenzie AE. 1994. Simpson–Golabi–Behmel syndrome associated with renal dysplasia and embryonal tumors: localization of the gene to Xqcen-q21. Am J Med Genet 30:428–435.

77. Neri G, Marini R, Cappa M, Borrelli P, Opitz JM. 1988. Simpson–Golabi–Behmel syndrome: an X-linked encephalo-troposchisis syndrome. Am J Med Genet 30:287–299.

78. Xuan JY, Besner A, Ireland M, Hughes-Benzie RM, MacKenzie AE. 1994. Mapping of Simpson–Golabi–Behmel syndrome to Xq25–q27. Hum Mol Genet 3:133–138.

79. Pilia G, Hughes-Benzie RM, MacKenzie A, Baybayan P, Chen EY, Huber R, Neri G, Cao A, Forabosco A, Schlessinger D. 1996. Mutations in *GPC3*, a glypican gene, cause the Simpson–Golabi–Behmel overgrowth syndrome. Nature Genet 12:241–247.

80. Neri G, Enrica Martini-Neri M, Katz BE, Opitz JM. 1984. The Perlman syndrome: familial renal dysplasia with Wilms' tumor, fetal gigantism and multiple congenital anomalies. Am J Med Genet 19:195–207.

81. Hartley AL, Birch JM, Tricker K, Wallace SA, Kelsey AM, Harris M, Jones PH. 1993. Wilms' tumor in the Li–Fraumeni cancer family syndrome. Cancer Genet Cytogenet 67:133–135.

82. Stay EJ, Vawter G. 1977. The relationship between nephroblastoma and neurofibromatosis. Cancer 39:2250–2255.

83. Szabo J, Heath B, Hill VM, Jackson CE, Zarbo RJ, Mallette LE, Chew SL, Besser GM, Thakker RV, Huff V, Leppert MF, Heath H III. 1994. Hereditary hyperparathyroidism — jaw tumor syndrome: the endocrine tumor gene HRPT2 maps to chromosome 1q21–q31. Am J Hum Genet 56:944–950.

84. Narod S. 1994. Genetics of breast and ovarian cancer. Br Med Bull 50:656–676.

85. Altura RA, Valentine M, Li H, Boyett JM, Shearer P, Grundy P, Shapiro DN, Look AT. 1996. Identification of novel regions of deletion in familial Wilms' tumor by comparative genomic hybridization. Cancer Res 56:3837–3841.

86. Mannens M, Devilee P, Bliek J, Mandjes I, De Kraker J, Heyting C, Slater RM, Westerveld A. 1990. Loss of heterozygosity in Wilms' tumors, studied for six putative tumor suppressor regions, is limited to chromosome 11. Cancer Res 50:3279–3283.

87. Grundy PE, Telzerow PE, Breslow N, Moksness J, Huff V, Paterson MC. 1994. Loss of heterozygosity for chromosomes 16q and 1p in Wilms' tumors predicts an adverse outcome. Cancer Res 54:2331–2333.

88. Huff V, Reeve AE, Leppert M, Strong LC, Douglass EC, Geiser CF, Li FP, Meadows A, Callen DF, Lenoir G, Saunders GF. 1992. Nonlinkage of 16q markers to familial predisposition to Wilms' tumor. Cancer Res 52:6117–6120.

89. Tsuda H, Zhang W, Shimosato Y, Yokota J, Terada M, Sugimura T, Miyamura T, Hirohashi S. 1990. Allele loss on chromosome 16 associated with progression of human hepatocellular carcinoma. Proc Natl Acad Sci USA 87:6791–6794.

90. Cleton-Jansen A-M, Moerland EW, Kuipers-Dijkshoorn NJ, Callen DF, Sutherland GR, Hansen B, Devilee P, Cornelisse CJ. 1994. At least two different regions are involved in allelic imbalance on chromosome arm 16q in breast cancer. Genes Chromosomes Cancer 9:101–107.

91. Kunimi K, Bergerheim USR, Larsson I, Ekman P, Collins VP. 1991. Allelotyping of human prostatic adenocarcinoma. Genomics 11:530–536.

92. Fong C-T, White PS, Peterson K, Sapienza C, Cavenee WK, Kern SE, Vogelstein B, Cantor AB, Look AT, Brodeur GM. 1992. Loss of heterozygosity for chromosomes 1 or 14 defines subsets of advanced neuroblastomas. Cancer Res 52:1780–1822.

93. Caron H, van Sluis P, van Hoeve M, De Kraker J, Bras J, Slater R, Mannens M, Voute PS, Westerveld A, Versteeg R. 1993. Allelic loss of chromosome 1p36 in neuroblastoma is of preferential maternal origin and correlates with *N-myc* amplification. Nature Genet 4:187–190.

94. Schwab M, Prami C, Amler LC. 1996. Genomic instability in 1p and human malignancies. Genes Chromosomes Cancer 16:211–229.

95. Rivera H. 1995. Constitutional and acquired rearrangements of chromosome 7 in Wilms tumor. Cancer Genet Cytogenet 81:97–98.

96. Wilmore HP, White GFJ, Howell RT, Brown KW. 1994. Germline and somatic abnormalities of chromosome 7 in Wilms' tumor. Cancer Genet Cytogenet 77:93–98.

97. Miozzo M, Perotti D, Minoletti F, et al. 1996. Mapping of a putative tumor suppressor locus to proximal 7p in Wilms tumors. Genomics 37:310–315.

98. Bardeesy N, Falkoff D, Petruzzi M-J, Nowak N, Zabel B, Adam M, Aguiar MC, Grundy P, Shows T, Pelletier J. 1994. Anaplastic Wilms' tumour, a subtype displaying poor prognosis, harbours p53 gene mutations. Nature Genet 7:91–97.

99. Malkin D, Sexsmith E, Yeger H, Williams BRG, Coppes MJ. 1994. Mutations of the *p53* tumor suppressor gene occur infrequently in Wilms' tumor. Cancer Res 54:2077–2079.

100. Bardeesy N, Beckwith JB, Pelletier J. 1995. Clonal expansion and attenuated apoptosis in Wilms' tumors are associated with *p53* gene mutations. Cancer Res 55:215–219.

101. Park S, Bernard A, Bove KE, Sens DA, Hazen-Martin DJ, Garvin J, Haber DA. 1993. Inactivation of WT1 in nephrogenic rests, genetic precursors to Wilms' tumour. Nature Genet 5:363–367.

102. Beckwith JB. 1993. Precursor lesions of Wilms tumor: clinical and biological implications. Med Pediatr Oncol 21:158–168.

5. Neuroblastoma: solving a biologic puzzle

Susan L. Cohn, Dafna Meitar, and Morris Kletzel

1. Introduction

Neuroblastoma, a childhood tumor arising in the adrenal medulla and sympathetic nervous system, presents an unusual challenge to pediatric oncologists. While virtually all patients with localized neuroblastoma can be cured by surgery alone, and most infants with disseminated disease are curable with chemotherapy, children with bone metastases usually have a fatal outcome [1–4]. Furthermore, in some patients the tumor undergoes spontaneous regression or differentiation [5,6]. This wide range of clinical behavior reflects the biologic heterogeneity of neuroblastoma. Much progress has been made recently in advancing our knowledge of human neuroblastoma at the cellular and molecular level, and specific genetic abnormalities have been identified that are characteristic of subsets of these tumors [7]. These transformation-linked genetic changes have contributed to our understanding of tumor predisposition, metastasis, treatment responsiveness, and prognosis. Continued study of these genetic abnormalities will hopefully lead to further insight into the molecular events associated with the malignant transformation of this heterogeneous tumor, and thereby provide clues for the development of specific therapy.

2. Incidence

Neuroblastoma is the most common tumor in infants younger than 1 year and the second most common solid tumor of childhood [8]. Approximately 500 new cases are diagnosed yearly in the United States. The overall incidence from birth to age 15 is 8.7 per million per year, with a slight predominance in Caucasians and males. The ratio of males to females is approximately 1.2:1. The median age at diagnosis is less than 2 years, with 35% of cases occurring under 1 year of age. The tumor may be congenital with metastases to the placenta [9]. Sixty percent of all cases present in children younger than 2 years, and 97% of cases occur in children younger than 10 years of age. Rare cases of adults with neuroblastoma have been reported, however [10].

D.O. Walterhouse and S.L. Cohn (eds), DIAGNOSTIC AND THERAPEUTIC ADVANCES IN PEDIATRIC ONCOLOGY. Copyright © 1997. Kluwer Academic Publishers, Boston. All rights reserved.

3. Etiology

The young age of most patients with neuroblastoma and the nondividing state of cells in the mature autonomic nervous system suggest that causative events occur prenatally or very early in life. Although no etiologic agent or genetic disease has been consistently linked with neuroblastoma, epidemiology studies have suggested a possible role for maternal exposure to alcohol, neurally active drugs, diuretics, and hair coloring and for paternal exposure to electromagnetic fields [11,12]. Case reports of neuroblastoma in patients with fetal hydantoin and fetal alcohol syndrome indicate that prenatal teratogenic insults may be involved in the pathogenesis of some cases [13]. Neuroblastoma has also been diagnosed in patients with other neurocristopathies, such as neurofibromatosis or aganglionic megacolon, suggesting a common genetic origin [14,15]. However, this occurs so rarely that a random association cannot be excluded.

Although rare, familial occurrence of neuroblastoma has been reported, suggesting that a recessive tumor suppressor gene may be involved in the mechanism of neuroblastoma tumorigenesis [16]. Affected individuals may have inherited germline mutations in a gene or genes that predispose them to an early onset and development of multiple primaries. In sporadic cases, the same or different genes may be involved, but the mutations are postzygotic events. In support of this hypothesis, Kushner and colleagues identified 55 patients in 23 families in a literature review of familial neuroblastoma; most were younger than 1 year at diagnosis, and eight patients had multiple primaries [16]. Recently, a constitutional deletion in chromosome 1p36 has been reported in one child with neuroblastoma, and a constitutional translocation involving chromosome 1p36 was observed in another patient with this tumor [17,18]. Efforts to identify a putative tumor suppressor gene in this region of chromosome 1 are ongoing.

4. Embryology

Neural crest cells are initially located along the sides of the embryonic neural tube [19]. During the development of the embryo, cells migrate from the neural tube along defined pathways, and subsequent commitment to cell fate occurs in response to environmental stimuli. The ventrally migrating cells develop into the spinal ganglia, the ganglia of the sympathetic side chain, the prevertebral ganglia, the paraganglia, and the chromaffin bodies. Visceral sympathetic ganglia are formed near the heart, lungs, gastrointestinal tract, and urogenital tract. In adults, these consist of ganglion cells and sporadic chromaffin cells, whereas in the fetus and newborn, cells of all stages of differentiation are seen.

Tumors that arise from this sympathetic blastema tissue include pheochromocytoma, ganglioneuroma, and neuroblastoma. The histologic correlation between the developmental stages of the sympathetic nervous and the various tumor types arising from this tissue was first noted over 100 years age [20]. Because neuroblastomas frequently consist of cells with divergent degrees of maturation, it was thought that these tumors were derived from a pluripotent neural crest cell. However, recent in situ hybridization studies suggest that neuroblastoma-associated Schwann cells are not malignant but rather normal cells [21]. Ambros and coworkers hypothesize that Schwann cells in maturing neuroblastomas are responding to one or more trophic signals that cause them to infiltrate the tumor. At the present time it is unclear what role, if any, Schwann cells have in the differentiation of neuroblastoma tumors.

5. Sites of disease

Because the sympathetic side chain extends from the posterior cranial fossa to the coccyx, neuroblastoma arises from a wide variety of sites. The most common site of primary disease is the abdomen, particularly the adrenal gland [22]. Approximately 30% of neuroblastomas originate in the cervical, thoracic, and pelvic side chains. Origins in the bladder wall, in the sciatic nerve, and in tissues adjacent to the testis have also been reported [23]. As mentioned previously, multiple primary tumors can occur, and these tumors may occur either simultaneously or sequentially [16,24]. Approximately two thirds of children will present with metastatic disease, and bone marrow, bone, liver and lymph nodes are the predominant metastatic sites. Rarely, the lung, pleura, and central nervous system are involved.

6. Clinical presentation

Clinical manifestations of neuroblastoma vary according to the location of the primary disease and the degree of dissemination (table 1). Neuroblastoma may be discovered as an abdominal or pelvic mass during examination of an asymptomatic child for a minor illness unrelated to the disease [25]. Thoracic tumors are often seen on chest roentgenograms done because of dyspnea or suspected pulmonary infection. Physical signs of tumor originating in the head and neck region include a palpable neck mass, Horner's syndrome, and heterochromia of the iris on the affected side. Tumors of the paraspinal area with intraspinal extension can lead to compression of the spinal cord, which, in turn, may cause localized back pain and tenderness, bladder and anal-sphincter dysfunction, disturbance of gait, paraplegia, hypotonia, areflexia, hyperreflexia, and spasticity [26].

Systemic symptoms include malaise, weight loss, anorexia, irritability, and fever. The most frequent symptoms of metastatic disease to bone and bone marrow are pain, limp, refusal to walk, and pallor [25]. The predilection for

127

Table 1. Neuroblastoma signs and symptoms

Primary cervical tumor	Cervical mass
	Horner's syndrome
	Heterochromia of the iris
	Superior Vena Cava syndrome
Primary thoracic tumor	Dyspnea
	Spinal cord compression
Primary abdominal tumor	Abdominal mass
	Spinal cord compression
	Abdominal pain
Primary pelvic tumor	Pelvic mass
	Spinal cord compression
	Hip and/or leg pain
Metastatic tumor	Lymphadenopathy
	Hepatomegaly
	Pallor
	Exophthalmos
	Eyelid ecchymosis
	Skull mass
	Bone pain
	Skin nodules
	Purpura
Systemic symptoms	Fever
	Weight loss
	Fatigue
	Hypertension
	Intractable diarrhea
	Opsoclonus/myoclonus

skeletal spread is particularly evident in the skull and facial bones, especially in the orbits. Orbital metastases can give rise to proptosis and to the character-istic ecchymoses in the upper eyelids. Lymph node metastases are also fre-quent, and enlarged cervical lymph nodes may be a presenting sign. Infants may have subcutaneous metastases that manifest as skin nodules, as well as diffuse metastatic spread to the liver that can lead to massive hepatomegaly and subsequent respiratory symptoms (figure 1). The tumor can also cause antenatal death as a result of severe anemia, hydramnios, or hydrops fetalis [27].

7. Rare systemic symptoms

In rare instances, a child with neuroblastoma may have hypertension caused by excessive tumor production of catecholamines [28]. However, marked par-oxysmal effects from catecholamine release, as seen in pheochromocytomas, are uncommon in neuroblastoma, most likely because the active metabolites are rapidly degraded. Intractable diarrhea due to tumor secretion of the pep-tide hormone vasoactive intestinal polypeptide (VIP) is another rare symptom

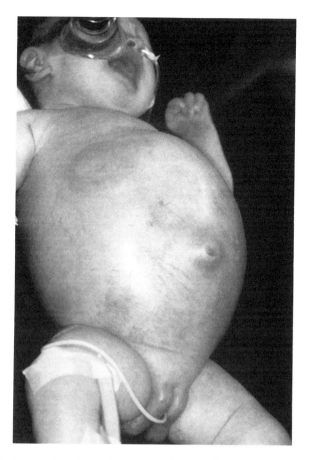

Figure 1. Infant with hepatomegaly and respiratory distress secondary to metastatic neuroblastoma.

[29]. VIP secretion is usually associated with more differentiated tumors such as ganglioneuroma or ganglioneuroblastoma [30].

Approximately 2% of patients with neuroblastoma will have acute cerebellar encephalopathy with opsoclonus, myoclonus, and ataxia [31]. Progressive ataxia and titubation of the head, myoclonic jerks, and chaotic conjugate jerking movements of the eyes can be prominent. Although the opsoclonus and myoclonus may abate in some patients after tumor removal, in some cases myoclonic encephalopathy has actually developed after tumor resection. This syndrome is more common in patients with localized disease, and almost all tumors have biologically favorable features [31–33]. More than 85% of these patients are long-term survivors, and in many patients the myoclonic symptoms will improve with steroid treatment or intravenous gammaglobulin [34,35]. However, successful treatment of the tumor or the movement disorder does not halt or reverse neurologic deterioration. Long-term follow-up studies have demonstrated that most patients have chronic neurologic deficits, including cognitive and motor delays, language deficits, and behavioral abnormalities [33,36,37].

The pathogenesis of this syndrome is not well understood, but it is believed that deregulation of the immune system plays a role [38]. Imaging studies and neuropathologic investigation have only inconsistently shown focal abnormalities in the brains of patients with neuroblastoma and opsoclonus–myoclonus [39]. Because the majority of patients continue to have long-term developmental and neurologic problems, early cognitive, developmental, and neurologic evaluation is indicated in all patients with this syndrome so that appropriate therapeutic and educational intervention may be instituted in an attempt to minimize or reverse deficits in these areas.

8. Diagnosis

The diagnosis of neuroblastoma may be established by unequivocal pathologic examination of tumor tissue. In most cases, a tissue diagnosis of neuroblastoma based on conventional staining (hematoxylin and eosin) is not difficult, especially if features suggestive of neuronal differentiation are present. However, in some cases, the neuroblasts exhibit little if any features of differentiation, and electron microscopy may be necessary to confirm the diagnosis. Alternatively, immunohistochemical, cytogenetic, and/or molecular analysis may be needed to help differentiate neuroblastoma from other small, round, blue cell tumors such as rhabdomyosarcoma, lymphoma, peripheral neuroepithelioma (also called primitive neuroectodermal tumor [PNET]), and Ewing's sarcoma [40–47]. For example, genetic features such as chromosome 1p deletion or amplification of the *MYCN* oncogene would support a diagnosis of neuroblastoma, whereas the presence of the chromosomal translocations t(11;22) or t(2;13) would be characteristic of Ewing's sarcoma/PNET and alveolar rhabdomyosarcoma, respectively.

The diagnosis may also be made by demonstrating unequivocal tumor cells in a bone marrow aspirate or biopsy combined with the detection of elevated urinary catecholamine excretion [48]. Excessive production of catecholamines is one of the most striking characteristics of neuroblasoma [49]. Sympathetic cells produce 3,4-dihydroxyphenylalanine (Dopa) by the enzyme tyrosine hydroxylase, and decarboxylation of Dopa results in the production of the first catecholamine, dopamine. Norepinephrine is formed by dopamine–beta hydroxylase, after which phenylethanolamine-N-methyl transferase forms epinephrine. Most of the excreted catecholamines are O-methylated by catechol-O-methyl transferase, and excretion of vanilglycolic acid (VGA), vanillylmandelic acid (VMA), vanil acetic acid (VAA), and homovanillic acid (HVA) can be measured for diagnostic purposes [23]. Using a cutoff of 3.0 standard deviations above the mean per milligram creatinine for age, approximately 92% of children with biopsy-proven neuroblastoma will have increased catecholamines at diagnosis.

A variety of serum markers, such as ferritin, lactic dehydrogenase (LDH), and neuron-specific enolase (NSE), have also been used to aid in the diagnosis of neuroblastoma and to follow response to treatment [48,50]. However, while ferritin and LDH may be useful prognostic markers for neuroblastoma at diagnosis, they lack sensitivity and specificity. Serum NSE is more specific, but this tumor marker is not as sensitive.

9. Evaluation of disease extent

Evaluation for extent of disease requires several studies (table 2). The primary site can be examined radiographically by plain films, computerized tomography (CT), magnetic resonance imaging (MRI), and radiolabeled meta-iodobenzylguanidine (MIBG). Bilateral bone marrow aspirates and biopsies should be performed to assess gross marrow involvement [48]. Lymph node involvement may be evaluated by radiographic studies as well as physical examination. At the time of surgery, representative biopsies of regional and any enlarged (>2 cm) nodes should be performed. A technetium diphosphonate bone scan is generally the most sensitive conventional modality for the detection of cortical bone involvement at the time of diagnosis [51]. Plain radiographs should be obtained of positive or suspicious lesions detected by bone scan to document bone abnormalities and to rule out other possible explanations for the abnormalities. There is controversy as to whether MIBG scans are as sensitive as technetium diphosphonate scans in detecting cortical bone disease [52]. Therefore, a technetium bone scan should always be performed if the MIBG scan is negative. Liver disease can be assessed with CT scan in most patients. However, in infants, liver involvement is often diffuse

Table 2. Evaluation of extent of disease

Tumor site	INSS recommended tests
Primary tumor	CT and/or MRI scan; MIBG scan, if available.
Metastatic sites	
Bone marrow	Bilateral posterior iliac crest marrow aspirates and trephine (core) bone marrow biopsies.
Bone	Bone scan and MIBG scan (if available); plain radiographs of positive lesions.
Lymph nodes	Clinical examination (palpable nodes), confirmed histologically. CT scan for nonpalpable nodes.
Abdomen/liver	CT and/or MRI scan.
Chest	AP and lateral chest radiographs. CT or MRI if chest radiograph positive.

Abbreviations: CT, computed tomography; MRI, magnetic resonance imaging; MIBG, meta-iodobenzylguanidine.

and may not be apparent by diagnostic imaging or by inspection of the liver at the time of surgery [53]. Therefore, it is recommended that a blind liver biopsy be performed to rule out liver involvement in infants with abdominal tumors [48]. A chest radiograph should be obtained to evaluate the presence of disease dissemination to the thorax. If the chest radiograph is positive, further evaluation with CT or MRI is indicated.

10. Differential diagnosis

The differential diagnosis of neuroblastoma includes a wide range of pediatric conditions. Because of the propensity to early and widespread metastases, neuroblastoma has been misdiagnosed as osteomyelitis, juvenile rheumatoid arthritis, storage disease, granulomatous processes, and leukemia. Patients presenting with orbital echymosis may be misdiagnosed as child abuse victims. Neoplastic processes from which neuroblastoma must be differentiated include Wilms' tumor of the extrarenal type, Ewing's sarcoma of the extraosseous type, and Ewing's of the vertebrae or ribs, teratomas, lymphomas, and peripheral neuroectodermal tumors (PNET).

11. Staging

Several different staging systems have been used to classify the extent of disease in neuroblastoma patients at the time of diagnosis, and all have prognostic value. The Evans system, which is currently used by the Children's Cancer Study Group (CCG), was initially described in 1971 [4]. The criteria for this system are clinical (table 3). A special category of disseminated neuroblastoma, stage IVS, was included in this staging system for a subset of patients with primary lesions that do not cross the midline and who have metastases limited to liver, skin, and/or bone marrow. Patients who meet the clinical criteria for this special stage are usually young, have a good prognosis despite extensive disease, and have a high rate of spontaneous remission. A surgicopathologic staging system was described by investigators from the St. Jude Children's Research Hospital [54], and a modified version of this system is currently used by the Pediatric Oncology Group (POG) (table 3) [1]. A third staging system, the tumor–node–metastasis (TNM) classification, has been devised under the auspices of the International Union Against Cancer, the International Society of Paediatric Oncology, and the American Joint Committee [55]. In general, the staging systems are comparable when distinguishing between patients with low-stage disease and good prognosis and those with advanced disease and poor prognosis. However, the differences between the staging systems for intermediate-stage disease are substantial.

Because the differences in these systems make it difficult to compare the results of clinical trials and biologic studies, an international consensus group

Table 3. Comparison of staging systems

Staging	Stage	Definition
Evans	I	Tumor confined to the organ or structure of origin.
	II	Tumor extending beyond the organ or structure but not crossing the midline.
	III	Tumor extending in continuity across the midline.
	IVS	Localized primary tumor (stage I or II) with dissemination limited to liver, skin, and/or bone marrow.
	IV	Any primary tumor with dissemination to distant lymph nodes, bone marrow, liver, skin, and/or other organs (except as defined for stage IVS)
POG	A	Complete gross resection of primary tumor. Attached lymph nodes may be positive. Distant nodes and liver negative.
	B	Grossly unresected tumor. Nodes and liver same as stage A
	C	Complete or incomplete resection. Unattached nodes positive.
	DS	Localized primary tumor (stage A or B) with dissemination limited to liver, skin, and/or bone marrow.
	D	Same as Evans stage IV.
INSS	1	Localized tumor with complete gross excision, with or without microscopic residual disease; representative ipsilateral lymph nodes negative for tumor microscopically (nodes attached to and removed with the primary tumor may be positive).
	2A	Localized tumor with incomplete gross excision; representative ipsilateral nonadherent lymph nodes negative for tumor microscopically.
	2B	Localized tumor with or without complete gross excision, with ipsilateral nonadherent lymph nodes positive for tumor. Enlarged contralateral lymph nodes must be negative microscopically.
	3	Unresectable unilateral tumor infiltrating across the midline, with or without regional lymph node involvement; or localized unilateral tumor with contralateral regional lymph node involvement; or midline tumor with bilateral extension by infiltration (unresectable) or by lymph node involvement.
	4S	Localized primary tumor (as defined for stage 1, 2A or 2B), with dissemination limited to skin, liver, and/or bone marrow (limited to infants <1 year of age; marrow involvement should be minimal, <10%).
	4	Same as Evans stage IV.

met in 1986 to establish international criteria for a common neuroblastoma staging system [56]. The staging system is known as the International Neuroblastoma Staging System (INSS), and most groups and countries have implemented the INSS in addition to, or instead of, the staging system they previously used (table 3). The INSS, which was revised in 1993 [48], categorizes patients according to the presence or absence of disease in the bone marrow, radiographic information, and surgical findings. Recently, the POG and CCG conducted a retrospective analysis that confirmed that the INSS definitions identified prognostic subsets of patients with neuroblastoma [57,58]. Further validation of the INSS criteria is ongoing in prospective POG and CCG studies.

12. Prognostic factors

12.1. Clinical factors

The only independent clinical prognostic factors in neuroblastoma are the stage of the disease and the age of the child at diagnosis [50]. As with most malignancies, stage of disease at diagnosis is the single most important prognostic factor in neuroblastoma. However, for all stages of disease beyond localized tumors, infants less than 1 year of age have a significantly better disease-free survival rate than older children with equivalent stage [59]. Survival of patients of any age with stage A disease approaches 100% [1]. Patients with widely disseminated neuroblastoma diagnosed at over 1 year of age do poorly, with less than a 20% rate of long-term survival despite aggressive multimodality treatments [3,60,61]. However, there is some suggestion that children over 5 years of age with metastatic neuroblastoma have a more indolent course resulting in prolonged survival [62]. Infants with metastatic disease have a significantly better outcome than children older than 1 year of age [3]. Biologic factors (discussed below) have provided critical insights regarding prognosis in this subset of patients and have had a major impact on management.

12.2. Tumor markers

Serum ferritin and lactic dehydrogenase (LDH) have been shown to be useful prognostic markers for neuroblastoma (table 4). Unfavorable outcomes are associated with elevated levels of serum ferritin (>142 ng/mL) and LDH (>1500 IU/L) [63,64]. Serum levels of neuron-specific enolase (NSE) above 100 ng/mL have been found more often in patients with advanced-stage disease than in those with localized disease [65]. Patients with regional and widely disseminated disease with normal NSE levels have been shown to have a better outcome than those with elevated NSE values [66].

12.3. Histology

The degree of maturation of neuroblastoma can vary from the most primitive form of undifferentiated neuroblastoma to primarily mature ganglioneuroma with only scattered nests of neuroblasts. In 1984 a classification scheme was devised by Shimada and colleagues that relates the pathologic features to clinical behavior [67]. Shimada classified tumors as favorable or unfavorable

134

Table 4. Prognostic factors in neuroblastoma

Prognostic factor	Favorable	Unfavorable
Clincial factors		
Stage	1,2A,2B,4S (INSS)	3,4 (INSS)
Age	≤12 months	>12 months
Tumor markers		
Ferritin	<142 ng/mL	>142 ng/mL
LDH	<1500 IU/L	>1500 IU/L
NSE	<100 ng/mL	>100 ng/mL
Biologic factors		
DNA Index	>1.0	1.0
MYCN	Normal	Amplified
Chromosome Ip	Normal	Deleted
TrKA	High levels of expression	Low levels of expression
MRP[a]	Low levels of expression	High levels of expression
CD44[a]	High levels of expression	Low levels of expression
Vascularity[a]	Low vascularity	High vascularity
Pathology		
Shimada classification	Favorable	Unfavorable
Joshi classification	Low-risk	High-risk

[a] Recently described prognostic factors: further studies needed to confirm results.

on the basis of neuroblast differentiation, stroma, mitosis–karyorrhexis index, and age at diagnosis. Joshi and coworkers proposed a modification of this classification using mitotic ratio (number of mitoses/10 high-power fields) and presence or absence of calcification. Three grades of tumor were defined as follows: grade 1, tumors with calcification and low mitotic ratio (≤10 mitoses/ 10 high-power fields); grade 2, tumors with either calcification or low mitotic ratio; and grade 3, tumors with high mitotic ratio and no calcification [68,69]. Patients of all ages with grade 1 tumors and patients 1 year of age or younger with grade 2 tumors were classified in the low-risk group. The high-risk group consisted of patients of all ages with grade 3 tumors and patients 1 year of age or older with grade 2 tumors. It is not known why unfavorable histology tumors are clinically more aggressive than favorable histology tumors. However, amplification of the *MYCN* oncogene has been shown to be strongly associated with unfavorable histology [70,71].

12.4. MYCN amplification

Cytogenetic analysis of human neuroblastomas frequently show either extra-chromosomal double-minute chromatin bodies or homogeneously staining regions [72,73]. Both abnormalities are cytogenetic manifestations of gene amplification. In 1983, Schwab and colleagues reported that an oncogene related to the viral oncogene *v-myc*, but distinct from *c-myc*, was amplified in 8 of the 9 neuroblastoma cell lines tested [74]. This amplified sequence, now known as *MYCN* [75], was mapped to homogeneously staining regions on

135

different chromosomes in neuroblastoma cell lines, and the normal single-copy locus was mapped to the distal short arm of chromosome 2 [76,77].

Brodeur and colleagues first reported the association between *MYCN* amplification and advanced-stage neuroblastoma in 1984 [78]. In 1985, Seeger and coworkers reported the association between *MYCN* amplification and rapid tumor progression and poor prognosis [60]. Brodeur and colleagues also analyzed *MYCN* copy number in multiple simultaneous or consecutive samples of neuroblastoma tissue from 60 patients and found a consistent copy number in different tumor samples taken from each patient [79]. No cases of neuroblastoma with a single copy of *MYCN* at the time of diagnosis developed amplification subsequently. These results suggest that *MYCN* amplification is an intrinsic biologic property of a subset of neuroblastomas and that tumors that develop *MYCN* amplification do so by the time of diagnosis. *MYCN* copy number has now been examined in more than 1200 patients with neuroblastoma enrolled in protocols of the CCG and POG, and the same associations are seen [7].

In vitro studies have supported the hypothesis that *MYCN* contributes to the biologic behavior of neuroblastoma. Enhanced *MYCN* expression through exogenous gene transfer has been associated with increased growth and metastatic potential in neuroblastoma cells [80,81]. In addition, decreased rates of proliferation and colony formation in soft agar have been seen with antisense *MYCN* expression [82–84], and downregulation of *MYCN* is seen in neuroblastoma cells chemically induced to differentiate [85]. Furthermore, constitutive expression of *MYCN* can block retinoic acid-induced differentiation [86].

MYCN is a member of the *MYC* family of genes. The gene encodes two polypeptides, with relative masses of 62 and 64 kDa, that result from alternative use of two translational start codons [87]. The two proteins are phosphorylated and localized to the nucleus. The encoded gene products of the *MYC* family share structural similarities in helix-loop-helix DNA-binding domains with other *trans*-acting differentiation factors such as MyoD and E2A [74,88]. This motif is thought to be responsible for both DNA binding and dimerization. The MYC proteins have been shown to form a sequence-specific DNA-binding complex with MAX, another helix-loop-helix leucine zipper [88,89]. It is, therefore, likely that *MYCN* is a *trans*-acting factor involved in controlling the expression of key cellular genes crucial for regulated cell growth and differentiation. In the same manner, high levels of *MYCN* expression subsequent to genomic amplification could result in altered cell growth and differentiation.

Because the *MYCN* amplicon ranges in size from 350 kb to more than 1 Mb [90], it is possible that the aggressive phenotype associated with *MYCN* amplification may be due to overexpression of additional genes within the amplicon. Recently, coamplification and concomitant high levels of expression of the DEAD (Asp-Glu-Ala-Asp) box gene *DDX1* with *MYCN* has been demonstrated in neuroblastoma tumors [91–93]. DEAD box proteins are putative RNA helicases that have ATP-dependent activities including modulation of RNA secondary structure [94]. It remains to be determined if *DDX1* amplification and overexpression contributes to the malignant phenotype of a subset of *MYCN* amplified tumors.

Only 5%–10% of patients with localized disease have tumors with *MYCN* amplification, whereas more than 30% of patients with advanced disease have tumors with amplification of this oncogene [60,95]. While *MYCN* amplification is strongly associated with poor outcome regardless of the clinical stage of the tumor, recently there have been reports suggesting that some children with localized *MYCN*-amplified tumors have a good prognosis [95,96]. Histologic analysis of these localized tumors suggests that the prognostic relevance of *MYCN* amplification may vary according to the histologic features of the tumor. Patients with favorable histology tumors do not appear to require aggressive multimodality therapy to be cured. However, the outcome of patients with localized, *MYCN*-amplified neuroblastomas with unfavorable histology is poor, similar to their counterparts with advanced stages of disease. Further elucidation of the biology of *MYCN*-amplified localized neuroblastomas may lead to the identity of the molecular events that are specific to this clinically favorable subset of tumors. Low levels of *MYCN* mRNA and protein have been demonstrated in one localized, *MYCN* amplified tumor [95]. Additional studies should be performed to determine if this finding is characteristic of localized, *MYCN*-amplified neuroblastomas with favorable histology.

Approximately 50% of patients with single-copy *MYCN* neuroblastomas will also die of disease [7]. At the present time, there are no specific biologic markers that consistently predict outcome for this group of patients. Although it is possible that activation of *MYCN* may occur by mechanisms other than amplification, higher levels of *MYCN* expression in single-copy tumors is not consistently correlated with unfavorable outcome [97–99]. Thus, another genetic lesion may contribute to the poor clinical outcome of this subset of patients.

Southern blot analysis was used to determined *MYCN* copy number in neuroblastoma in most of the clinical studies discussed in this chapter. However, several cooperative groups are now using florescence in situ hybridization (FISH) to measure *MYCN* copy number (figure 2) [100]. While both techniques can be used to accurately determine gene amplification, there are several advantages to the FISH technique. First, results can be obtained more rapidly with FISH, and second, only small numbers of tumor cells are required to perform the analysis. *MYCN* copy number can be accurately determined in tissue that contains only small numbers of infiltrating tumor cells, whereas false-negative results are often obtained when Southern blot analysis is performed with this type of tumor sample. In addition, with FISH it is possible to distinguish low levels of *MYCN* amplification from hyperdiploidy of chromosome 2.

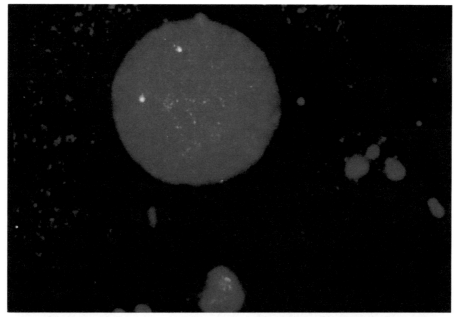

a

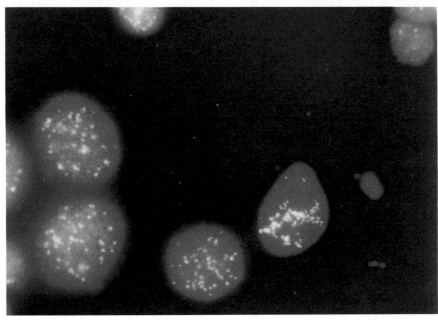

b

Figure 2. A cosmid clone containing the *MYCN* gene is shown hybridized to interphase nuclei from (**a**) a neuroblastoma lacking *MYCN* amplification; (**b**) a neuroblastoma tumor containing double-minute chromatin bodies containing increased copy number of this locus of *MYCN*; and (**c**) a neuroblastoma containing homogeneously staining regions containing increased copy number of this locus of *MYCN*. (Photographs are courtesy of Dr. A. Thomas Look and Susan Rowe from the POG Neuroblastoma Reference Laboratory, St. Judes Children's Research Hospital, Memphis, TN.)

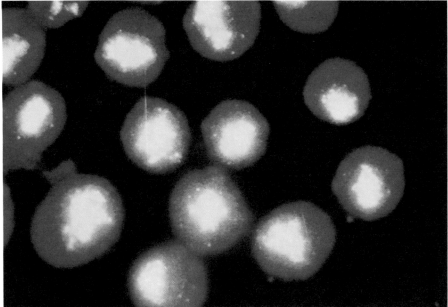

c

Figure 2 (continued)

12.5. Tumor cell ploidy

Flow-cytometric analysis of the DNA content of human neuroblastoma cells was first reported in a series of 35 infants [101]. In this analysis, diploidy was more common in infants with widely disseminated disease. Furthermore, all 17 evaluable patients with unresectable hyperdiploid tumors had either a complete or a partial response to cyclophosphamide and doxorubicin, while six with diploid tumors failed to respond. Subsequent studies have confirmed the prognostic importance of flow-cytometric measurement of DNA content, particularly in patients less than 12 months of age [3,102–105]. Several studies comparing tumor cell ploidy and *MYCN* amplification have shown that a correlation between amplification and diploidy exists, although the association is not absolute [71,106,107]. Thus, *MYCN* copy number and tumor cell ploidy provide complementary prognostic information.

12.6. Deletion or loss of heterozygosity of the short arm of chromosome 1

Deletion of the short arm of chromosome 1 is the most characteristic cytogenetic abnormality in primary human neuroblastomas and tumor-derived cell lines [7,72,73]. Most commonly, chromosome 1p deletions are seen in near-diploid neuroblastomas and cell lines, while tumors with modal chromosome numbers in the triploid range rarely have deletions or rearrangements of the

139

short arm of chromosome 1 [108]. The region most commonly deleted is between 1p32 and 1pter. This deletion is thought to represent the loss of a neuroblastoma suppressor gene [72]. In support of this hypothesis, there have been recent reports of neuroblastoma patients with germline deletions or translocations in the 1p chromosome [17,18].

Similar to the cytogenetic analyses, molecular studies using chromosome-1-specific DNA probes that identify restriction fragment length polymorphisms along the short and long arms of chromosome 1 have also shown a high incidence of 1p deletion in neuroblastoma. Fong and coworkers analyzed 45 primary neuroblastomas and reported that 13 of the 47 cases (28%) showed loss of heterozygosity (LOH) at one or more loci [109]. The common region of LOH was at the distal end of chromosome 1p from 1p36.1 to 1p36.3. Others have reported similar results [110–113]. Mutation in the critical 1p36 locus on one chromosome, followed by deletion of the same region on the homologous chromosome (manifested by LOH), may be an important mechanism in the malignant transformation or progression of neuroblastoma. Several investigators are currently mapping chromosome 1p in an effort to identify the putative neuroblastoma suppressor gene.

Several studies have demonstrated that chromosome 1p loss is strongly correlated with poor clinical outcome. In a large series reported by Maris and coworkers, 1p LOH was detected in 30 of 156 (19%) neuroblastoma tumor samples [114]. Loss of chromosome 1p was strongly associated with advanced-stage disease, elevated LDH ($>1500 IU/L$), and *MYCN* amplification. While 1p LOH was also strongly predictive of poor outcome, its prognostic value was equivocal when stratified for amplification of the *MYCN* oncogene. Others have reported similar findings [115]. However, a recent study by Caron and colleagues suggests that 1p loss has prognostic value independent of *MYCN* amplification [116]. Among patients with favorable-stage tumors that lack amplification of the *MYCN* oncogene, loss of chromosome 1p identified those in whom standard treatment was most likely to fail (three-year event-free survival, 34 ± 15%). Furthermore, outcome was significantly better for patients with advanced-stage tumors that lacked 1p deletions (three-year event-free survival, 53 ± 10%) than for those with neuroblastomas with 1p loss (three-year event-free survival, 0%).

12.7. Defects of the nerve growth factor receptor (NGFR) pathway

Nerve growth factor (NGF) is a peptide hormone required for the survival of sympathetic and sensory neurons, and its effects are mediated through a specific cell surface receptor, nerve growth factor receptor (NGFR) [117]. This peptide is known to cause differentiation of the rat pheochromocytoma cell line PC12 into cells resembling sympathetic neurons. NGF also induces neurite extension in a few receptor-positive neuroblastoma cell lines, although most neuroblastoma cell lines fail to respond [118,119]. Multiple defects in the NGFR pathway in neuroblastoma lines have been detected, including 1) absence of NGFR mRNA or protein expression, 2) expression of only a low-affinity receptor, and 3) inability of the high-affinity receptor to mediate a response to NGF. While it is possible that these defects may be involved in the maintenance of an undifferentiated phenotype, the role of the NGFR pathway in the pathogenesis of neuroblastoma remains unclear.

There are two classes of NGFRs, namely, high and low affinity [120]. The low-affinity NGFR gene encodes a transmembrane protein, which is glycosylated so that it yields a protein of about 75 kDa. No known biologic responses are mediated solely by the low-affinity receptor. The high-affinity NGF receptor, p140$^{proto-TRK}$, is encoded by the proto-oncogene TrkA. This transmembrane glycoprotein is a tyrosine kinase that is expressed selectively in the developing nervous system [121]. The biologic responsiveness to NGF depends on interactions with the high-affinity receptor [122]. Neurite extensions have been seen in primary cultures of neuroblastomas from patients with high levels of expression of both TrkA and the low-affinity NGFR after treatment with NGF [123]. In addition, prolonged survival was seen in cells treated with NGF compared to tumor cells cultured in standard medium or in NGF-depleted medium, suggesting that some neuroblastoma cells are dependent on NGF for survival and deprivation of neurotrophic factor may lead to programmed cell death. Other neuroblastomas have defects within the NGFR-pathway and are therefore not responsive to NGF nor dependent on it for survival. However, transfection of TrkA cDNA into neuroblastoma cells that are not responsive to NGF treatment is sufficient to generate a functional NGF receptor complex that leads to growth arrest and differentiation in the presence of NGF [124,125].

TrkA is expressed in a substantial number of primary neuroblastomas of all stages. However, significantly higher levels of TrkA mRNA expression are present in localized and stage 4S tumors than in advanced-stage tumors (stages 3 and 4) [123,126–128]. TrkA expression is also inversely associated with amplification of *MYCN*; extremely low levels of TrkA are observed in the vast majority of amplified tumors. The expression of TrkA is also associated with survival. Nakagawara reported a five-year cumulative-survival rate of patients with a high level of TrkA expression of 86% [123]. The survival rate for the group of patients with a low level of TrkA expression was 14%. A five-year survival rate of 87% was seen for the 62 patients who had tumors with high levels of TrkA expression and normal *MYCN* copy number. Overall survival of the four patients with tumors with normal *MYCN* copy number and low levels of TrkA expression was 50%. All 11 patients with *MYCN* amplification and low level TrkA expression died within two years after diagnosis. Although TrkA was statistically predictive of outcome in a univariate analysis, when outcome was adjusted for the effect of *MYCN* amplification, TrkA expression was no longer significant among the patients studied. Similar results have been reported by others [126–128]. Nevertheless, both *MYCN* and TrkA appear to play a role in the pathogenesis of neuroblastoma, and it is likely that they will provide complementary prognostic information.

Multidrug resistance contributes to treatment failure of a variety of cancers. Among the underlying mechanisms, the best known involves the MDR1 gene, which encodes P-glycoprotein [129]. This 170-kDa plasma membrane protein has homology to bacterial-transport proteins and is thought to cause cross-resistance to structurally unrelated anticancer drugs by functioning as an ATP-dependent drug-efflux pump of broad specificity. Although high levels of P-glycoprotein may be found in cells from many human malignant tumors, controversy exists regarding the role P-glycoprotein plays in determining the multidrug-resistance phenotype in neuroblastoma. Chan and colleagues found a strong correlation between increased expression of this protein and failure of chemotherapy in a retrospective study of sequential tumor samples from 67 children with neuroblastoma [130]. While P-glycoprotein was not detected in pretreatment samples from any child with stage I, II, or IVS disease, 1 of 17 patients with stage III disease and 12 of 19 patients with stage IV disease had tumors with P-glycoprotein expression. When outcome was stratified for age and stage, the group that was negative for P-glycoprotein had a significantly longer relapse-free survival and overall survival rate than the group that was positive. However, others have shown that P-glycoprotein is not predictive of outcome. Favrot and coworkers reported that expression of P-glycoprotein was restricted to normal cells in neuroblastoma biopsies [131], and Nakagawara and colleagues found an inverse correlation between expression of P-glycoprotein and the unfavorable prognostic factor *MYCN* amplification [132]. Similarly, no difference in either survival or event-free survival was seen with respect to the level of expression of MDR1 in a series of 60 patients with neuroblastoma reported by Norris and coworkers [133].

Another gene, the multidrug-resistance-associated protein (MRP), has been found to confer a multidrug-resistant phenotype in vitro [134,135]. The MRP gene is located on chromosome 16p13.1 [136], and encodes a 190-kd membrane-bound glycoprotein [134,137]. Like P-glycoprotein, MRP mediates resistance to a range of drugs including the vinca alkaloids, anthracyclines, and epipodophyllotoxins. High levels of MRP expression are correlated with amplification of *MYCN* in neuroblastoma [138]. In addition, downregulation of both MRP and *MYCN* is seen in neuroblastoma cell lines chemically induced to differentiate with retinoic acid, suggesting that expression of the two genes may be linked. In a recent retrospective study, Norris and colleagues reported that high levels of MRP expression are predictive of poor outcome in patients with neuroblastoma [133]. When tumors were divided into quartiles according to ascending levels of MRP expression, the cumulative rates of event-free survival for the quartiles were 93%, 87%, 72%, and 38%, respectively, indicating a correlation between increasing levels of MRP expression and the increasing risk of poor outcome. High MRP expression was also associated with a worse outcome in subsets of patients such as those with tumors without *MYCN* amplification and those with localized disease. Multivariate analysis demonstrated that MRP expression remained prognostic after adjustment for the effect of *MYCN* amplification. Although these results need to be confirmed in large prospective studies, these data suggest that MRP expression may play an important role in determining the clinical behavior of neuroblastoma. At the present time, it is not clear how MRP influences outcome in patients with neuroblastoma.

12.9. Angiogenesis

All malignant solid tumors depend on neovascularization for their progressive growth to a clinically relevant size and for metastasis [139,140]. Angiogenic factors are produced by cells in progressively growing solid tumors that directly or indirectly activate endothelial cells, stimulating them to sprout into vessels that grow toward the developing tumor [141]. The clinical outcome of adults with a variety of cancers can be predicted by the degree of tumor angiogenesis [142–146]. To date, there has been one study that suggests that vascular density may also be predictive of outcome in patients with neuroblastoma [147]. Meitar and coworkers evaluated the vascularity of neuroblastoma tumors from 50 patients by counting vessels in tumor tissue sections. In addition, tumors were classified histologically according to the criteria of Shimada, and *MYCN* copy number was determined by Southern blot analysis. Higher vascular density was strongly correlated with widely disseminated disease, *MYCN* amplification, and poor outcome. Thus, angiogenesis appears to be another important factor in determining neuroblastoma phenotype.

12.10. CD44

The cell-surface glycoprotein CD44 is the principle receptor for hyaluronate [148]. In addition, CD44 is involved in the homing process [149], cell–cell and cell–extracellular matrix interactions [150], lymphocyte activation [151], and induction of homotypic cell aggregation [152]. While overexpression of CD44 or its variants has been correlated with enhanced tumorigenicity and metastatic behavior [153,154] in breast cancer, colon cancer, and lymphoma, several studies have shown that repression of CD44 in neuroblastoma tumors is highly predictive of poor prognosis [155–158]. Recently, Combaret and colleagues analyzed CD44 expression in tumors from a cohort of 121 neuroblastoma patients treated with the same well-standardized protocols [156]. Only disease stage and CD44 expression remained statistically independent prognostic markers in a multivariate analysis of the prognostic factors stage, age, *MYCN* amplification, tumor histology, and CD44 expression. Because the assessment of CD44 expression by immunostaining is a rapid and easily standardized method, CD44 can be routinely evaluated at diagnosis. If prospective studies confirm the clinical relevance of CD44 expression, it may be useful to analyze CD44 for estimating the risk of disease recurrence in neuroblastoma patients.

13. Screening

A number of mass screening programs for neuroblastoma have been established over the past ten years, with the goal of detecting the tumors at a relatively early stage of disease. Mass screening for neuroblastoma originated in Kyoto, Japan, and since 1985 this program has become nationally supported by the Japanese Welfare Ministry [159–161]. Because most of the reports from the Japanese screening projects refer only to survival data, it is difficult to draw conclusions regarding the impact of screening on mortality. However, a recent study from Saitama Prefecture, which did provide population incidence data, demonstrated that the incidence rate for infants increased with mass screening while no corresponding decrease in the rate for children at older ages was seen [162]. Several other investigators have reported cases of fatal neuroblastoma that were not detected by the screening program [163–166], further suggesting that screening at the age of 6 months may not alter mortality.

Several population-based incidence screening programs are in progress outside of Japan in areas such the United Kingdom, France, Austria, Australia, Italy, Norway, Germany, and Canada [167–170]. To date, data from these screening studies are similar to that of Saitama Prefecture. Neuroblastoma screening before the age of 6 months is feasible, but no significant reduction in mortality has been demonstrated. Furthermore, the tumors from most of the cases diagnosed by screening have been shown to have favorable histologic and biologic features [164,171]. Several investigators have suggested that screening at a later age, such as 1 year, may lead to the early detection of poor-prognosis neuroblastomas [170,172]. The SENSE Group (Study for the Evaluation of Neuroblastoma Screening in Europe), in cooperation with the International Agency for Research on Cancer (Lyon, France), is working on an enormous scale to develop a screening program for 1-year-old children that will include an equally large control group [170,173]. Results of such a study should determine whether screening for neuroblastoma at a later age can lead to a reduction in mortality and whether it will be worthwhile to recommend screening for the general population.

14. Treatment

Because of the clinical heterogeneity of this disease, treatment of neuroblastoma is tailored for the age of the patient, stage of disease, and biology of the tumor. At the present time, most cooperative groups utilize a variety of clinical and biologic factors to define risk groups, and treatment is determined accordingly. Although these risk groups currently differ somewhat among various cooperative groups around the world, there is general agreement that patients with localized disease can be cured with minimal therapy, whereas children over 1 year of age with widely disseminated disease require intensive, multimodality therapy to achieve remission. Efforts are ongoing in the POG and CCG to unify the criteria for each neuroblastoma risk group so that intergroup clinical trials can be conducted.

14.1. Localized neuroblastoma (all ages)

The treatment of localized tumors is primarily surgical [1,174]. For all age groups, surgery alone has been shown to be effective therapy for patients with completely resected neuroblastomas in whom regional lymph nodes are free of tumor. Furthermore, Matthay and coworkers found no significant difference in outcome between 40 patients with gross or microscopic residual disease treated with surgery alone and 59 patients with residual disease who also received radiation [2]. Although most patients had 10% or less gross residual disease, these data suggest that surgery alone, even if complete resection is not achieved, is sufficient therapy for most patients with localized neuroblastomas. Similarly, De Bernardi and coworkers reported overall survival and event-free survival rates of 94% and 90%, respectively, for patients with completely resected localized tumors (stage 1) treated with surgery alone [175]. Patients with minimal residual tumor and/or tumor infiltration of regional lymph nodes and/or tumor rupture were classified as stage 2. Stage 2 patients less than 12 months of age and older children with negative lymph nodes and no tumor rupture received no adjuvant therapy. This group had a 96% overall survival rate and 85% event-free survival rate. Stage 2 patients over the age of 12 months with positive lymph nodes and/or tumor rupture received adjuvant chemotherapy for 6 months. An 87% overall survival rate and a 61% event-free survival rate was achieved in this high-risk subset of stage 2 patients, indicating that this group of patients may require more intensive adjuvant therapy.

Although others have also suggested that the presence of tumor infiltration of regional lymph nodes is associated with a worse prognosis [54,176], the prognostic value of positive lymph nodes remains controversial. In a series of 22 patients with INSS 2A, 2B, 3, and 4S disease, Kushner and coworkers reported that neuroblastoma in lymph nodes had no prognostic significance [177]. Regardless of stage, cytotoxic therapy was not given initially to any of the patients in this study. Six of the 22 patients developed recurrent or enlarging tumors; two regressed spontaneously, and four were excised 5 to 39 months after diagnosis. Only one patient received adjuvant chemotherapy. All the tumors lacked *MYCN* amplification, and all 22 patients remain alive 24 to 98 months from diagnosis. Although this is a small study from a single institution, it appears that a subset of patients with regional disease can be successfully treated with surgery alone even when regional lymph nodes are involved. If these results are confirmed in a large prospective study, it may be possible to avoid the acute and long-term sequelae of cytotoxic therapy in the subset of patients with non-stage 4 favorable biology neuroblastomas.

14.2. Stage 4S neuroblastoma (infants ≤ 12 months)

Infants with this special stage of neuroblastoma often undergo spontaneous regression of their tumors, and these patients have a survival of 75% to 90% [4–6]. Many of these patients may be treated with supportive care only, without cytotoxic therapy [178]. However, infants younger than 6 weeks at diagnosis are at higher risk of death due to respiratory complications from hepatic enlargement. In young infants, therapy should be directed toward control of the symptoms caused by the tumor through the use of either low-dose chemotherapy or limited hepatic irradiation. Rarely, *MYCN* amplification is detected in the tumors of patients who present clinically with stage 4S disease [179]. In most cases, these amplified tumors are clinically aggressive, and the patients have a poor outcome despite treatment with adjuvant chemotherapy.

14.3. Regional and disseminated disease (infants ≤ 12 months)

It is well known that infants with regional and disseminated disease have a significantly better response to chemotherapy than older children with metastatic disease [3,4]. In an effort to further tailor therapy for this subset of patients, the POG conducted a clinical trial, which began in 1987, in which therapy was based on the DNA index of the tumor. All infants with unresectable hyperdiploid tumors were initially treated with low-dose oral cyclophosphamide and adriamycin [180]. Outcome for this group of patients was excellent, with three-year survival estimates of more than 90%. There were four patients with hyperdiploid tumors and *MYCN* amplification, three of whom developed progressive disease and died. Infants with unresectable diploid tumors were treated with cisplatin and teniposide because previous studies had demonstrated that diploid tumors are not responsive to low-dose oral cyclophosphamide and doxorubicin [101]. The actuarial three-year survival estimate for this subset of patients was 55% ± 8%. Only 1 of 9 infants with *MYCN*-amplified diploid tumors was alive at the time of the report, whereas 14 of 20 infants with diploid tumors that lacked *MYCN* amplification were alive. Based on these results, only infants with hyperdiploid neuroblastomas with normal *MYCN* copy number were treated with cyclophosphamide and adriamycin in the subsequent POG clinical trial. In an effort to improve survival in infants with unfavorable biology tumors, all infants with *MYCN*-amplified and/or diploid tumors were treated more intensively with alternating cycles of carboplatin/etoposide and ifosfamide/etoposide. Early results of this trial show excellent response rates to this treatment.

14.4. Regional disease (patients >1 year)

The outlook for children with extensive local and regional neuroblastoma is better than that of children with distant metastatic disease. Clinical trials from the 1970s and early 1980s have demonstrated that some children older than 1 year with Evans stage III neuroblastoma can be cured with surgery and moderately intensive chemotherapy. Evans and coworkers reported a 44% disease-free survival rate using a combination of vincristine and cyclophosphamide, and a nearly 50% disease-free survival with the addition of imidazolecarboxamide [181,182]. Using more intensive chemotherapy, surgery, and radiation, West and colleagues recently reported a 72% event-free survival (median follow-up of 85 months) for 25 patients with Evans stage III disease over the age of 1 year [183]. In that study, children with favorable histology tumors according to the criteria of Shimada had a better prognosis than those with unfavorable histologic features. *MYCN* copy number was analyzed in 16 tumors, and amplification was associated with a poor outcome: 4 of the 6 with *MYCN* amplified neuroblastomas relapsed. One of the two patients who remain disease-free had a tumor with favorable histologic features. Castleberry and colleagues reported a three-year survival rate of 72% for patients over the age of 1 with stage C disease treated with chemotherapy, radiation, and surgery [184]. Patients who did not receive radiation achieved only a 46% complete response rate. Thus, in this study, radiation therapy clearly improved outcome. However, it is not clear whether more aggressive multidrug chemotherapy would blunt the efficacy of radiation. A large randomized prospective clinical trial will need to be performed to answer this question.

14.5. Disseminated disease (patients >1 year)

The long-term outcome of children over 1 year of age with stage 4 neuroblastoma remains dismal, with survival rates ranging from less than 10% to 30% [185,186]. Improved response rates and survival have been seen with increased dose intensity of the most active agents, such as cisplatin, carboplatin, etoposide, doxorubicin, cyclophosphamide, and ifosfamide [187–190]. In addition, aggressive surgical approaches have also been shown to improve patient outcome when used in combination with intensive chemotherapy capable of inducing effective responses at primary and metastatic sites [191]. However, even though more than 80% of children achieve complete or partial response to modern multimodality therapy, more than half of these patients will recur within the first two years of treatment [187,190,192].

The dose-responsiveness of neuroblastoma provided the rationale for the use of myeloablative treatment with bone marrow transplantation for consolidating remission status. Using this approach, some studies have shown improved progression-free survival rates compared to historical controls [186,193–203]. Table 5 lists the results of several clinical trials in which autologous bone marrow transplantation was used as consolidation therapy in children older than 1 year of age with stage 4 neuroblastoma. Many of the studies must be interpreted with caution because only those patients who achieved a good response to induction chemotherapy were included, the patient number is small, and the follow-up is short. However, the LCME1 study included an

Table 5. Clinical trials using autologous bone marrow transplantation as consolidation therapy in metastatic neuroblastoma

Series (ref.)	Patient no.	PFS	Regimen	Bone marrow purging
CCG (197)	46	40% @ 4 years	VAMP, TBI	Yes
AIEOP (198)	53	29% @ 5 years	VAMP, TBI	No
MSKCC (202)	28	6% @ 2 years	MLP, TBI	Yes
LMCE (186)	62	39% @ 2 years 20% @ 5 years 13% @ 7 years	VCR, MLP, TBI	Yes
LMCE (199)	17	50% @ 2 years	Double graft	Yes
French Multicenter (200)	33	40% @ 2 years	MLP, VM26, BCNU	Yes
POG (194)	54	CR1: 32% @ 2 years PR1: 43% @ 2 years	MLP, TBI	Yes
Australia (203)	17	94% @ 2 years 87% @ 5 years	VAMP, TBI	No

Abbreviations: No., number; PFS, progression-free survival; VAMP, teniposide, doxorubicin, melphalan, cisplatin; TBI, total body irradiation; MLP, melphalan; VCR, vincristine; CR1, first complete remission; PR1, first partial remission.

unselected group of patients, and the strategy for megatherapy and autologous bone marrow transplant purging was constant over a six-year period [186]. Progression-free survival for the 62 patients who were transplanted in this trial was 39% at two years, 20% at four years, and 13% at seven years. Interestingly, patients who had healing bone metastases before bone marrow transplant had a 30% progression-free survival at five years, suggesting that there is a subgroup of patients who may achieve long-term remission with megatherapy followed by autologous bone marrow transplant.

At the present time, it is not clear if the source of stem cells will affect outcome. Allogeneic bone marrow transplant does not appear to offer any significant survival advantage compared to autologous bone marrow transplant [204,205]. Recently, autologous peripheral blood stem cells (PBSCs) have been used to rescue neuroblastoma patients in lieu of bone marrow stem cells [206,207]. This approach has several advantages over autologous bone marrow stem cell transplant: 1) general anesthesia is not required, 2) there is less discomfort for the patient, and 3) hematopoietic recovery occurs more rapidly. The average length of hospital stay for a patient undergoing PBSC transplant is 22 days compared to 29 days for unpurged marrow transplants and 34 days for purged marrow transplants (personal communication, Dr. Morris Kletzel).

Two studies comparing outcome after megatherapy followed by autologous bone marrow to a concomitant group of children treated with chemotherapy only did not show significant differences in overall progression-free survival [192,208]. Furthermore, myeloablative regimens have not improved the outcome of patients with refractory or gross disease, and have only rarely resulted in long-term survival of patients in second remission [194,195,209]. Thus, at the present time, the impact of myeloablative treatments on the cure rate of patients with high-risk neuroblastoma remains uncertain. CCG is currently conducting a prospective, randomized clinical trial comparing myeloablative therapy followed by autologous bone marrow transplantation to conventional intensive chemotherapy. Results from this trial should determine the relative efficacy of these two approaches. Other issues that remain to be resolved include the clinical significance of residual neuroblastoma in bone marrow or peripheral stem cell harvests and the efficacy of purging [207,210–215].

15. Novel treatment approaches

As mentioned in the previous section, more than 50% of high-risk neuroblastoma patients will develop tumor recurrence after achieving a complete or partial response to intensive multimodality therapy. Thus, alternative therapeutic strategies are desperately needed for this subset of patients. Targeted radiotherapy, immunotherapy, and biological response modifiers are promising novel treatments for neuroblastoma.

15.1. MIBG treatment

MIBG, a guanethidine analogue, was initially developed as an adrenal-medullary imaging agent with ^{131}I radiolabeling. The agent is bound at the cell membrane and, in the majority of neuroblastoma tumors, is actively transported into cells, providing the opportunity for selective high levels of radiation of both primary and metastatic disease [216,217]. Initial studies demonstrated activity of ^{131}I MIBG in heavily pretreated neuroblastoma patients with refractory or relapsed disease [217–223]. More recently, promising results have been seen in clinical trials that have incorporated ^{131}I MIBG in treatment regimens of newly diagnosed patients [217,224]. De Kraker and colleagues used ^{131}I MIBG as first-line therapy for 31 stage 4 patients with unresectable primary neuroblastomas [225]. After treatment, 70% of the evaluable patients either had a complete response to treatment and did not require surgery or were able to undergo more than 95% resection of their primary tumor.

[131]I MIBG has also been used in combination with hyperbaric oxygen. This approach is based on the finding that oxygen possesses the highest enhancement ratio for radiation [226]. Several investigators have shown that hyperbaric oxygen increases tumor oxygenation [227,228] and decreases radioresistance in tumors [227,229]. Voute and coworkers used the combination of ^{131}I MIBG and hyperbaric oxygen in 27 heavily pretreated neuroblastoma patients [226]. Remarkably, the estimated survival of this very unfavorable group of patients was 32% with 28 months follow-up. Because there is heterogeneity of uptake among tumor sites in the same patient

[230,231], it is unlikely that ^{131}I MIBG will be curative as a single agent. However, this treatment modality may prove to be effective in combination with other treatment modalities.

15.2. Pentetreotide

Pentetreotide is an eight-amino-acid peptide analogue of the neuropeptide somatostatin. Pentetreotide is bound by high-affinity somatostatin receptors on the surface of tumor cell membranes including neuroblastoma, and ^{111}In-pentetreotide has been used for tumor imaging. It has been suggested that radiolabeled pentetreotide may be useful in the treatment of neuroblastoma [232], although to date this has not been demonstrated.

15.3. Monoclonal antibodies

Monoclonal antibodies to the GD2 ganglioside have been used in phase I clinical trials with neuroblastoma patients [233–236], and variable responses have been observed. Cheung and colleagues conducted a phase II trial in which 16 stage IV neuroblastoma patients were treated with the 3F8 mono-clonal antibody daily for five days per cycle [237]. Although 10 patients developed progressive disease, responses were observed in five patients. To enhance these promising responses, cytokines such as granulocyte-macrophage colony-stimulating factor and interleukin-2 (IL-2) are being administered in combination with the monoclonal antibodies to further stimulate host immune response [238]. Concerns remain about the development of antimouse or anti-idiotype responses.

15.4. Immunotherapy

In general, neuroblastoma cells are resistant to cytotoxic T lymphocytes, but sensitive to killing by natural killer (NK) cells [239]. This cytotoxicity can be further augmented in vitro with IL-2 or interferon γ. In a Lyon–Marseille–Curie–East of France Group Study, high-dose recombinant IL-2 was administered to neuroblastoma patients achieving only partial remission after induction chemotherapy [240]. Although antitumor response was observed in 3 of 15 evaluable patients, a survival advantage was not seen with this therapy in the posttransplant setting. Similar results have been reported in other studies using IL-2, interferon γ, or lymphokine-activated killer cells [241–244].

15.5. Retinoic acid

Retinoic acid is known to inhibit neuroblastoma growth and induce differentiation in vitro. In clinical trials, objective responses have been observed with this agent in some children with recurrent neuroblastoma [245–247]. Because retinoic acid may be most effective in cases without bulky disease, CCG is conducting a randomized phase III trial of retinoic acid in the setting of minimal residual disease, following bone marrow transplant.

15.6. Future therapies

The identification of biologic prognostic factors has greatly facilitated the rational choice of therapies for individual patients. Low-risk patients are currently treated with minimal therapy and thus are spared the toxic effects of high-dose chemotherapy and radiation. However, effective therapy is still needed for high-risk patients. It is likely that future laboratory investigations will lead to the development of effective biology-based treatment for this subset of neuroblastoma patients. Hopefully, treatment regimens that include anti-angiogenic drugs, agents that reverse the drug-resistant phenotype, gene therapy, or other biologic techniques will result in improved survival of high-risk neuroblastoma patients.

References

1. Nitschke R, Smith EI, Shochat S, et al. 1988. Localized neuroblastoma treated by surgery: a Pediatric Oncology Group Study. J Clin Oncol 6:1271–1279.
2. Matthay KK, Sather HN, Seeger RC, Haase GM, Hammond GD. 1989. Excellent outcome of stage II neuroblastoma is independent of residual disease and radiation therapy. J Clin Oncol 7:236–244.
3. Look AT, Hayes FA, Shuster JJ, et al. 1991. Clinical relevance of tumor cell ploidy and N-myc gene amplification in childhood neuroblastoma: a Pediatric Oncology Group study. J Clin Oncol 9:581–591.
4. Evans AE, D'Angio GJ, Randolph J. 1971. A proposed staging for children with neuroblastoma. Children's Cancer Study Group A. Cancer 27:374–378.
5. Evans AE, Gerson J, Schnaufer L. 1976. Spontaneous regression of neuroblastoma. Natl Cancer Inst Monogr 44:49–54.
6. D'Angio GJ, Evans AE, Koop CE. 1971. Special pattern of widespread neuroblastoma with a favourable prognosis. Lancet 1:1046–1049.
7. Brodeur GM, Azar C, Brother M, et al. 1992. Neuroblastoma. Effect of genetic factors on prognosis and treatment. Cancer 70:1685–1694.
8. Young JL, Jr., Miller RW. 1975. Incidence of malignant tumors in U.S. children. J Pediatr 86:254–258.
9. Perkins DG, Koop CM, Haust MD. 1980. Placental infiltration in congenital neuroblastoma. Histopathology 4:383.
10. Lopez R, Karakousis C, Rad U. 1980. Treatment of adult neuroblastoma. Cancer 45:840.
11. Bunin GR, Ward E, Kramer S, Rhee CA, Meadows AT. 1990. Neuroblastoma and parental occupation. Am J Epidemiol 131:776–780.
12. Kramer S, Ward E, Meadows AT, Malone KE. 1987. Medical and drug risk factors associated with neuroblastoma: a case–control study. J Natl Cancer Inst 78:797–804.
13. Kinney H, Faix R, Brazy J. 1980. The fetal alcohol syndrome and neuroblastoma. Pediatrics 66:130–132.
14. Kushner BH, Hajdu SI, Helson L. 1985. Synchronous neuroblastoma and von Recklinghausen's disease: a review of the literature. J Clin Oncol 3:117–120.
15. Carachi R, Auldist AW, Chow CW. 1982. Neuroblastoma and Hirschsprung's disease. Z Kinderchir 35:24–25.

16. Kushner BH, Gilbert F, Helson L. 1986. Familial neuroblastoma. Case reports, literature review, and etiologic considerations. Cancer 57:1887–1893.

17. Laureys G, Speleman F, Opdenakker G, Benoit Y, Leroy J. 1990. Constitutional translocation t(1;17)(p36;q12–21) in a patient with neuroblastoma. Genes Chromosomes Cancer 2:252–254.

18. Biegel JA, White PS, Marshall HN, et al. 1993. Constitutional 1p36 deletion in a child with neuroblastoma. Am J Hum Genet 52:176–182.

19. Bronner-Fraser M. 1995. Origins and developmental potential of the neural crest. Exp Cell Biol 218:405–417.

20. Landau M. 1912. Die maligne neuroblastoma des sympathicus, frank. Z Pathol 11:26.

21. Ambros IM, Zellner A, Roald B, et al. 1996. Role of ploidy, chromosome 1p, and Schwann cells in the maturation of neuroblastoma. N Engl J Med 334:1505–1511.

22. Lopez-Ibor B, Schwartz AD. 1985. Neuroblastoma. Pediatr Clin North Am 32:755–778.

23. Voute PA. 1984. Neuroblastoma. In Sutow WW, Fernbach DJ, Vietti TJ (eds.). Clinical Pediatric Oncology. St. Louis: The C.V. Mosby Company, pp. 559–587.

24. Gonzalez-Crussi F, Hsueh W. 1988. Bilateral adrenal ganglioneuroblastoma with neuromelanin. Clinical and pathologic observations. Cancer 61:1159–1166.

25. Broduer GM, Castelberry RP. 1993. Neuroblastoma. In Pizzo PA, Poplack DG (eds.). Principles and Practice of Pediatric Oncology. J.B. Lippincott Co., pp. 739–767.

26. Hayes FA, Thompson EI, Hvizdala E, O'Connor D, Green AA. 1984. Chemotherapy as an alternative to laminectomy and radiation in the management of epidural tumor. J Pediatr 104:221–224.

27. van der Slikke JW, Balk AG. 1980. Hydramnios and hydrops fetalis and disseminated fetal neuroblastoma. Obstet Gynecol 55:250.

28. Weinblatt ME, Heisel MA, Siegel SE. 1983. Hypertension in children with neurogenic tumors. Pediatrics 71:947–951.

29. Mitchell CH, Sinatra FR, Crast FW, Griffin R, Sunshine P. 1976. Intractable watery diarrhea, ganglioneuroblastoma, and vasoactive intestinal peptide. J Pediatr 89:593–595.

30. Mendelsohn G, Eggleston JC, Olson JL, Said SI, Baylin SB. 1979. Vasoactive intestinal peptide and its relationship to ganglion cell differentiation in neuroblastic tumors. Lab Invest 41:144–149.

31. Altman AJ, Baehner RL. 1976. Favorable prognosis for survival in children with coincident opso-myoclonus and neuroblastoma. Cancer 37:846–852.

32. Cohn SL, Salwen H, Herst CV, et al. 1988. Single copies of the N-*myc* oncogene in neuroblastomas from children presenting with the syndrome of opsoclonus–myoclonus. Cancer 62:723–726.

33. Koh PS, Raffensperger JG, Berry S, et al. 1994. Long-term outcome in children with opsoclonus–myoclonus and ataxia and coincident neuroblastoma. J Pediatr 125:712–716.

34. Nickerson BG, Hutter JJ. 1979. Opsoclonus and neuroblastoma: response to ACTH. Clin Pediatr 18:446–448.

35. Petruzzi MJ, de Alarcon PA. 1995. Neuroblastoma-associated opsoclonus–myoclonus treated with intravenously administered immune globulin G. J Pediatr 127:328–329.

36. Telander RL, Smithson WA, Groover RV. 1989. Clinical outcome in children with acute cerebellar encephalopathy and neuroblastoma. J Pediatr Surg 24:11–14.

37. Mitchell WG, Snodgrass SR. 1990. Opsoclonus–ataxia due to childhood neural crest tumors: a chronic neurologic syndrome. J Child Neurol 5:153–158.

38. Pranzatelli MR. 1992. The neurobiology of the opsoclonus–myoclonus syndrome. Clin Neuropharmacol 15:186–228.

39. Ziter FA, Brav PF, Cancilla PA. 1979. Neuropathologic findings in a patient with neuroblastoma and myoclonic encephalopathy. Arch Neurol 36:51.

40. Donner L, Triche TJ, Israel MA, Seeger RC, Reynolds CP. 1985. A panel of monoclonal antibodies which discriminate neuroblastoma from Ewing's sarcoma, rhabdomyosarcoma, neuroepithelioma, and hematopoietic malignancies. Prog Clin Biol Res 175:347–366.

41. Israel MA, Thiele C, Whang-Peng J, Kao-Shan CS, Triche TJ, Miser J. 1985. Peripheral neuroepithelioma: genetic analysis of tumor derived cell lines. Prog Clin Biol Res 175:161–170.

42. Triche TJ, Askin FB. 1983. Neuroblastoma and the differential diagnosis of small-, round-, blue-cell tumors. Hum Pathol 14:569–595.

43. Whang-Peng J, Triche TJ, Knutsen T, Miser J, Douglass EC, Israel MA. 1984. Chromosome translocation in peripheral neuroepithelioma. N Engl J Med 311:584–585.

44. Triche TJ. 1982. Round cell tumors in childhood: the application of newer techniques to the differential diagnosis. Persp Pediatr Pathol 7:279–322.

45. Biegel JA, Nycum LM, Valentine V, Barr FG, Shapiro DN. 1995. Detection of the t(2;13)(q35;q14) and PAX3-FKHR fusion in alveolar rhabdomyosarcoma by fluorescence in situ hybridization. Genes Chromosomes Cancer 12:186–192.

46. Shapiro DN, Sublett JE, Li B, Downing JR, Naeve CW. 1993. Fusion of PAX3 to a member of the forkhead family of transcription factors in human alveolar rhabdomyosarcoma. Cancer Res 53:5108–5112.

47. Douglass EC, Shapiro DN, Valentine M, et al. 1993. Alveolar rhabdomyosarcoma with the t(2;13): cytogenetic findings and clinicopathologic correlations. Med Pediatr Oncol 21:83–87.

48. Brodeur GM, Pritchard J, Berthold F, et al. 1993. Revisions of the international criteria for neuroblastoma diagnosis, staging, and response to treatment. J Clin Oncol 11:1466–1477.

49. Bertani-Dziedzic L, Dziedzic SW, Gitlow SE. 1990. Catecholamine metabolism in neuroblastoma. In Pochedly C (ed.). Neuroblastoma: Tumor Biology and Therapy. Boca Raton: CRC, pp. 69–91.

50. Evans AE, D'Angio GJ, Propert K, Anderson J, Hann HL. 1987. Prognostic factors in neuroblastoma. Cancer 59:1853–1859.

51. Heisel MA, Miller JH, Reid BS, Siegel SE. 1983. Radionuclide bone scan in neuroblastoma. Pediatrics 71:206–209.

52. Gordon I, Peters AM, Gutman A, Morony S, Dicks-Mireaux C, Pritchard J. 1990. Skeletal assessment in neuroblastoma—the pitfalls of iodine-123-MIBG scans. J Nucl Med 31:129–134.

53. Smith EI, Castelberry RP. 1990. Neuroblastoma. Curr Prob Surg 27:573–620.

54. Hayes FA, Green A, Hustu HO, Kumar M. 1983. Surgicopathologic staging of neuroblastoma: prognostic significance of regional lymph node metastases. J Pediatr 102:59–62.

55. American Joint Committee on Cancer. 1983. Neuroblastoma. Manual for Staging of Cancer. Philadelphia: J.B. Lippincott, p. 237.

56. Brodeur GM, Seeger RC, Barrett A, et al. 1988. International criteria for diagnosis, staging, and response to treatment in patients with neuroblastoma. J Clin Oncol 6:1874–1881.

57. Castleberry RP, Shuster JJ, Smith EI, Member Institutions of Pediatric Oncology Group. 1994. The Pediatric Oncology Group experience with the International Staging System criteria for neuroblastoma. J Clin Oncol 12:2378-2381.

58. Haase GM, Atkinson JB, Stram DO, Lukens JN, Matthay KK. 1995. Surgical management and outcome of locoregional neuroblastoma: comparison of the Childrens Cancer Group and the international staging systems. J Pediatr Surg 30:289–294.

59. Breslow N, McCann B. 1971. Statistical estimation of prognosis for children with neuroblastoma. Cancer Res 31:2098–2103.

60. Seeger RC, Brodeur GM, Sather H, et al. 1985. Association of multiple copies of the N-*myc* oncogene with repid progression of neuroblastomas. N Engl J Med 313:1111–1116.

61. Philip T. 1992. Overview of current treatment of neuroblastoma. Am J Pediatr Hematol Oncol 14:97–102.

62. Finklestein JZ, Klemperer MR, Evans A, et al. 1979. Multiagent chemotherapy for children with metastatic neuroblastoma: a report from Childrens Cancer Study Group. Med Pediatr Oncol 6:179–188.

63. Hann HW, Levy HM, Evans AE. 1980. Serum ferritin as a guide to therapy in neuroblastoma. Cancer Res 40:1411–1413.

64. Quinn JJ, Altman AJ, Frantz CN. 1980. Serum lactic dehydrogenase, an indicator of tumor activity in neuroblastoma. J Pediatr 97:89–91.
65. Zeltzer PM, Marangos PJ, Parma AM, et al. 1983. Raised neuron-specific enolase in serum of children with metastatic neuroblastoma. A report from the Children's Cancer Study Group. Lancet 2:361–363.
66. Zeltzer PM, Marangos PJ, Sather H, et al. 1985. Prognostic importance of serum neuron specific enolase in local and widespread neuroblastoma. Prog Clin Biol Res 175:319–329.
67. Shimada H, Chatten J, Newton WA Jr, et al. 1984. Histopathologic prognostic factors in neuroblastic tumors: definition of subtypes of ganglioneuroblastoma and an age-linked classification of neuroblastomas. J Natl Cancer Inst 73:405–416.
68. Joshi VV, Cantor AB, Altshuler G, et al. 1992. Recommendations for modification of terminology of neuroblastic tumors and prognostic significance of Shimada classification. A clinicopathologic study of 213 cases from the Pediatric Oncology Group. Cancer 69:2183–2196.
69. Joshi VV, Cantor AB, Altshuler G, et al. 1992. Age-linked prognostic categorization based on a new histologic grading system of neuroblastomas. A clinicopathologic study of 211 cases from the Pediatric Oncology Group. Cancer 69:2197–2211.
70. Shimada H, Stram DO, Chatten J, et al. 1995. Identification of subsets of neuroblastomas by combined histopathologic and N-*myc* analysis. J Natl Cancer Inst 87:1470–1476.
71. Cohn SL, Rademaker AW, Salwen HR, et al. 1990. Analysis of DNA ploidy and proliferative activity in relation to histology and N-*myc* amplification in neuroblastoma. Am J Pathol 136:1043–1052.
72. Brodeur GM, Fong CT. 1989. Molecular biology and genetics of human neuroblastoma. Cancer Genet Cytogenet 41:153–174.
73. Brodeur GM, Green AA, Hayes FA, Williams KJ, Williams DL, Tsiatis AA. 1981. Cytogenetic features of human neuroblastomas and cell lines. Cancer Res 41:4678–4686.
74. Schwab M, Alitalo K, Klempnauer KH, et al. 1983. Amplified DNA with limited homology to *myc* cellular oncogene is shared by human neuroblastoma cell lines and a neuroblastoma tumour. Nature 305:245–248.
75. Human gene mapping. London Conference, 1991. Eleventh International Workshop on Human Gene Mapping. Cytogenet Cell Genet 58:1–984.
76. Schwab M, Varmus HE, Bishop JM, et al. 1984. Chromosome localization in normal human cells and neuroblastomas of a gene related to c-*myc*. Nature 308:288–291.
77. Kohl NE, Kanda N, Schreck RR, et al. 1983. Transposition and amplification of oncogene-related sequences in human neuroblastomas. Cell 35:359–367.
78. Brodeur GM, Seeger RC, Schwab M, Varmus HE, Bishop JM. 1984. Amplification of N-*myc* in untreated human neuroblastomas correlates with advanced disease stage. Science 224:1121–1124.
79. Brodeur GM, Hayes FA, Green AA, et al. 1987. Consistent N-*myc* copy number in simultaneous or consecutive neuroblastoma samples from sixty individual patients. Cancer Res 47:4248–4253.
80. Schweigerer L, Breit S, Wenzel A, Tsunamoto K, Ludwig R, Schwab M. 1990. Augmented *MYCN* expression advances the malignant phenotype of human neuroblastoma cells: evidence for induction of autocrine growth factor activity. Cancer Res 50:4411–4416.
81. Bernards R, Dessain SK, Weinberg RA. 1986. N-*myc* amplification causes down-modulation of MHC class I antigen expression in neuroblastoma. Cell 47:667–674.
82. Schmidt ML, Salwen HR, Manohar CF, Ikegaki N, Cohn SL. 1994. The biologic effects of antisense N-*myc* expression in human neuroblastoma. Cell Growth Differ 5:171–178.
83. Negroni A, Scarpa S, Romeo A, Ferrari S, Modesti A, Raschella G. 1991. Decrease of proliferation rate and induction of differentiation by a *MYCN* antisense DNA oligomer in a human neuroblastoma cell line. Cell Growth Differ 2:511–518.
84. Whitesell L, Rosolen A, Neckers LM. 1991. Episome-generated N-*myc* antisense RNA restricts the differentiation potential of primitive neuroectodermal cell lines. Mol Cell Biol 11:1360–1371.

154

85. Thiele CJ, Reynolds CP, Israel MA. 1985. Decreased expression of N-*myc* precedes retinoic acid-induced morphological differentiation of human neuroblastoma. Nature 313:404–406.

86. Thiele CJ, Israel MA. 1988. Regulation of N-*myc* expression is a critical event controlling the ability of human neuroblasts to differentiate. Exp Cell Biol 56:321–333.

87. Ikegaki N, Bukovsky J, Kennett RH. 1986. Identification and characterization of the N-*myc* gene product in human neuroblastoma cells by monoclonal antibodies with defined specificities. Proc Natl Acad Sci USA 83:5929–5933.

88. Blackwood EM, Eisenman RN. 1991. Max: a helix-loop-helix zipper protein that forms a sequence-specific DNA-binding complex with Myc. Science 251:1211–1217.

89. Blackwell TK, Kretzner L, Blackwood EM, Eisenman RN, Weintraub H. 1990. Sequence-specific DNA binding by the c-Myc protein. Science 250:1149–1151.

90. Schneider SS, Hiemstra JL, Zehnbauer BA, et al. 1992. Isolation and structural analysis of a 1.2-megabase N-*myc* amplicon from a human neuroblastoma. Mol Cell Biol 12:5563–5570.

91. Manohar CF, Salwen HR, Brodeur GM, Cohn SL. 1995. Co-amplification and concomitant high levels of expression of a DEAD box gene with *MYCN* in human neuroblastoma. Genes Chromosomes Cancer 14:196–203.

92. Squire JA, Thorner PS, Weitzman S, et al. 1995. Co-amplification of *MYCN* and a DEAD box gene (*DDX1*) in primary neuroblastoma. Oncogene 10:1417–1422.

93. George RE, Kenyon RM, McGuckin AG, et al. 1996. Investigation of co-amplification of the candidate genes ornithine decarboxylase, ribonucleotide reductase, syndecan-1 and a DEAD box gene, *DDX1*, with N-*myc* in neuroblastoma. Oncogene 12:1583–1587.

94. Schmid SR, Linder P. 1992. D-E-A-D protein family of putative RNA helicases. Mol Microbiol 6(3):283–291.

95. Cohn SL, Look AT, Joshi VV, et al. 1995. Lack of correlation of N-*myc* gene amplification with prognosis in localized neuroblastoma: a Pediatric Oncology Group Study. Cancer Res 55:721–726.

96. Fabbretti G, Valenti C, Loda M, et al. 1993. N-*myc* gene amplification/expression in localized stroma-rich neuroblastoma (ganglioneuroblastoma). Hum Pathol 24:294–297.

97. Nisen PD, Waber PG, Rich MA, et al. 1988. N-*myc* oncogene RNA expression in neuroblastoma. J Natl Cancer Inst 80:1633–1637.

98. Slavc I, Ellenbogen R, Jung WH, et al. 1990. *myc* gene amplification and expression in primary human neuroblastoma. Cancer Res 50:1459–1463.

99. Grady-Leopardi EF, Schwab M, Ablin AR, Rosenau W. 1986. Detection of N-*myc* oncogene expression in human neuroblastoma by in situ hybridization and blot analysis: relationship to clinical outcome. Cancer Res 46:3196–3199.

100. Shapiro DN, Valentine MB, Rowe ST, et al. 1993. Detection of N-*myc* gene amplification by fluorescence in situ hybridization. Diagnostic utility for neuroblastoma. Am J Pathol 142:1339–1346.

101. Look AT, Hayes FA, Nitschke R, McWilliams NB, Green AA. 1984. Cellular DNA content as a predictor of response to chemotherapy in infants with unresectable neuroblastoma. N Engl J Med 311:231–235.

102. Taylor SR, Locker J. 1990. A comparative analysis of nuclear DNA content and N-*myc* gene amplification in neuroblastoma. Cancer 65:1360–1366.

103. Oppedal BR, Storm-Mathisen I, Lie SO, Brandtzaeg P. 1988. Prognostic factors in neuroblastoma. Clinical, histopathologic, and immunohistochemical features and DNA ploidy in relation to prognosis. Cancer 62:722–780.

104. Taylor SR, Blatt J, Costantino JP, Roederer M, Murphy RF. 1988. Flow cytometric DNA analysis of neuroblastoma and ganglioneuroma. A 10-year retrospective study. Cancer 62:749–754.

105. Gansler T, Chatten J, Varello M, Bunin GR, Atkinson B. 1986. Flow cytometric DNA analysis of neuroblastoma. Correlation with histology and clinical outcome. Cancer 58:2453–2458.

106. Bourhis J, DeVathaire F, Wilson GD, et al. 1991. Combined analysis of DNA ploidy index and N-*myc* genomic content in enuroblastoma. Cancer Res 51:33–36.

155

107. Oppedal BR, Oien O, Jahnsen T, Brandtzaeg P. 1989. N-*myc* amplification in neuoblastomas: histopathological, NDA ploidy, and clinical variables. J Clin Pathol 42:1148–1152.

108. Kaneko Y, Kanda N, Maseki N, et al. 1987. Different karyotypic patterns in early and advanced stage neuroblastomas. Cancer Res 47:311–318.

109. Fong CT, Dracopoli NC, White PS, et al. 1989. Loss of heterozygosity for the short arm of chromosome 1 in human neuroblastomas: correlation with N-*myc* amplification. Proc Natl Acad Sci USA 86:3753–3757.

110. Weith A, Martinsson T, Cziepluch C, et al. 1989. Neuroblastoma Consensus deletion maps to 1p36.1–2. Genes Chromosomes Cancer 1:159–166.

111. Takeda O, Homma C, Maseki N, et al. 1994. There may be two tumor suppressor genes on chromosome arm 1p closely associated with biologically distinct subtypes of neuroblastoma. Genes Chromosomes Cancer 10:30–39.

112. Schleiermacher G, Peter M, Michon J, et al. 1994. Two distinct deleted regions on the short arm of chromosome 1 in neuroblastoma. Genes Chromosomes Cancer 10:275–281.

113. White PS, Maris JM, Beltinger C, et al. 1995. A region of consistent deletion in neuroblastoma maps within human chromosome 1p36.2–36.3 Proc Natl Acad Sci USA 92:5520–5524.

114. Maris JM, White PS, Beltinger CP, et al. 1995. Significance of chromosome 1p loss of heterozygosity in neuroblastoma. Cancer Res 55:4664–4669.

115. Gehring M, Berthold F, Edler L, Schwab M, Amler LC. 1995. The 1p deletion is not a reliable marker for the prognosis of patients with neuroblastoma. Cancer Res 55:5366–5369.

116. Caron H, van Sluis P, de Kraker J, et al. 1996. Allelic loss of chromosome 1p as a predictor of unfavorable outcome in patients with neuroblastoma. N Engl J Med 334:225–230.

117. Thoenen H, Barde YA. 1980. Physiology of nerve growth factor. Physiol Rev 60:1284–1335.

118. Chen J, Chattopadhyay B, Venkatakrishnan G, Ross AH. 1990. Nerve growth factor-induced differentiation of human neuroblastoma and neuroepithelioma celll lines. Cell Growth Differ 1:79–85.

119. Azar CG, Scavarda NJ, Reynolds CP, Brodeur GM. 1990. Multiple defects of the nerve growth factor receptor in human neuroblastomas. Cell Growth Differ 1:421–428.

120. Green SH, Greene LA. 1986. A single Mr approximately 103,000 ^{125}I-beta-nerve growth factor- affinity-labeled species represents both the low and high affinity forms of the nerve growth factor receptor. J Biol Chem 261:15316–15326.

121. Martin-Zanca D, Barbacid M, Parada LF. 1990. Expression of the trk proto-oncogene is restricted to the sensory cranial and spinal ganglia of neural crest origin in mouse development. Genes Dev 4:683–694.

122. Kaplan DR, Martin-Zanca D, Parada LF. 1991. Tyrosine phosphorylation and tyrosine kinase activity of the *trk* proto-oncogene product induced by NGF. Nature 350:158–160.

123. Nakagawara A, Arima-Nakagawara M, Scavarda NJ, Azar CG, Cantor AB, Brodeur GM. 1993. Association between high levels of expression of the TRK gene and favorable outcome in human neuroblastoma. N Engl J Med 328:847–854.

124. Lavenius E, Gestblom C, Johansson I, Nanberg E, Pahlman S. 1995. Transfection of TRK-A into human neuroblastoma cells restores their ability to differentiate in response to nerve growth factor. Cell Growth Differ 6:727–736.

125. Matsushima H, Bogenmann E. 1993. Expression of trkA cDNA in neuroblastomas mediates differentiation in vitro an in vivo. Mol Cell Biol 13:7447–7456.

126. Kogner P, Barbany G, Dominici C, Castello MA, Raschella G, Persson H. 1993. Coexpression of messenger RNA for TRK protooncogene and low affinity nerve growth factor receptor in neuroblastoma with favorable prognosis. Cancer Res 53:2044–2050.

127. Borrello MG, Bongarzone I, Pierotti MA, et al. 1993. TRK and RET protooncogene expression in human neuroblastoma specimens: high-frequency of TRK expression in non-advanced stages. Int J Cancer 54:540–545.

128. Suzuki T, Bogenmann E, Shimada H, Stram D, Seeger RC. 1993. Lack of high-affinity nerve growth factor receptors in aggressive neuroblastomas. J Natl Cancer Inst 85:337–384.

156

129. 1991. Molecular and Cellular Biology of Multidrug Resistance in Tumor Cells. New York: Editor Roninson, IB. Plenum Press.
130. Chan HSL, Haddad G, Thorner PS, et al. 1991. P-glycoprotein expression as a predictor of the outcome of therapy for neuroblastoma. N Engl J Med 325:1608–1614.
131. Favrot M, Combaret V, Goillot E, et al. 1991. Expression of P-glycoprotein restricted to normal cells in neuroblastoma biopsies. Br J Cancer 64:233–238.
132. Nakagawara A, Kadomatsu K, Sato S, et al. 1990. Inverse conrrelation between expression of multidrug resistance gene and N-*myc* oncogene in human neuroblastomas. Cancer Res 50:3043–3047.
133. Norris MD, Bordow SB, Marshall GM, Haber PS, Cohn SL, Haber M. 1996. Expression of the gene for multidrug-resistance-associated protein and outcome in patients with neuroblastoma. N Engl J Med 334:231–238.
134. Grant CE, Valdimarsson G, Hipfner DR, Almquist KC, Cole SP, Deeley RG. 1994. Overexpression of multidrug resistance-associated protein (MRP) increases resistance to natural product drugs. Cancer Res 54:357–361.
135. Cole SP, Bhardwaj G, Gerlach JH, et al. 1992. Overexpression of a transporter gene in a multidrug-resistant human lung cancer cell line. Science 258:1650–1654.
136. Slovak ML, Ho JP, Bhardwaj G, Kurz EU, Deeley RG, Cole SP. 1993. Localization of a novel multidrug resistance-associated gene in the HT1080/DR4 and H69AR human tumor cell lines. Cancer Res 53:3221–3225.
137. Zaman GJ, Flens MJ, van Leusden MR, et al. 1994. The human multidrug resistance-associated protein MRP is a plasma membrane drug-efflux pump. Proc Natl Acad Sci U S A 91:8822–8826.
138. Bordow SB, Haber M, Madafiglio J, Cheung B, Marshall GM, Norris MD. 1994. Expression of the multidrug resistance-associated protein (MRP) gene correlates with amplification and overexpression of the N-*myc* oncogene I childhood neuroblastoma. Cancer Res 54:5036–5040.
139. Folkman J. 1990. What is the evidence that tumors are angiogenesis dependent? J Natl Cancer Inst 82:4–6.
140. Folkman J. 1995. Angiogenesis in cancer, vascular, rheumatoid and other disease. Nature Med 1:27–31.
141. Weinstat-Saslow D, Steeg PS, 1994. Angiogenesis and colonization in the tumor metastatic process: basic and applied advances. FASEB J 8:401–407.
142. Weidner N, Folkman J, Pozza F, et al. 1992. Tumor angiogenesis: a new significant and independent prognostic indicator in early-stage breast carcinoma. J Natl Cancer Inst 84:1875–1887.
143. Weidner N, Carroll PR, Flax J, Blumenfeld W, Folkman J. 1993. Tumor angiogenesis correlates with metastasis in invasive prostate carcinoma. Am J Pathol 143:401–409.
144. Toi M, Kashitani J, Tominaga T. 1993. Tumor angiogenesis is an independent prognostic indicator in primary breast carcinoma. Int J Cancer 55:371–374.
145. Macchiarini P, Fontanini G, Hardin MJ, Squartini F, Angeletti CA. 1992. Relation of neovascularisation to metastasis of non-small-cell lung cancer. Lancet 340:145–146.
146. Maeda K, Chung Y, Takatsuka S, et al. 1995. Tumor angiogenesis as a predictor of recurrence in gastric carcinoma. J Clin Oncol 13:477–481.
147. Meitar D, Crawford SE, Rademaker AW, Cohn SL. 1996. Tumor angiogenesis correlates with metastatic disease, N-*myc* amplification, and poor outcome in human neuroblastoma. J Clin Oncol 14:405–414.
148. Aruffo A, Stamenkovic I, Melnick M, Underhill CB, Seed B. 1990. CD44 is the principal cell surface receptor for hyaluronate. Cell 61:1303–1313.
149. Jalkanen ST, Bargatze RF, Herron LR, Butcher EC. 1986. A lymphoid cell surface glycoprotein involved in endothelial cell recognition and lymphocyte homing in man. Eur J Immunol 15:1195–1202.
150. Miyake K, Underhill CB, Lesley J, Kincade PW. 1990. Hyaluronate can function as a cell adhesion molecule and CD44 participates in hyaluronate recognition. J EXT Med 172:69–75.

157

151. Huet S, Groux H, Caillou B, Valentin H, Prieur AM, Bernard A. 1989. CD44 contributes to T cell activation. J Immunol 143:798–801.

152. St. John T, Meyer J, Idzerda R, Gallatin WM. 1990. Expression of CD44 confers a new adhesive phenotype on transfected cells. Cell 60:45–52.

153. Jalkanen S, Joensuu H, Soderstrom KO, Klemi P. 1991. Lymphocyte homing and clinical behavior of non-Hodgkin's lymphoma. J Clin Invest 87:1835–1840.

154. Matsumura Y, Tarin D. 1992. Significance of CD44 gene products for cancer diagnosis and disease evaluation. Lancet 340:1053–1058.

155. Favrot MC, Combaret V, Lasset C. 1993. CD44 — a new prognostic marker for neuroblastoma. N Engl J Med 329:1965.

156. Combaret V, Gross N, Lasset C, et al. 1996. Clinical relevance of CD44 cell-surface expression and N-*myc* gene amplification in a multicentric analysis of 121 pediatric neuroblastomas. J Clin Oncol 14:25–34.

157. Combaret V, Lasset C, Frappaz D, et al. 1995. Evaluation of CD44 prognostic value in neuroblastoma: comparison with the other prognostic factors. Eur J Cancer 31A:545–549.

158. Gross N, Beretta C, Peruisseau G, Jackson D, Simmons D, Beck D. 1994. CD44H expression by human neuroblastoma cells: relation to *MYCN* amplification and lineage differentiation. Cancer Res 54:4238–4242.

159. Kodama K, Nakata T, Ishii J, et al. 1985. VMA mass screening program of neuroblastoma for infants in Nagoya City, Japan. Am J Public Health 75:173–175.

160. Sawada T, Kidowaki T, Sakamoto I, et al. 1984. Neuroblastoma. Mass screening for early detection and its prognosis. Cancer 53:2731–2735.

161. Nishi M, Miyake H, Takeda T, et al. 1992. Mass screening of neuroblastoma in Sapporo City, Japan. Am J Pediatr Hematol Oncol 14:327–331.

162. Yamamoto K, Hayashi Y, Hanada R, et al. 1995. Mass screening and age-specific incidence of neuroblastoma in Saitama Prefecture, Japan. J Clin Oncol 13:2033–2038.

163. Ishimoto K, Kiyokawa N, Fujita H, et al. 1990. Problems of mass screening for neuroblastoma: analysis of false-negative cases. J Pediatr Surg 25:398–401.

164. Nakagawara A, Zaizen Y, Ikeda K, et al. 1991. Different genomic and metabolic patterns between mass screening-positive and mass screening-negative later-presenting neuroblastomas. Cancer 68:2037–2044.

165. Kaneko Y, Kanda N, Maseki N, et al. 1990. Current urinary mass screening for catecholamine metabolites at 6 months of age may be detecting only a small portion of high-risk neuroblastomas: a chromosome and N-*myc* amplification study. J Clin Oncol 8:2005–2013.

166. Bessho F, Hashizume K, Nakajo T, Kamoshita S. 1991. Mass screening in Japan increased the detection of infants with neuroblastoma without a decrease in cases in older children. J Pediatr 119:237–241.

167. Craft AW, Parker L, Dale G, et al. 1992. A pilot study of screening for neuroblastoma in the north of England. Am J Pediatr Hematol Oncol 14:337–341.

168. Woods WG, Tuchman M, Bernstein ML, et al. 1992. Screening for neuroblastoma in North America. 2-year results from the Quebec Project. Am J Pediatr Hematol Oncol 14:312–319.

169. Schilling FH, Erttmann R, Dohrmann S, et al. 1992. Early neuroblastoma detection in Germany. On the status of the Hamburg–Stuttgart cooperative pilot study. Klin Padiatr 204:282–287.

170. Treuner J, Schilling FH. 1995. Neuroblastoma mass screening: the arguments for and against. Eur J Cancer 31A:565–568.

171. Takeuchi LA, Hachitanda Y, Woods WG, et al. 1995. Screening for neuroblastoma in North America: preliminary results of a pathology review from the Quebec project. Cancer 76:2363–2371.

172. Murphy SB, Cohn SL, Craft AW, et al. 1991. Do children benefit from mass screening for neuroblastoma? Consensus Statement from the American Cancer Society Workshop on Neuroblastoma Screening. Lancet 337:344–346.

158

173. Esteve J. 1994. Some remarks on power calculation for neuroblastoma screening. In Sawada T, Matsumura T, Kizaki Z (eds.). Proceedings of the 3rd International Symposium on Neuroblastoma Screening. Kyoto: Kyoto Prefectural Unviersity of Medicine, pp. 47–51.

174. Evans AE, Albo V, D'Angio GJ, et al. 1976. Factors influencing survival of children with nonmetastatic neuroblastoma. Cancer 38:661–666.

175. De Bernardi B, Conte M, Mancini A, et al. 1995. Localized resectable neuroblastoma: results of the second study of the Italian Cooperative Group for Neuroblastoma. J Clin Oncol 13:884–893.

176. Ninane J, Pritchard J, Morris Jones PH, Mann JR, Malpas JS. 1982. Stage II neuroblastoma. Adverse prognostic significance of lymph node involvement. Arch Dis Child 57:438–442.

177. Kushner BH, Cheung NV, LaQuaglia MP, et al. 1996. Survival from locally invasive or widespread neuroblastoma without cytotoxic therapy. J Clin Oncol 14:373–381.

178. Evans AE, Baum E, Chard R. 1981. Do infants with stage IV-S neuroblastoma need treatment? Arch Dis Child 56:271–274.

179. Cohn SL, Herst CV, Maurer HS, Rosen ST. 1987. N-*myc* amplification in an infant with stage IVS neuroblastoma. J Clin Oncol 5:1441–1444.

180. Bowman L, Castleberry R, Altshuler G, et al. 1992. Therapy based on DNA index (DI) for infants with unresectable and disseminated neuroblastoma (NB): The Pediatric Oncology Group 'better risk' study. Proc Am Soc Clin Oncol 11:365.

181. Evans AE, D'Angio GJ, Koop CE. 1984. The role of multimodal therapy in patients with local and regional neuroblastoma. J Pediatr Surg 19:77–80.

182. Evans AE, Brand W, de Lorimier A, et al. 1984. Results in children with local and regional neuroblastoma managed with and without vincristine, cyclophosphamide, and imidazolecarboxamide. A report from the Children's Cancer Study Group. Am J Clin Oncol 7:3–7.

183. West DC, Shamberger RC, Macklis RM, et al. 1993. Stage III neuroblastoma over 1 year of age at diagnosis: improved survival with intensive multimodality therapy including multiple alkylating agents. J Clin Oncol 11:84–90.

184. Castleberry RP, Kun LE, Shuster JJ, et al. 1991. Radiotherapy improves the outlook for patients older than 1 year with Pediatric Oncology Group stage C neuroblastoma. J Clin Oncol 9:789–795.

185. Bowman LC, Hancock ML, Santana VM, et al. 1991. Impact of intensified therapy on clinical outcome in infants ad children with neuroblastoma: the St. Jude Children's Research Hospital experience, 1962 to 1988. J Clin Oncol 9:1599–1608.

186. Philip T, Zucker JM, Bernard JL, et al. 1991. Improved survival at 2 and 5 years in the LMCE1 unselected group of 72 children with stage IV neuroblastoma older than 1 year of age at diagnosis: is cure possible in a small subgroup? J Clin Oncol 9:1037–1044.

187. Cheung NK, Heller G. 1991. Chemotherapy dose intensity conrrelates strongly with response, median survival, and median progression-free survival in metastatic neuroblastoma. J Clin Oncol 9:1050–1058.

188. Bernard JL, Philip T, Zucker JM, et al. 1987. Sequential cisplatin/VM-26 and vincristine/cyclophosphamide/doxorubicin in metastatic neuroblastoma: an effective alternating non-cross-resistant regimen? J Clin Oncol 5:1952–1959.

189. Campbell IA, Seeger RC, Harris RE, Villablanca JG, Matthay KK. 1993. Escalating dose of continuous infusion combination chemotherapy for refractory neuroblastoma. J Clin Oncol 11:623–629.

190. Kushner BH, LaQuaglia MP, Bonilla MA, et al. 1994. Highly effective induction therapy for stage 4 neuroblastoma in children over 1 year of age. J Clin Oncol 12:2607–2613.

191. Haase GM, O'Leary MC, Ramsay NKC, et al. 1991. Aggressive surgery combined with intensive chemotherapy improves survival in poor-risk neuroblastoma. J Pediatr Surg 26:1119–1124.

192. Stram DO, Matthay KK, O'Leary M, Reynolds CP, Seeger RC. 1994. Myeloablative chemoradiotherapy versus continued chemotherapy for high risk neuroblastoma. Prog Clin Biol Res 385:287–291.

159

193. Seeger RC, Villablanca JG, Matthay KK, et al. 1991. Intensive chemoradiotherapy and autologous bone marrow transplantation for poor prognosis neuroblastoma. Prog Clin Biol Res 366:527–533.

194. Pole JG, Casper J, Elfenbein G, et al. 1991. High-dose chemoradiotherapy supported by marrow infusions for advanced neuroblastoma: a Pediatric Oncology Group study. J Clin Oncol 9:152–158.

195. Kushner BH, O'Reilly RJ, Mandell LR, Gulati SC, LaQuaglia M, Cheung NK. 1991. Myeloablative combination chemotherapy without total body irradiation for neuroblastoma. J Clin Oncol 9:274–279.

196. Dini G, Lanino E, Garaventa A, et al. 1991. Myeloablative therapy and unpurged autologous bone marrow transplantation for poor-prognosis neuroblastoma: report of 34 cases. J Clin Oncol 9:962–969.

197. Seeger RC, Matthay KK, Villablanca JG, et al. 1991. Intensive chemoradiotherapy and autologous bone marrow transplantation (ABMT) for high risk neuroblastoma. Proc Am Soc Clin Oncol 10:310.

198. Dini G, Lanino E, Garaventa A, et al. 1991. Unpurged ABMT for neuroblastoma: AIEOPBMT experience. Bone Marrow Transplant 7 (Suppl. 2):92.

199. Zucker JM, Philip T, Bernard JL, et al. 1991. Single or double consolidation treatment according to remission status after initial therapy in metastatic neuroblastoma: first results of LMCE3 study in 40 patients. Bone Marrow Transplant 7 (Suppl. 2):91.

200. Hartmann O, Benhamou E, Beaujean F, et al. 1987. Repeated high-dose chemotherapy followed by purged autologous bone marrow transplantation as consolidation therapy in metastatic neuroblastoma. J Clin Oncol 5:1205–1211.

201. August CS, Serota FT, Koch PA, et al. 1984. Treatment of advanced neuroblastoma with supralethal chemotherapy, radiation, and allogeneic or autologous marrow reconstitution. J Clin Oncol 2:609–616.

202. Kushner BH, Gulati SC, Kwon JH, O'Reilly RJ, Exelby PR, Cheung NK. 1991. High-dose melphalan with 6-hydroxydopamine-purged autologous bone marrow transplantation for poor-risk neuroblastoma. Cancer 68:242–247.

203. McCowage GB, Vowels MR, Shaw PJ, Lockwood L, Mameghan H. 1995. Autologous bone marrow transplantation for advanced neuroblastoma using teniposide, doxorubicin, melphalan, cisplatin, and total-body irradiation. J Clin Oncol 13:2789–2795.

204. Matthay KK, Atkinson JB, Stram DO, Selch M, Reynolds CP, Seeger RC. 1993. Patterns of relatpse after autologous purged bone marrow transplantation for neuroblastoma: a Childrens Cancer Group pilot study. J Clin Oncol 11:2226–2233.

205. Pole JG. 1991. Autologous marrow transplantation in pediatric tumors. In Gale RP, Champlin RE (eds.). New Strategies in BMT. New York: Wiley Liss, pp. 413–422.

206. Di Caro A, Bostrom B, Moss TJ, et al. 1994. Autologous peripheral blood cell transplantation in the treatment of advanced neuroblastoma. Am J Pediatr Hematol Oncol 16:200–206.

207. Kletzel M, Longino R, Danner K, Olszewski M, Moss T. 1994. Peripheral Blood stem cell rescue in children with advanced stage IV neuroblastoma. Prog Clin Biol Res 389:513–519.

208. Shuster JJ, Cantor AB, McWilliams N, et al. 1991. The prognostic significance of autologous bone marrow transplant in advanced neuroblastoma. J Clin Oncol 9:1045–1049.

209. Pinkerton CR, Philip T, Biron P, et al. 1987. High-dose melphalan, vincristine, and total-body irradiation with autologous bone marrow transplantation in children with relapsed neuroblastoma: a phase II study. Med Pediatr Oncol 15:236–240.

210. Reynolds CP, Seeger RC, Vo DD, Black AT, Wells J, Ugelstad J. 1986. Model system for removing neuroblastoma cells from bone marrow using monoclonal antibodies and magnetic immunobeads. Cancer Res 46:5882–5886.

211. Moss TJ, Cairo M, Santana VM, Weinthal J, Hurvitz C, Bostrom B. 1994. Clonogenicity of circulating neuroblastoma cells: implications regarding peripheral blood stem cell transplantation. Blood 83:3085–3089.

212. Brenner MK, Rill DR, Moen RC, et al. 1994. Gene marking and autologous bone marrow transplantation. Ann N Y Acad Sci 716:204–214.
213. Moss TJ, Ross AA. 1992. The risk of tumor cell contamination in peripheral blood stem cell collections. J Hematother 1:225–232.
214. Moss TJ, Reynolds CP, Sather HN, Romansky SG, Hammond GD, Seeger RC. 1991. Prognostic value of immunocytologic detection of bone marrow metastases in neuroblastoma. N Engl J Med 324:219–226.
215. Moss TJ, Sanders DG, Lasky LC, Bostrom B. 1990. Contamination of peripheral blood stem cell harvests by circulating neuroblastoma cells. Blood 76:1879–1883.
216. Wiseman GA, Kvols LK. 1995. Therapy of neuroendocrine tumors with radiolabeled MIBG and somatostatin analogues. Semin Nucl Med 25:272–278.
217. Gaze MN, Wheldon TE. 1996. Radiolabelled mIBG in the treatment of neuroblastoma. Eur J Cancer 32A:93–96.
218. Garaventa A, Guerra P, Arrighini A, et al. 1991. Treatment of advanced neuroblastoma with I-131 meta-iodobenzylguanidine. Cancer 67:922–928.
219. Voute PA, Hoefnagel CA, de Kraker J, Valdes Olmos R, Bakker DJ, van de Kleij AJ. 1991. Results of treatment with 131 I-metaiodobenzylguanidine (131 I-MIBG) in patients with neuroblastoma. Future prospects of zetotherapy. Prog Clin Biol Res 366:439–445.
220. Lashford LS, Lewis IJ, Fielding SL, et al. 1992. Phase I/II study of iodine 131 metaiodobenzylguanidine in chemoresistant neuroblastoma: a United Kingdom Chidren's Cancer Study Group investigation. J Clin Oncol 10:1889–1896.
221. Matthay KK, Huberty JP, Hattner RS, et al. 1991. Efficacy and safety of [131I]metaiodobenzylguanidine therapy for patients with refractory neuroblastoma. J Nucl Biol Med 35:244–247.
222. Mastrangelo R, Tornesello A, Riccardi R, et al. 1995. A new approach in the treatment of stage IV neuroblastoma using a combination of [131I]meta-iodobenzylguanidine (MIBG) and cisplatin. Eur J Cancer 31A:606–611.
223. Pritchard J, Kiely E, Rogers DW, et al. 1987. Long-term survival after advanced neuroblastoma. N Engl J Med 317:1026–1027.
224. Hoefnagel CA, de Kraker J, Valdes Olmos RA, Voute PA. 1994. 131I-MIBG as a first-line treatment in high-risk neuroblastoma patients. Nucl Med Commun 15:712–717.
225. de Kraker J, Hoefnagel CA, Caron H, et al. 1995. First line targeted radiotherapy, a new concept in the treatment of advanced stage neuroblastoma. Eur J Cancer 31A:600–602.
226. Voute PA, van der Kleij AJ, de Kraker J, Hoefnagel CA, Tiel-van Buul MM, Van Gennip H. 1995. Clinical experience with radiation enhancement by hyperbaric oxygen in children with recurrent neuroblastoma stage IV. Eur J Cancer 31A:596–600.
227. Mueller-Klieser W, Vaupel P, Manz R. 1983. Tumour oxygenation under normobaric and hyperbaric conditions. Br J Radiol 56:559–564.
228. Sostman HD, Rockwell S, Sylvia AL, et al. 1991. Evaluaton of BA1112 rhabdomyosarcoma oxygenation with microelectrodes, optical spectrophotometry, radiosensitivity, and magnetic resonance spectroscopy. Magn Reson Med 20:253–267.
229. Fujimura E. 1974. Experimental studies on radiation effects under high pressure oxygen. Osaka Daigaku Shigaku Zasshi 19:100–108.
230. Yeh SD, Larson SM, Burch L, et al. 1991. Radioimmunodetection of neuroblastoma with iodine-131-3F8: correlation with biopsy, iodine-131-metaiodobenzylguanidine and standard diagnostic modalities. J Nucl Med 32:769–776.
231. Moyes JS, Babich JW, Carter R, Meller ST, Agrawal M, McElwain TJ. 1989. Quantitative study of radioiodinated metaiodobenzylguanidine uptake in children with enuroblastoma: correlation with tumor histopathology. J Nucl Med 30:474–480.
232. Srkalovic G, Cai RZ, Schally AV. 1990. Evaluation of receptors for somatostatin in various tumors using different analogs. J Clin Endocrinol Metab 70:661–669.
233. Mujoo K, Cheresh DA, Yang HM, Reisfeld RA. 1987. Disialoganglioside GD2 on human neuroblastoma cells: target antigen for monoclonal antibody-mediated cytolysis and suppression of tumor growth. Cancer Res 47:1098–1104.

161

234. Cheung NK, Lazarus H, Miraldi FD, et al. 1987. Ganglioside GD2 specific monoclonal antibody 3F8: a phase I study in patients with neuroblastoma and malignant melanoma. J Clin Oncol 5:1430–1440.

235. Murray JL, Cunningham JE, Brewer H, et al. 1994. Phase I trial of murine monoclonal antibody 14G2a administered by prolonged intravenous infusion in patients with neuroectodermal tumors. J Clin Oncol 12:184–193.

236. Reisfeld RA, Mueller BM, Handgretinger R, Yu AL, Gillies SD. 1994. Potential of genetically engineered anti-ganglioside GD2 antibodies for cancer immunotherapy. Prog Brain Res 101:201–212.

237. Cheung NK, Kushner BH, Yeh SJ, Larson SM. 1994. 3F8 monoclonal antibody treatment of patients with stage IV neuroblastoma: a phase II study. Prog Clin Biol Res 385:319–328.

238. Hank JA, Surfus J, Gan J, et al. 1994. Treatment of neuroblastoma patients with antiganglioside GD2 antibody plus interleukin-2 induces antibody-dependent cellular cytotoxicity against neuroblastoma detected in vitro. J Immunother 15:29–37.

239. Main EK, Lampson LA, Hart MK, Kornbluth J, Wilson DB. 1985. Human neuroblastoma cell lines are susceptible to lysis by natural killer cells but not by cytotoxic T lymphocytes. J Immunol 135:242–246.

240. Michon J, Negrier S, Coze C, et al. 1994. Administration of high-dose recombinant interleukin 2 after autologous bone marrow transplantation in patients with neuroblastoma: toxicity, efficacy and survival. A Lyon–Marseille–Curie–East of France Group Study. Prog Clin Biol Res 385:293–300.

241. Negrier S, Michon J, Floret D, et al. 1991. Interleukin-2 and lymphokine-activated killer cells in 15 children with advanced metastatic neuroblastoma. J Clin Oncol 9:1363–1370.

242. Favrot MC, Floret D, Negrier S, et al. 1989. Systemic interleukin-2 therapy in children with progressive neuroblastoma after high dose chemotherapy and bone marrow transplantation. Bone Marrow Transplant 4:499–503.

243. Bauer M, Reaman GH, Hank JA, et al. 1995. A phase II trial of human recombinant interleukin-2 administered as a 4-day continuous infusion for children with refractory neuroblastoma, non-Hodgkin's lymphoma, sarcoma, renal cell carcinoma, and malignant melanoma. A Childrens Cancer Group study. Cancer 75:2959–2965.

244. Evans A, Main E, Zier K, et al. 1989. The effects of gamma interferon on the natural killer and tumor cells of children with neuroblastoma. A preliminary report. Cancer 64:1383–1387.

245. Villablanca JG, Khan AA, Avramis VI, et al. 1995. Phase I trial of 13-cis-retinoic acid in children with neuroblastoma following bone marrow transplantation. J Clin Oncol 13:894–901.

246. Finklestein JZ, Krailo MD, Lenarsky C, et al. 1992. 13-cis-retinoic acid (NSC 122758) in the treatment of children with metastatic neuroblastoma unresponsive to conventional chemotherapy: report from the Childrens Cancer Study Group. Med Pediatr Oncol 20:307–311.

247. Adamson PC. 1994. Clinical and pharmacokinetic studies of all-trans-retinoic acid in pediatric patients with cancer. Leukemia 8 (Suppl 3):22–25.

6. Pediatric germ cell tumors

Elizabeth J. Perlman and Cynthia Kretschmar

1. Introduction

Germ cell tumors historically have been considered to be a single nosologic category comprising tumors with different histologic manifestations and different degrees of malignancy and arising at different sites of origin. Only in the last decade has the biologic heterogeneity of germ cell tumors been recognized and addressed. Therapy tailored for the many biologically distinct subsets of germ cell tumors has yet to be defined. Because many categories exclusively involve children, this challenge has been assumed by pediatric oncologists, resulting in the multi-institutional and multinational cooperative studies currently in progress. Current protocols utilize regimens that have been effective in adult germ cell tumors. The probability that the biologically unique pediatric subsets may be best treated by other regimens awaits future protocols.

The overall incidence of germ cell tumors in children is difficult to assess due to the large contribution of benign tumors that are unreported. The incidence of malignant germ cell tumors at all ages in the United States is 2–3 per 1,000,000 births. Listed in table 1 are the site, sex, and histology from a representative large study of pediatric germ cell tumors [1]. The subclassification of germ cell tumors that will be utilized in this chapter, outlined in table 2, is based on these demographic data as well as additional biologic parameters. In summary, the broad group of germ cell tumors shows a clear biphasic distribution with regard to age. One population peaks at 1–2 years of age, and a second population peaks at 15–25 years. Tumors belonging to these two groups show biologic and clinical differences, as will be discussed. Within this dichotomy, the tumors are subdivided according to site, with the common sites being ovarian, testicular, and extragonadal. The subcategorization by site reflects less significant biologic distinction than the categorization by age. Following an overview of germ cell embryology and histogenesis, and the pathology of germ cell tumors, each category will be considered separately.

D.O. Walterhouse and S.L. Cohn (eds), DIAGNOSTIC AND THERAPEUTIC ADVANCES IN PEDIATRIC ONCOLOGY. Copyright © 1997. Kluwer Academic Publishers, Boston. All rights reserved.

Table 1. Site, sex, and histology of pediatric germ cell tumors [1]

	Male	Female	Benign	Immature	Malignant	Total
Ovary	0	73	56	4	13	73 (39%)
Testis	13	0	3	1	9	13 (7%)
Intracranial	9	1	1	2	7	10 (5%)
Mediastinal	6	2	2	2	4	8 (4%)
Sacrococcygeal	24	43	33	14	20	67 (36%)
Other	7	10	11	5	1	17 (9%)
Total	59 (31%)	129 (69%)	106 (56%)	28 (15%)	54 (29%)	188

Table 2. Classification of germ cell tumors

A. Germ cell tumors of young children
   1. Testicular
      Teratoma (mature, immature)
      Endodermal sinus tumor
   2. Extragonadal
      Teratoma (mature, immature)
      Endodermal sinus tumor
B. Germ cell tumors of adolescents and young adults
   1. Testicular
      Seminoma
      Nonseminomatous germ cell tumor
   2. Ovarian
      Mature teratoma
      Immature teratoma
      Dysgerminoma
      Endodermal sinus tumor
      Mixed malignant germ cell tumor
      Gonadoblastoma
   3. Extragonadal (mediastinal, central nervous system)
      Teratoma
      Immature teratoma
      Germinoma
      Nongerminomatous germ cell tumor

2. Embryology and histogenesis

Primordial germ cells segregate from somatic cells very early in gestation and reside in the extraembryonic yolk sac. At about five weeks gestation, they migrate to the gonadal ridge by way of the dorsal mesentery, a process that appears to be governed by c-kit receptor and its ligand, stem cell factor. The primordial germ cells express the c-kit receptor on their cell membrane; the soft tissue in the migration pathway expresses the c-kit ligand, commonly called stem cell factor, in an increasing gradient. This gradient guides the germ cells toward the gonad where the sex cords express stem cell factor at the highest concentration. The c-kit–stem cell factor receptor–ligand pair is responsible for the viability and proliferative ability of the germ cells during migration [2–4]. C-kit is also considered an oncogene, and has been shown to be expressed in several human malignancies, including adult and ovarian germ cell tumors [5,6]. The role of these proteins in the development or progression of germ cell neoplasia has not been defined.

In males, the primordial germ cells arrive in the gonad concomitant with testicular determination. Upon arrival they become surrounded by Sertoli cells, which likely play an important regulatory role. After a short period of continued c-kit-dependent proliferation, the primordial germ cells undergo mitotic arrest, which persists until birth. The germ cells slowly divide during the first decade of life, keeping pace with the growth of the gonad. Approaching puberty, germ cell proliferation (c-kit dependent) increases dramatically; following puberty, spermatogonia begin to undergo meiosis. This overview provides an explanation for the observation that all male germ cell tumors arise in cells that are premeiotic. In the absence of the Y chromosome, in females, the primordial germ cells populate the gonadal ridge and continue to proliferate (and express c-kit) for an extended period of time. At about 14 weeks gestation, the germ cells begin to undergo DNA replication and enter into the prophase of meiosis I, where they are arrested. Unlike mitotic arrest in the testis, meiotic arrest in the ovary is a gradual process that is not completed until after birth. The germ cells remain arrested in meiosis I until puberty, and meiosis is not completed until fertilization occurs. This overview suggests that the cell of origin of ovarian germ cell tumors may differ from those in the testis by showing genetic evidence of entry into meiosis I, which is indeed the case for most [7–9].

Many germ cell tumors in children do not arise in gonads but in extragonadal sites. These tumors are presumed to arise in ectopic germ cells that have abberantly migrated. However, very few ectopic germ cells have been described in humans, and ectopic germ cells have never been described in the sites most common for adolescent/adult extragonadal germ cell tumors, namely, the brain and mediastinum [10]. Instead, human ectopic germ cells are most often found in the adrenal gland, where they disappear completely by 18 weeks gestation [11]. In mice, ectopic germ cells are less rare, and in both males and females these germ cells enter into meiosis in phase with normal oocytes and largely disappear in the early postnatal period [12,13]. Therefore, if extragonadal germ cell tumors are truly derived from germ cells, like ovarian germ cell tumors they would be expected to show evidence of meiotic recombination *unless* they arise prior to entry into meiosis. Numerous extragonadal childhood germ cell tumors have been analyzed, and all studies agree that these tumors arise from premeiotic cells [14–17]. In addition, thus far no heterosexual (46, XX) germ cell tumors have been seen in males. Therefore, if extragonadal germ cell tumors arose from germ cells, all such tumors must arise prior to 12–18 weeks gestation. The occurrence of large bulky lesions in infants suggests that this may indeed be the case for early childhood extragonadal germ cell tumors. However, those extragonadal tumors that present later in life are more difficult to reconcile with this pathway. An alternate hypothesis is that extragonadal germ cell tumors may arise from

165

totipotent embryonic cells [18]. This hypothesis is attractive in that it explains the midline predisposition of adolescent/adult tumors and also accounts for the similarities to teratoma development in mice at the site of injection with embryonal stem cells.

3. Pathology

The histologic appearance of the different subtypes of germ cell tumors is largely independent of the site and age of presentation. Therefore, the pathology of all germ cell tumors will be briefly discussed. The clinical and biologic implications for each histologic type, however, are highly dependent on the site and age. Therefore, following a discussion of the pathology, each subtype within the classification will be considered separately.

3.1. Mature teratoma

Teratomas are neoplasms containing a haphazard growth of one or more types of tissue derived from the three embryonic layers (ectoderm, mesoderm and endoderm). While rigid criteria require representatives from each embryonic layer, the existence of monodermal and bidermal teratomas is now accepted, including struma ovarii and strumal carcinoids of the ovary. Full pathologic descriptions of teratomas may be obtained from many sources. Teratomas have been described in virtually every location and may contain virtually every tissue type [18–20]. The biologic implications of mature teratoma depend on the age and site of presentation; ovarian lesions are entirely benign, whereas those in the adolescent testis are potentially malignant.

The development of a somatic malignancy within a teratoma has been referred to as *teratocarcinoma* or *malignant teratoma*, terms that are confusing and best avoided. The types of nongerm cell malignancies most commonly encountered are sarcomas, nephroblastoma, neuroblastoma, rhabdomyosarcoma, and glioblastoma [21,22]. The vast majority of these arise in tumors of adolescents and not in early childhood. This malignant transformation is usually associated with teratomatous foci and is thought to be derived from teratomatous elements rather than from totipotent embryonal cells. The development of nongerm cell malignancy is associated with a worse prognosis due to poor response to therapy. The degree of reduction in survival depends on the nature of the nongerm cell malignancy. The development of an embryonal rhabdomyosarcoma is associated with a dismal prognosis, while the development of other sarcomas is associated with a somewhat better prognosis [21].

3.2. Immature teratoma

Immature teratomas are teratomas in which at least one element shows histologic immaturity. Terms such as *malignant teratoma* and *teratocarcinoma* have

166

also been applied to immature teratoma and should be avoided. Immature teratomas can be graded histologically according to the quantity of immature elements, most commonly the quantity of immature neuroectoderm (table 3, figure 1) [20,23,24]. Many variants of this grading system have been proposed; however, the differences are not substantive. Grade 1 lesions are those with immature tissue limited to rare low-magnification fields, with not more than one field in any one slide. Grade 2 lesions contain immature neuroectoderm not exceeding three low-power fields per slide. Grade 3 tumors show extensive immature neural epithelium in more than four low-power fields per slide. While this grading system based on the presence of immature neuroectoderm

Table 3. Grading of immature teratomas

Grade 1:	Immature tissue present in less than one low-power field[a] per slide
Grade 2:	Immature tissue comprising 1–3 low-power fields per slide
Grade 3:	Immature tissue in four or more low-power fields per slide

[a] Low-power fields vary in the magnification used by different authors. Most common is the 10X objective with a 4X–10X ocular for a total magnification of 40–100X.

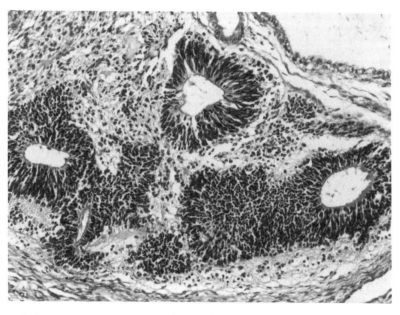

Figure 1. Immature teratomas are characterized by varying quantities of immature neuroectoderm. This routine hematoxylin- and eosin-stained field shows several immature neural tubules.

167

is accepted, the significance of immaturity of nonneural elements (embryonal muscle, cartilage, or kidney) is somewhat controversial. In practice, this seldom presents difficulties, since the immature elements are almost invariably accompanied by immature neural elements. This grading system has been most successfully applied to ovarian immature teratomas, where the grade correlates with metastatic potential as well as with behavior [25]. Similar correlations have been difficult to demonstrate at extraovarian sites, and the ability of pathologists to predict behavior in these indeterminant tumors is limited.

In the pediatric age group, the most significant pathologic event occurring within an immature teratoma is the development of endodermal sinus tumor. Such occurrences may be multifocal and may be difficult to identify. A valuable indicator of this event is an elevated serum alpha-feto protein (AFP) level. Most observers attribute elevated AFP in immature teratomas to unrecognized, small foci of endodermal sinus tumor. However, some reports of carefully examined tumors have suggested that immature neural tissue or intestinal tissue may be a source of elevated AFP [26–28]. This suggestion is supported by the immunoreactivity of these tissue types with AFP. The judgment of most experienced observers has been that while these tissue elements may, in a minority of cases, explain a small, stable increase in serum AFP, a large or rapidly increasing elevation in a patient without liver failure must be assumed to represent the presence of endodermal sinus tumor [18,29].

3.3. Germinoma (seminoma and dysgerminoma)

Germinomas in the pediatric age group are primarily restricted to the ovary and pineal region; those in the testis are uncommon under the age of 18 due to their slower growth and later detection in adulthood. Most germinomas are pure and are composed of aggregates or nests of uniform neoplastic cells with distinct, nonoverlapping cellular borders (figure 2). Germinomas often show a lymphocytic infiltrate and occasionally multinucleated giant cells. While anaplastic variants of germinoma have been rarely reported, these foci may represent areas of solid embryonal carcinoma. No pathologic features (such as mitotic rate) have been shown to identify prospectively subpopulations of germinomas that have different clinical outcome [30]. Synciotrophoblastic cells may be scattered individually throughout germinomas, and may be responsible for HCG production, but do not represent choriocarcinoma and have no effect on prognosis [31]. Immunohistochemically, the majority of germinomas are positive for placental-like alkaline phosphatase (PLAP), a cell surface glycoprotein [32–35]. While PLAP is a valuable marker for germinomas, it may also be present focally in embryonal carcinomas and endodermal sinus tumors, as well as in a wide variety of somatic tumors [32–34,36].

168

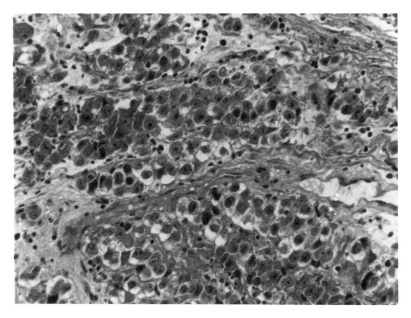

Figure 2. Germinomas (including dysgerminoma, seminoma, and extragonadal germinoma) are composed of uniform cells with distinct cell borders and a prominent nucleolus.

3.4. Endodermal sinus tumor (yolk sac tumor)

The most common malignant germ cell tumor in prepubertal children, and virtually the only histologic form of malignant germ cell tumor found in children less than 4 years of age, is the endodermal sinus tumor or yolk sac tumor. As mentioned before, these neoplasms are often associated with teratomas. Endodermal sinus tumor has only been reliably distinguished from other patterns of malignant germ cell tumor for the last two decades. Therefore, caution is advised when evaluating earlier studies that may equate endodermal sinus tumor with embryonal carcinoma. The histology and cytology of endodermal sinus tumors vary widely, often causing difficulty in diagnosis. For detailed description of the protean manifestations of endodermal sinus tumor, many excellent reviews are available [18,20,37–39]. Several histologic subtypes of endodermal sinus tumor have been described; most tumors contain several subtypes, and none of these divisions has prognostic implication. Small foci of this histologically variable neoplasm in the midst of an immature teratoma may be extraordinarily difficult to identify. The prototypic Schiller–Duvall bodies of endodermal sinus tumors (figure 3) are present in 50%–75% of tumors. Endodermal sinus tumors are commonly associated with highly elevated serum alpha-feto protein levels, which may be monitored clinically for recurrence and/or metastasis [40,41]. However, AFP levels may be misleading in the newborn and in patients with liver injury.

169

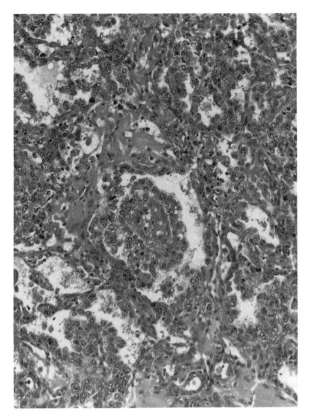

Figure 3. Endodermal sinus tumors are most commonly papillary lesions. Of these 50%–70% show Schiller–Duval bodies, which are illustrated in this field. These are characterized by a glomeruloid structure with a central vessel surrounded by epithelial tumor cells that project into a sinusoidal space, which is in turn lined by tumor cells.

3.5. Embryonal carcinoma

Pure embryonal carcinomas are seldom seen in the pediatric age group; this histologic type is most often seen as a component of a mixed malignant germ cell tumor of the adolescent ovary or testis. Like endodermal sinus tumors, embryonal carcinomas may show papillary, glandular, and solid areas. The cells are large, epitheliod, and often anaplastic, with large nucleoli, abundant mitotic activity, hemorrhage and necrosis (figure 4). As with germinomas, syncytiotrophoblasts may be seen and may produce HCG, but these do not indicate the presence of choriocarcinoma unless they are accompanied by cytotrophoblastic cells. Embryonal carcinomas show immunoreactivity for cytokeratin but not for epithelial membrane antigen, a feature that may help to distinguish embryonal carcinoma from other epithelial neoplasms [42]. A minority of embryonal carcinomas show focal, weak immunoreactivity for

170

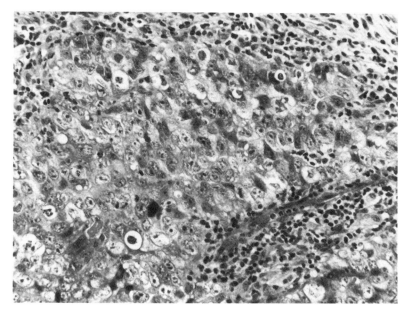

Figure 4. The cells of embryonal carcinomas are large and anaplastic, with abundant mitoses.

PLAP, as well as for AFP [33,43]. More recently, it has been noted that embryonal carcinomas, but not other germ cell tumor histologic types, show immunopositivity for CD30, a marker more conventionally utilized for Hodgkin's disease [44].

3.6. Choriocarcinoma

Choriocarcinoma is rare in children and is usually seen as a minor component of mixed germ cell tumors in adolescents. In addition, adolescence is a period of high risk for gestational trophoblastic neoplasms. Choriocarcinoma may rarely be seen as a pure form in infants, but in these cases it virtually always represents metastatic gestational trophoblastic tumor [45]. Choriocarcinomas are composed of both medium-sized cytotrophlastic and multinucleate syncytiotrophoblastic cells with frequent evidence of hemorrhage. Immuno-histochemical stains for HCG identify syncytiotrophoblastic cells, with unreliable staining of cytotrophoblasts.

4. Serologic markers

Serum and CSF concentrations of alpha-feto protein (AFP) and of human chorionic gonadotropin (HCG) are useful as markers of certain types of germ cell tumors. AFP is a major serum protein of the human fetus and is produced

171

Table 4. Alpha-feto protein levels in infants

AGE	MEAN ± SD (ng/mL)
Premature	134,734.0 ± 41,444.0
Newborn	48,406.0 ± 34,718.0
Newborn to two weeks	33,113.0 ± 32,503.0
Newborn to one month	9,452.0 ± 12,610.0
Two weeks to one month	2,654.0 ± 3,080.0
Two months	323.0 ± 278.0
Three months	88.0 ± 87.0
Four months	74.0 ± 56.0
Five months	46.5 ± 19.0
Six months	12.5 ± 9.8
Seven months	9.7 ± 7.1
Eight months	8.5 ± 5.5

in the embryonic liver and GI tract [46]. It is expressed at high levels by over 85% of endodermal sinus tumors [47] and at lower levels in other histologic types. Its predominate utility is for monitoring for recurrence or metastasis in AFP-secreting tumors. The utility of AFP is diminished in infants less than 8 months of age; however, AFP levels may be quite high in this group, and the half-life is quite variable (table 4) [48]. After the newborn period, the half-life of AFP is 5–7 days. In young children whose AFP returns to normal after therapy, there may be no need for second-look surgery [49]. Other neoplastic and nonneoplastic disorders may result in elevation of AFP, e.g., hepatitis, cirrhosis, and other malignancies.

The beta subunit of human chorionic gonadotropin (HCG) is secreted by the syncytiotrophoblastic cells of the placenta and thus is characteristically markedly elevated in choriocarcinomas. However, virtually all histologic subtypes of malignant germ cell tumors may show rare or scattered syncytiotrophoblastic cells that may result in mildly elevated HCG but do not indicate a worse prognosis. Elevations above 100 ng/mL are unusual and suggest the true presence of choriocarcinoma. The half-life of HCG is approximately 20–30 hours.

5. Germ cell tumors of young children

Germ cell tumors in children less than 5 years of age are almost exclusively composed of teratomas (mature or immature) and/or endodermal sinus tumors. These may arise in the testis, in a wide variety of extragonadal sites, and only rarely in the ovary. By far the most common extragonadal site of presentation in young children is the sacrococcygeal region, for unknown reasons. The evidence available to date suggests that the biology of these lesions does not differ by site.

172

5.1.1. Sacrococcygeal teratomas. Teratomas arising in the sacrococcygeal region represent the most common tumor of newborns. These are usually large midline and protuberant masses with a broad-based attachment in the region of the coccyx (figure 5). A striking female predominance remains unexplained [50–55]. Developmental anomalies secondary to the mass effect of the bulky sacrococcygeal tumors may be present but are seldom life-threatening. Examples include sacral scoliosis, spina bifida, imperforate anus, and hip dislocation [55]. High-output cardiac failure may be seen and is attributed to intratumoral vascular shunting [50]. Sacrococcygeal lesions have been classified according to the location of the tumor relative to the sacrum. Type I lesions have minimal presacral (intra-abdominal) growth; type II tumors are

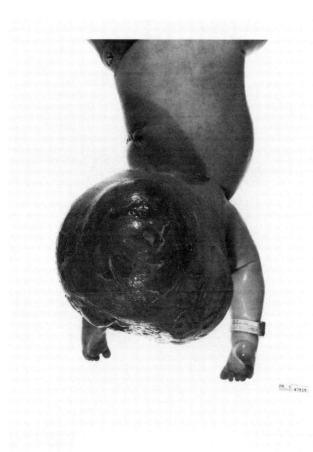

Figure 5. Sacrococcygeal teratomas are commonly bulky, disforming lesions present at birth.

173

predominantly external but have a definitive intra-abdominal extension; type III are predominately intra-abdominal but have a small external component; and type IV are entirely presacral with no external component [55]. This classification scheme has been shown to correlate with risk of endodermal sinus tumor development; 2 of 28 type I, 5 of 18 types II or III, and 4 of 5 type IV tumors developed endodermal sinus tumor histology [52]. This outcome may be related to the older age at presentation of the intra-abdominal type IV tumors and to difficulty of total excision. Sacrococcygeal teratomas should be excised to prevent transformation into endodermal sinus tumor. Currently, the surgical practice is to remove the coccyx at the time of excision — a practice that has markedly reduced the frequency of recurrence. This practice has been extant for only two decades, and much of the survival information in the literature rely on data derived from less complete surgical excision.

5.1.2. Sacrococcygeal immature teratomas. Histologically, most sacrococcygeal teratomas are composed of many tissue types that show maturity of the degree expected at the patient's age, and are classified as mature teratoma. However, many show varying degrees of immature somatic tissue, of uncertain implications. Attempts have been made to apply a grading system to sacrococcygeal lesions similar to that of ovarian immature teratomas [51,53,54,56]. These studies, summarized in table 5, have shown that up to 30% of all sacrococcygeal teratomas lacking endodermal sinus tumor show some degree of immaturity at the time of initial resection. Of the completely mature teratomas, recurrences were due to failure to completely excise the lesion; those that recurred did so only once and did not develop an endodermal sinus tumor component. Of 49 sacrococcygeal teratomas containing immature elements, five recurred as endodermal sinus tumor, four recurred locally as immature teratoma, and three recurred with metastatic immature teratoma [51,53,54,56]. There was no clear evidence of an increased frequency of recurrence with increased grade. It may be concluded that the presence of immature elements is associated with an increased risk of developing endodermal sinus tumor as well as local recurrence of immature teratoma, and that immature teratoma itself is potentially malignant. However, these data are difficult to apply to current practice, since many of the recurrent/metastatic tumors reported were initially incompletely excised due to less aggressive surgical

Table 5. Recurrences of metastases in sacrococcygeal teratomas (recurrence or metastases/total in category)

	Crussi et al. [53]	Kooijman [51]	Tapper [56]	Valdiseri [54]	Total
Mature	4/22	?/36	2/73	?/37	
Grade 1	0/3	1/3	1/5	0	2/11
Grade 2	2/5	2/3	1/8	0/2	5/18
Grade 3	2/3	1/4	3/7	0/6	6/20

practices. On the other hand, three of the grade 2–3 tumors were clearly incompletely excised yet did not recur. Regardless of the degree of immaturity, once the mass is completely resected (including the coccyx), current management includes careful radiographic monitoring for recurrence and serial measurements of serum alpha-feto protein. Preliminary results from cooperative studies that have used modern surgical guidelines and performed postoperative AFP monitoring include 23 infantile extragonadal immature teratomas (six grade 1, eight grade 2, nine grade 3), with seven containing small foci of endodermal sinus tumor that were initially undetected. Of these 24 tumors treated with surgical excision alone, with a follow-up of 6–57 months, there was only one local recurrence of a lesion that initially contained a small focus of endodermal sinus tumor [57]. This finding suggests that surgery alone may be sufficient treatment for infantile extragonadal immature teratomas. The appropriate treatment for immature teratomas containing small foci of endodermal sinus tumor remains controversial.

In the majority of immature teratomas, the immature elements identified are neural. Rare cases have been reported that show immature nephrogenic tissue supportive of a nephroblastoma, without immature neural elements [54]. No such case has been reported to recur or metastasize. Cases of 'extrarenal Wilms' tumors arising in a sacrococcygeal teratoma have been described, although their malignant potential remains to be proven [58]. Other malignancies arising in the setting of a sacrococcygeal teratomas were reported prior to the recognition of the many histologic manifestations of endodermal sinus tumor, which they are now thought to represent.

5.1.3. Sacrococcygeal endodermal sinus tumor. The development of endodermal sinus tumor within a sacrococcygeal teratoma may occur in up to 20% of cases. This development is more common in tumors that arise in, or recur in, older infants. Prior to the advent of modern chemotherapy regimens, the survival of children with endodermal sinus tumor was only 10–20% after surgery alone or in combination with radiotherapy. The introduction of regimens that include cisplatin, etoposide, and bleomycin has resulted in a dramatic improvement in outcome, with a two-year survival of over 60% for stage III and IV patients with sacrococcygeal endodermal sinus tumor [49,59,60]. Unanswered therapeutic questions revolve around the treatment of sacrococcygeal lesions that are predominately teratomatous with only small foci of endodermal sinus tumor, and the treatment of those patients with mature or immature teratoma alone by histology who have elevated AFP. The answer to such questions are often determined by the completeness of the excision.

5.1.4. Early childhood germ cell tumors at other extragonadal sites. Teratomas and endodermal sinus tumors in young children have also been described in a wide variety of extragonadal sites other than the sacrococcygeal region, such as the head and neck region [41,61–63], retroperitoneum [64], stomach [51,65,66], liver [67,68], central nervous system [62,69], and vagina

Table 6. Staging for extragonadal tumors

Stage I
    Localized disease completely resected (includes coccygectomy
    for sacral lesions); tumor markers return to baseline following
    resection
Stage II
    Microscopic residual disease or persistent elevation of tumor
    markers; capsular invasion; microscopic lymph node
    involvement
Stage III
    Gross residual disease or positive ascitic or pleural fluid
Stage IV
    Distant metastases

[41,60,70–72]. Tumors at these sites are histologically, biologically, and clinically similar to those in the sacrococcygeal region. The prognosis for these often large, bulky lesions depends on where they are located, what structures are involved, and the degree of resection. A recent report of early childhood extragonadal endodermal sinus tumors suggests that radical excision may not be required, and that biopsy may be successfully followed by cisplatin-based chemotherapy with a two-year survival of 67% [60]. Like those in the sacrococcygeal region, histologic immaturity in extragonadal teratomas has not been shown to clearly affect prognosis. The staging of all extragonadal germ cell tumors is based on tumor extent, degree of surgical excision, and AFP determination (table 6).

5.2. Testicular germ cell tumors in infants

5.2.1. Testicular teratomas. Testicular germ cell tumors of children less than 5 years of age, like those in extragonadal sites, are all teratomas or endodermal sinus tumors [73]. Unlike those in the sacrococcygeal regions, testicular teratomas in young children are much less frequent than endodermal sinus tumors and are usually small, measuring less than 2–4 cm. Over 50% are completely mature, and the presence of immature elements does not seem to adversely effect the benign prognosis [1,50,51,74]. Bilateral testicular teratomas have been reported but are quite rare [75]. Primitive neural tumors may arise in testicular teratomas of young boys, as may small foci of endodermal sinus tumor. However, these events are quite rare and poorly understood.

5.2.2. Testicular endodermal sinus tumor. Testicular endodermal sinus tumors in infants represent the most common malignant tumor of the testis in pediatric patients. The mean age of presentation is 24 months, with rare bilateral involvement (1%). Associated malformations (ventricular septal defects, Down's syndrome, and undescended testis) have been reported in up to 11% of these patients [40]. Over 80% are stage I at diagnosis, with excellent survival after surgical excision alone [40,47]. Early studies suggest that age at

Table 7. Staging for testicular germ cell tumors

Stage I
  Tumor confined to the testis, completely resected by high
  inguinal orchiectomy, serum markers return to normal
Stage II
  Tumor confined to testis; transcrotal orchiectomy; microscopic
  disease high in spermatic cord; microscopic disease in
  retroperitoneal lymph nodes
Stage III
  Increased tumor markers; macroscopic retroperitoneal lymph
  node involvement
Stage IV
  Distant metastasis

---

presentation may be an important prognostic factor. Relapse-free survival of children with local tumors who underwent surgical excision was 70%–77% for children 0–12 months, 65%–72% for children 13–24 months, and 30%–54% for children over 24 months of age [52,73]. Studies of patients treated with more current cisplatin-based therapeutic protocols have not shown age to be prognostically significant, with over 90% progression-free survival for all stages [47,59]. Historically, the treatment of testicular germ cell tumors involved high inguinal orchiectomy and retroperitoneal lymph node dissection. The latter staging procedure carries much morbidity, and its necessity has been questioned in adult patients. Retroperitoneal lymph node dissection in young boys is now controversial, since survival for those undergoing lymph node dissection shows no significant improvement [40,47]. Lymph node dissection may, however, be indicated in those patients who did not have a preorchiectomy AFP level, or in the up to 15% of patients who have a normal preorchiectomy AFP [47]. Current investigational protocols recommend lymph node sampling with resection of at least 13 lymph nodes, and resection of all lymph nodes greater than 3 cm. Many different staging systems are applied to testicular germ cell tumors; one staging system used in current pediatric protocols is outlined in table 7.

5.3. Genetic studies of early childhood germ cell tumors

Cytogenic and DNA content studies performed on a large number of sacrococcygeal and testicular teratomas of young children have shown the vast majority to be diploid; numeric and structural abnormalities are rare even in immature teratomas [16,76,77]. Genetic studies of early childhood endodermal sinus tumors, extragonadal and testicular, strongly point to a genetic change within a teratoma that results in the development of endodermal sinus tumor. The DNA content of endodermal sinus tumors is often tetraploid or aneuploid, and cytogenetic analysis shows recurrent, nonrandom chromosomal abnormalities that differ from those seen in adolescent and adult germ cell tumors [16,77]. Deletion of the terminal portion of the short arm of

177

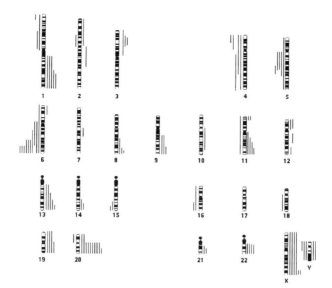

Figure 6. Schematic diagram of genetic gains (lines to right of chromosome) and losses (lines to left of chromosomes) detected in 16 childhood endodermal sinus tumors by comparative genomic hybridization.

chromosome 1 has been documented by classic cytogenetic analysis, fluorescence in situ hybridization, and comparative genomic hybridization [78–81]. Unlike similar analyses of neuroblastoma, the majority of childhood endodermal sinus tumors showing 1p deletion show loss of very small regions on distal 1p including 1p36. Thus far, deletion of 1p36 has not demonstrated prognostic associations. More frequent than deletion of 1p is deletion of 6q, and the common region of deletion by classic cytogenetics and comparative genomic hybridization appears to reside in the terminal region of 6q25–6qter [78,81]. Gain of 12p material, characteristic of adult germ cell tumors, is present in rare cases. Genetic abnormalities seen in endodermal sinus tumor are summarized in figure 6.

6. Germ cell tumors of adolescents and young adults

6.1. Adolescent testicular germ cell tumors

Tumors arising in the adolescent and adult testis are by far the most common subtype of germ cell tumors. These have shown an increase in incidence in the last few decades [82], although there has been a concomitant decline in mortality due to therapeutic advances. Unlike the testicular germ cell tumors of young children, those in adolescents and adults arise from a precursor lesion known as intratubular germ cell neoplasia [83,84]. This lesion is characterized by seminiferous tubules containing neoplastic germ cells (figure 7). Intratubular germ cell neoplasia is present with increased frequency in patients at risk for germ cell tumors, prior to the development of an invasive lesion, and is present adjacent to almost all sufficiently sampled adolescent and adult testicular germ cell tumors [85,86]. Recognition of this lesion is aided by positivity of the malignant cells for placental-like alkaline phosphatase [33,35,87,88]. The presence of intratubular germ cell neoplasia heralds the development of an invasive tumor within five years in 50% of patients [83]. The use of testicular biopsy to identify intratubular germ cell neoplasia in patients at risk for future development of a germ cell tumor is highly controversial and, while actively utilized in other countries, is currently not routinely performed in the United States [89]. This is largely due to the high degree of response of these tumors to chemotherapy and radiation therapy, reducing the benefit of surveillance.

The most frequent histologic subtype of germ cell tumor in the pediatric group is mixed malignant germ cell tumor. The histologic types most commonly seen in mixed germ cell tumors are embryonal carcinoma (present in 87%), followed by endodermal sinus tumor (22%), teratoma (55%) and choriocarcinoma (17%). The most common type of postpubertal testicular germ cell tumor is seminoma; however, because this subtype is slowly growing, it presents at a later age and is rarely seen in the pediatric age group.

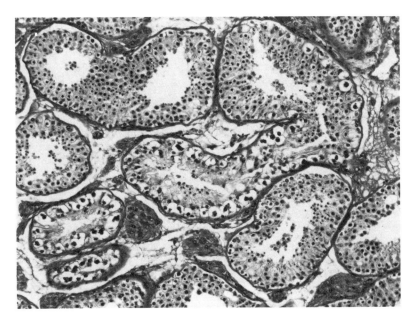

Figure 7. Seminiferous tubules with central tubule containing enlarged, atypical germ cells, consistent with intratubular germ cell neoplasia.

The standard initial treatment of all adolescent testicular germ cell tumors is high inguinal orchiectomy. Other surgical approaches that involve scrotal incisions are avoided, since local recurrences are increased [90]. Following orchiectomy, the histology and stage of the tumor determines whether or not adjuvant treatment is utilized. The introduction in 1974 of the Einhorn regimen for germ cell tumors, which included vinblastin, cisplatin, and bleomycin, dramatically improved the survival rate for patients with of all subtypes of germ cell tumors [91]. The cure rate of disseminated testicular germ cell tumors is now 60%–90% with regimens that have evolved from the Einhorn regimen. Modifications to this regimen include the replacement of vinblastin by etoposide to decrease neurotoxicity, omission of bleomycin to avoid pulmonary toxicity, and replacement of cisplatin with high-dose cisplatin or with carboplatin [91–96]. In addition to considerations of toxicity, other studies have consistently shown a dose-related 45%–50% rate of oligospermia and 20% rate of azospermia two years following chemotherapy [97].

The success of cisplatin-based chemotherapy has resulted in modification of the surgical staging of testicular germ cell tumors. Historically, all testicular germ cell tumors were managed with high inguinal orchiectomy followed by retroperitoneal lymph node dissection. Currently, the need for retroperitoneal lymph node dissection is controversial. Pure seminomas are treated with surgery, followed by adjuvant chemotherapy only in stages III and IV, resulting in complete or partial response of greater than 90% of patients with advanced-stage seminoma [98]. Clinical stage I nonseminomatous germ cell tumors are now managed with orchiectomy followed either by serologic surveillance or by retroperitoneal lymph node dissection. With intensive surveillance and early cisplatin-based chemotherapy for relapsing patients, both management plans provide cure rates of greater than 95%. The chief advantage of surveillance alone is that it prevents the morbidity associated with retroperitoneal node dissection, which provides therapeutic benefit to only 10% of clinical stage I patients. Pathologic features that have been associated with adverse outcome include lymphatic or vascular invasion, invasion of the tunica albuginea, rete testis or epidydimis, and a high percentage of embryonal carcinoma [92,99–107]. Patients with clinical stage I tumors showing these histologic features who are then treated with two courses of BEP show a greater than 90% relapse-free survival with minimal toxicity. Patients with stage I nonseminomatous germ cell tumors who show persistent elevation of serum tumor markers with negative radiographic imaging studies following orchiectomy may also be treated with adjuvant chemotherapy, with successful normalization of markers [108].

Patients with less than five retroperitoneal lymph nodes involved, and all nodes less than 2 cm, may be carefully watched following node sampling, as these patients have a low risk of relapse. Those with greater lymph node involvement have a high risk of relapse without adjuvant therapy and are treated with cisplatin-containing adjuvant chemotherapy, resulting in a greater than 95% relapse-free survival [93].

Patients with stage IV nonseminomatous germ cell tumors show a 70%–80% relapse-free survival following cisplatin-containing adjuvant chemotherapy. For the 20%–30% refractory to this therapy, salvage regimens have been studied that include additional agents (etoposide, ifosphomide, cisplatin, vinblastin, bleomycin), resulting in a 45%–65% disease-free survival, although with significant toxicity [109,110]. High-dose chemotherapy followed by the reinfusion of hematopoetic progenitor cells can also be used in relapsed or refractory germ cell tumors that have failed to respond to conventional-dose salvage regimens, resulting in a failure-free survival of 20%–30% [111–113].

It should be noted that teratomas in the postpubertal testis are most commonly seen as components of malignant germ cell tumors and only rarely occur alone. These are potentially malignant tumors at risk for metastases [114–116]. For these reasons, it is important to distinguish these aneuploid teratomas from epidermoid or dermoid cysts, which are benign.

6.1.1. Genetic studies of adolescent testicular germ cell tumors. Postpubertal testicular tumors represent the most extensively studied subgroup of germ cell tumors. DNA content analysis has shown all tumors in this category to be aneuploid in the triploid to hypotetraploid range [117–119]. Mathematical analyses of such studies have further suggested that all postpubertal testicular germ cell tumors arise in a tetraploid precursor stem line that is seminomatous, with subsequent nonrandom chromosomal loss associated with the development of other histologic subtypes [118,120]. Cytogenetic analysis has consistently shown the characteristic isochromosome 12p, i(12p), in 75%–80% of all postpubertal testicular germ cell tumors [121–128]. The i(12p) is composed of two mirror-image copies of the short arm of chromosome 12, of uniparental origin, with retention of 12q heterozygosity [129]. The presence of the i(12p) has also been documented by fluorescence in situ hybridization in intratubular germ cell neoplasia [130]. It has been suggested that patients with more than three copies of the i(12p) have a worse prognosis [123]. Comparative genomic hybridization has been successful in identifying a small region of high-level amplification at 12p11.2–12.1, providing an important clue to the localization of candidate proto-oncogenes on 12p [131,132]. Those tumors that lack the i(12p) often show deletion of 12q, and molecular studies suggest there are two deleted regions, at 12q13 and 12q22 [133]. The genes involved at these loci have not yet been identified.

6.2. Ovarian germ cell tumors

While epithelial malignancies represent the most common type of ovarian tumor in adults, germ cell tumors comprise 80% of ovarian tumors in children. Germ cell tumors in children show a higher frequency of malignancy than those in adults [134]. The vast majority of ovarian germ cell tumors are diagnosed in peripubertal and postpubertal children and adolescents; malignant germ cell tumors in the ovaries of very young children are exceedingly

Table 8. Federation of International Gynecologist and Obstetricians (FIGO) staging of ovarian carcinoma [209]

I.	Tumor limited to ovaries
	IA. Tumor limited to one ovary; no ascites
	i. Capsule intact
	ii. Capsule ruptured or tumor present on the external surface
	IB. Tumor limited to both ovaries; no ascites
	i. Capsule intact
	ii. Capsule ruptured or tumor present on the external surface
	IC. Tumor limited to ovaries; ascites present or positive peritoneal washings
II.	Tumor involving ovaries with pelvic extension
	IIA. Extension and/or metastases to uterus and/or tubes; no ascites
	IIB. Extension to other pelvic tissues; no ascites
	IIC. Tumor either IIA or IIB with ascites or positive peritoneal washings
III.	Tumor involving ovaries with intraperitoneal metastases outside the pelvis and/or positive retroperitoneal lymph nodes
IV.	Distant metastasis, including parenchymal liver metastasis

rare. Children with ovarian germ cell tumors often present with acute abdominal pain similar to appendicitis, frequently resulting in emergent laparotomy. Recent advances in the classification, management, and therapy of these tumors have resulted in increased cure rates and preservation of future fertility. The staging of ovarian lesions is indicated in table 8. Ovarian germ cell tumors show a biologic and clinical heterogeneity not seen in their testicular or extragonadal counterparts, with at least four distinct subgroups. These include mature teratomas, immature teratomas, malignant germ cell tumors similar to those seen in the testis, and germ cell tumors arising in dysgenetic gonads.

6.2.1. Mature teratomas. Mature ovarian teratomas in children most commonly present at 13–15 years of age, with a 10% incidence of bilaterality. Mature teratomas can be subdivided into those that are predominately cystic and those that are predominately solid. Cystic teratomas may contain the copious hair and sebaceous material characteristic of those in adults, but this type is less common in children. Immature elements are very rarely found in predominately cystic teratomas, and their malignant potential is minimal unless the child has a constitutional genetic abnormality resulting in increased risk of development of neoplasms (such as Li–Fraumeni syndrome). Similarly, malignant degeneration (including the development of squamous carcinoma, adenocarcinoma, and melanoma, a phenomenon that occurs in up to 2% of adult mature cystic teratomas) seldom occurs in children. The solid mature teratoma is one of the least common ovarian germ cell tumors. These are biologically closer to immature teratomas than to cystic mature teratomas and should be carefully sectioned to exclude immature elements. Glial tissue is the predominant component in these lesions. Small capsular ruptures may result in small gray-white nodules of mature glial tissue on peritoneal surfaces, representing gliomatosis peritonei [27]. It is important that these peritoneal nodules be adequately examined to identify foci of immaturity. Mature nodules, whether peritoneal or in lymph nodes, may require additional surgery but have no adverse prognostic significance [66,135–137].

6.2.2. Immature teratomas. Immature teratomas of the ovary are most common in children and adolescents and are the third most common germ cell tumor seen in adolescent females. Immature teratomas rarely metastasize and are considered intermediate lesions. The study of immature teratomas has been confused by the lack of consistency in terminology and in their histologic description, making interpretation of the literature difficult at times. Immature teratomas are predominately solid tumors that may be quite large and are most often confined to the ovary. These lesions have been graded histologically according to the amount of immature tissue present, discussed previously in the pathology section. Immature teratomas are rarely bilateral (less than 1% of cases), and the treatment of choice is unilateral oopherectomy. If a frozen section performed at the time of excision shows an immature teratoma, staging should be performed. Without adjuvant chemotherapy, the post-resection prognosis of immature teratomas depends on the histologic grade of the tumor, the size of the tumor, the age of the patient, and the stage at presentation [25]. Stage Ia, grade 1 immature teratomas are often treated with surgery alone, with reports of 13/14 recurrence-free survival. However, survival for grades 2 and 3 lesions approximates to 60% and 30%, respectively, when treated by surgery alone [25]. This benign experience with stage Ia tumors is not uniform. Piver reported five stage Ia immature teratomas surgically resected without adjuvant chemotherapy; all five developed abdominal recurrences within 10 months of surgery [138]. In 1986, Gershenson et al. reported 41 patients with ovarian immature teratoma; 15 of 16 stage I (mostly grade I) patients treated with surgery alone developed recurrent disease, and 11 of these are surviving with subsequent therapy. Of 21 others that received adjuvant chemotherapy, 18 are alive and well [139]. Subsequent studies showed sustained remission in over 80% of immature teratomas following vincristin, dactinomycin, and cyclophosphamide (VAC) chemotherapy. The Einhorn regimen has subsequently proven successful in the treatment of ovarian germ cell tumors, although most studies include few patients with immature teratoma [140].

The benefit of adjuvant chemotherapy for ovarian immature teratomas in the pediatric age group has not been determined. Preliminary analysis of the outcome of 41 ovarian immature teratomas treated by surgery alone (19 grade 1, 13 grade 2, and 9 grade 3), 10 of which also showed small foci of endodermal sinus tumor (EST), noted only one recurrence of a grade 1 lesion that contained EST in the initial tumor [57]. Other recent reports also suggest that low-stage immature ovarian teratomas do not require chemotherapy [141,142]. The chief diagnostic and therapeutic difficulty of immature teratomas is the presence of small foci of endodermal sinus tumor. As discussed in the pathology section, such foci may be exceedingly difficult to recognize even by experienced pathologists. Furthermore, it is not clear what impact their presence should have on the subsequent management.

The role of second-look laparotomy in patients receiving adjuvant chemotherapy in the management of immature teratoma remains unclear. Most observers suggest that second-look laparotomy should be performed only in patients with high-stage disease [139]. However, it is clear that second-look laparotomy may clarify the histology of residual nodules [143].

6.2.3. Ovarian dysgerminoma. Dysgerminoma is the most common malignant germ cell tumor in the ovary, composing 48% of such lesions. It is the most common ovarian malignancy in children and adolescents. There is a 10%–15% incidence of bilaterality. The majority of dysgerminomas (70%–80%) present as stage I [144,145]. Dysgerminomas are exquisitely radiosensitive, and five-year survivals with radiotherapy range from 90% in stage I disease to 60%–90% in patients with more advanced disease [146]. Properly evaluated patients with stage Ia ovarian pure dysgerminoma who desire fertility can be safely treated without radiotherapy by unilateral oophorectomy after careful lymph node sampling alone. Of these patients, 17% subsequently recur, but over 90% of these may be successfully treated with chemotherapy [144]. Other experienced observers have opted for adjuvant treatment for patients with apparent stage I disease, especially those that have not been surgically staged [145]. For higher-stage tumors, and for recurrences, chemotherapy regimens including bleomycin, etoposide, and cisplatin may result in comparable or superior outcome to radiotherapy while preserving reproductive capacity [140,147–149]. Bilateral dysgerminoma may be treated with bilateral oopherectomy and chemotherapy, with the uterus left in situ for future embryo transfer. Radiation in these cases is reserved for salvage therapy. As with most other forms of ovarian germ cell tumor, the utility of second-look laparotomy is marginal [143,150].

6.2.4. Nongerminomatous germ cell tumors. Like tumors of the adolescent and adult testis, for management purposes those of the ovary are divided into germinomatous and nongerminomatous tumors. However, the lack of a testicular counterpart to the ovarian immature teratoma/endodermal sinus tumor merits emphasis.

6.2.4.1. Endodermal sinus tumor. The second most common histologic subtype of malignant ovarian germ cell tumor in children (22%) is endodermal sinus tumor, also called *yolk sac tumor.* It is important to evaluate ovarian endodermal sinus tumor separately from ovarian mixed germ cell tumors in the event that these represent biologically distinct entities with consequent therapeutic and prognostic differences. The understanding of this histologic subtype has been plagued by inconsistent terminology and by the relatively recent full recognition of its histologic spectrum and separation from embryonal carcinoma. Rarely bilateral, these tumors are rapidly growing, yet most

184

present as stage Ia tumors [37]. Prior to the advent of multiagent chemotherapy, fewer than 20% of children with stage Ia tumors treated by surgery alone survived. As with other germ cell tumor categories, the initial adjuvant chemotherapy utilized vincristin, actinomycin-D, and cyclophosphamide (VAC) but was replaced by the Einhorn regimen of bleomycin, etoposide, and cisplatin (BEP) following the appreciation of the superior long-term relapse-free survival [59,140,151]. VAC remains of utility for patients who fail to respond to BEP. The vast majority of endodermal sinus tumors are associated with high serum levels of AFP [142]. Aggressive monitoring of serum AFP levels constitutes one of the important improvements in the management of patients with germ cell tumor, particularly those with endodermal sinus tumor. The AFP should fall into the normal range 5–7 weeks following surgery if resection of the tumor is complete.

6.2.4.2. Other histologic types of nongerminomatous tumors. Pure embryonal carcinomas are rare ovarian neoplasms (4%) that should be differentiated from the more common endodermal sinus tumor. These are more commonly seen as a minor component of a mixed germ cell tumor. Similarly, ovarian choriocarcinoma is rarely seen as the sole histologic type but may constitute a minor component within a mixed germ cell tumor. Precocious puberty is evident in one third of prepubertal children with malignant mixed germ cell tumor.

The prognosis of nongerminomatous germ cell tumors prior to the chemotherapy era was dismal. With the advent of bleomycin, etoposide, and cisplatin protocols, survival rates of 70%–90% have been reported [59,139,140,152]. The Gynecologic Oncology Group reported that 50 of 52 patients with stage I–III disease following complete resection were disease free after three cycles of BEP [153]. Others have suggested substituting carboplatin for cisplatin and eliminating bleomycin to reduce pulmonary toxicity. For patients with recurrent malignant germ cell tumor after failure on BEP, VAC chemotherapy may salvage 40% of patients.

As with other ovarian germ cell tumors, second-look laparotomy remains controversial; most patients have negative findings on second-look laparotomy. However, patients with advanced disease (stage II–IV) are more likely to show persistent disease at laparotomy and may benefit from a different chemotherapy regimen. In most cases, surveillance of tumor markers may substitute for laparotomy if such markers normalize following treatment. Second-look laparotomy may be indicated in patients with negative markers at the start of chemotherapy.

6.2.5. Ovarian germ cell tumors arising in dysgenetic gonads. Gonadoblastoma is a rare tumor that arises in the dysgenetic gonads of phenotypic females having Y chromosomal determinants [154,155]. It is virtually never seen in normal males or females, in 46,XY males with undescended but well developed testes, or in 47,XXY or 46,XX phenotypic males.

Gonadoblastomas can develop quite early in life and have been reported in infants [156]. Gonadoblastomas are benign tumors; however, 50% of patients with gonadoblastoma will develop a dysgerminoma [154,155,157]. Therefore, early gonadectomy is indicated in patients with gonadal dysgenesis who contain the Y chromosome, and examination of the opposite gonad must be performed in every patient with an ovarian germ cell tumor.

Gonadoblastomas are usually quite small and recognizable only on microscopic examination. Histologically, gonadoblastomas are characterized by nests containing both germ cells and stromal cells. Calcifications are common in gonadoblastoma and likely represent regression. Numerous calcifications within a dysgerminoma should suggest the possibility that the patient may have gonadal dysgenesis and may be at a high risk for developing a contralateral dysgerminoma. Approximately 5% of dysgerminomas are found in phenotypic females with chromosomal abnormalities such as 46,XY or mosaic 45, X/46,XY. While dysgerminoma is the most common histologic subtype of malignancy following gonadoblastoma, endodermal sinus tumor and embryonal carcinoma are also reported. Little is known of the biology of gonadoblastomas. Because gonadoblastomas are present almost exclusively in patients with 46,XY gonadal dysgenesis, it has been suggested that a gene residing on the long arm of the Y chromosome codes for an oncogene that results in gonadoblastoma when exposed to the environment of a dysgenetic gonad [158].

6.2.6. Genetic studies of ovarian germ cell tumors. Ovarian mature teratomas have been the most thoroughly studied biologically due to their abundant numbers. Over 325 cases have been cytogenetically analyzed, demonstrating 95% to be karyotypically normal and the remainder to show nonrecurrent numerical abnormalities [8,159–161]. Studies of molecular loci show that the majority of mature ovarian teratomas have entered, but have not completed, meiosis [8,9]. These studies suggest that mature ovarian teratomas arise from germ cells arrested in meiosis I.

Ovarian immature teratomas are genetically heterogeneous, with evidence of a meiotic stem cell origin in some and mitotic origins in others [7]. DNA fingerprinting studies suggest that immature teratomas arise from postmeiotic germ cells [9]. Cytogenetic studies show a higher frequency of chromosomal abnormalities in immature teratomas (60%) when compared to mature teratomas; however, no consistent abnormalities have been identified. No evidence of the i(12p) has been reported in pure immature teratomas [7,162–164]. Most immature ovarian teratomas are diploid; however, occasional tumors are aneuploid in the triploid to tetraploid range. Most of these high-level aneuploid tumors harbor foci of endodermal sinus tumor [165]. There also appears to be a relationship between grade of teratoma, prognosis, and low-level aneuploidy [77,162,165]. However, these studies involve small numbers of patients, and the independent prognostic value of DNA content determination has yet to be demonstrated.

Genetic studies of malignant ovarian germ cell tumors involving normal gonads, which are scant, show no difference from their testicular counterparts. Most malignant ovarian germ cell tumors are aneuploid or near-tetraploid. Most contain the i(12p) by classic cytogenetics and amplification of 12p by comparative genomic hybridization [16,166–168]. As previously mentioned, endodermal sinus tumors frequently develop in the context of immature teratomas. The biologic changes associated with this histologic transformation have not been adequately studied; however, ploidy analyses have suggested that a genetic change is associated with the histologic transformation [165]. The absence of the i(12p) in immature teratomas and the presence of the i(12p) in endodermal sinus tumors associated with immature teratomas suggest that one genetic change may be the acquisition of the i(12p) [167–169].

6.3. Extragonadal germ cell tumors of adolescents

6.3.1. Mediastinum. The most common site of extragonadal germ cell tumors is the mediatinium. These account for 6%–7% of all germ cell tumors in children and range from benign, incidentally discovered tumors to malignant tumors presenting with chest pain and dyspnea. Benign teratomas may not recurr if they are able to be totally excised. Mediastinal immature teratomas are quite rare, and the prognostic significance of assessing the quantity of immature elements has not been established. Malignant mediastinal germ cell tumors in adolescents and adults may show any histologic subtype. Metastases are present at the time of diagnosis in 60%–70% of germinomatous and 85%–95% of nongerminomatous mediastinal germ cell tumors [170]. Therefore, complete surgical excision is seldom possible in mediastinal malignant germ cell tumors.

Prior to 1975, the prognosis for mediastinal germ cell tumors was abysmal. With the administration of cisplatin-based chemotherapy following surgery, however, the survival of patients with nongerminomatous and germinomatous mediastinal germ cell tumors is now 50% and 94%, respectively [95,171]. In the largest reported series, Nichols reported 18 of 31 patients with non-germinomatous mediastinal germ cell tumors who were disease free after initial therapy. Of these, 11 remained continuously free of disease, two showed mature teratomatous recurrences which were resected, three relapsed with recurrent germ cell tumor (one of these was successfully salvaged), and three developed hematologic malignancies. Of 24 patients referred for salvage therapy following relapse, four (17%) achieved complete remission and four partial remission. There was no statistically significant relationship between outcome and histologic type, marker elevation, or treatment [95]. Other studies likewise show that patients requiring salvage treatment for refractory or relapsed extragonadal nongerminomatous germ cell tumors carry a poor prognosis [171,172]. The decreased survival of patients with mediastinal malignant germ cell tumors, when compared to their testicular counterparts, has been attributed to an increased prevalence of AFP-producing tumors, to more advanced stage, and to intrinsic biologic differences. The addition of etoposide may yield better outcomes [94,95,171]. In contrast, extragonadal germinomas carry a better prognosis. While radiotherapy can lead to a long-term disease-free survival, at present most investigators favor high-dose cisplatin-based chemotherapy as first-line treatment, which results in 83% long-term disease-free survivors [170].

Frequently, a mass remains following therapy and requires additional surgery. Approximately one third of mediastinal germ cell tumors require postchemotherapy surgery due to a persistent mass. Of these, 40% show mature teratoma, 20% show malignant nongerm cell elements, 20% show necrosis only, and 20% show residual viable germ cell tumor [95].

6.3.2. Genetic studies of mediastinal germ cell tumors.
Mediastinal germ cell tumors are complex biologically. Ploidy analysis has suggested that mediastinal germ cell tumors are diploid or tetraploid, in contrast with the aneuploid adolescent testicular tumors [173]. However, cases have been reported that show the i(12p) characteristic of testicular germ cell tumors [174]. Other studies have shown an association between extragonadal germ cell tumors, most commonly mediastinal, and Klinefelter's syndrome, with up to 20% of patients with mediastinal nongerminomatous germ cell tumors having a constitutional 47,XXY karyotype [15,175,176].

6.3.3. Retroperitoneal germ cell tumors.
A minority of adolescent and adult extragonadal germ cell tumors arise in the retroperitoneum. The suspicion that these tumors largely represent metastases from an occult testicular origin remains prevalent. This is supported by the finding of testicular fibrous scars in such patients, the development of a testicular tumor following presentation with an retroperitoneal tumor [171], and the finding of in situ neoplasia on testicular biopsy in 42% of patients with retroperitoneal tumors [177]. Testicular ultrasound is indicated to rule out an unsuspected testicular primary when a patient presents with a retroperitoneal germ cell tumor.

6.3.4. Germ cell tumors of the brain.
Germ cell tumors compose approximately 10% of pediatric central nervous system tumors [178]. A small number of these involve young infants and were discussed earlier. Germ cell tumors of older children most often arise in the region of the pineal gland, with a 2–4-fold increased frequency in males [58,178,179]. The clinical parameters of intracranial germ cell tumors are represented in table 9 [26,69,180]. The signs and symptoms of tumors in the pineal region are commonly those of obstruction of the third ventricle, including acute hydrocephalus with headaches, papilledema, nausea, vomiting, and lethargy. Compression of the midbrain may result in Parinaud's syndrome, with paralysis of upward gaze, diminished pupillary response to light, and nystagmus. Those tumors arising in the suprasellar region cause hypothalamic or pituitary dysfunction including diabetes insipidus, delayed or precocious puberty, or growth failure. These symp-

Table 9. Primary intracranial germ cell tumors [26]

	Number	Median age	Sex ratio
Germinoma	30 (59%)	16 (4–64 yrs)	21 M : 9 F
Teratoma	8 (16%)	4 (2 mo–13 yrs)	8 M : 0 F
Endodermal sinus tumor	5 (10%)	10 (8–11 yrs)	1 M : 4 F
Choriocarcinoma	2 (4%)	23 (17–28 yrs)	1 M : 1 F
Mixed germ cell tumor	6 (12%)	13 (7–26 yrs)	6 M : 0 F

toms may predate the neuroradiologic diagnosis by months or even years [180]. The evaluation of pineal or suprasellar lesions must include the craniospinal axis to detect metastatic seeding, which may be present in 10%–15% of cases [181,182]. CSF should be obtained for cytologic analysis and AFP and HCG measurements at the time of initial surgery or shunt placement. Metastases outside the CNS at diagnosis are rare; systemic radiologic evaluation is not indicated unless suggested by symptoms. Fuller reported 9 of 233 patients who developed pulmonary or abdominal metastases, but all were associated with retroperitoneal shunts, which have been demonstrated by others to result in spread of disease [178]. Patients with choriocarcinoma have a higher frequency (31%) of extraneural recurrences [183].

The specific diagnosis and therapy for germ cell tumors depends on histologic sampling. Historically, the operative morbidity or mortality for pineal region biopsy was 30%–60%, resulting in the use of empiric radiation therapy [179]. Current surgical practices have improved operative mortality to less than 2%–5% [184–186], and initial tissue diagnosis of pineal–suprasellar lesions is now strongly recommended. This approach enables the correct diagnosis of pineal lesions that are not germinomas (approximately 40%), avoids unnecessary CNS radiation for a benign lesion, and may improve outcome if the tumor can be resected [187]. While stereotactic biopsy has a low morbidity [181], open biopsy is generally preferred to achieve greater sampling in these histologically heterogeneous tumors [179,184].

For many years, the standard treatment for CNS germ cell tumors was whole-brain radiation [178]. The success of this therapy is somewhat difficult to evaluate, since only about half of all patients were biopsied. Radiation of the brain of young children causes impairment of brain development and intelligence and is usually contraindicated in children less than 3 years of age [188–190]. Most current treatment protocols administer initial systemic chemotherapy in an effort to postpone or reduce radiation fields for children with good-risk tumors. The impetus for chemotherapeutic treatment of CNS germ cell tumors is driven by the successful treatment of testicular germ cell tumors with cisplatin-based therapy [91]. There have been numerous case reports and several small series of patients with recurrent CNS germ cell tumors treated with chemotherapy [180,184]. In 1987, the Japanese Intracranial Germ Cell Tumor Study Group reported 30 patients treated with vincristine, cisplatin and bleomycin; the response rate was 71%, with a two-year survival of 67.7%,

189

while the control patients who received radiation alone showed a two-year survival rate of 46.5% [191]. This study was followed by a smaller series of four patients with germinomas and eight patients with nongerminomatous tumors who were treated either at recurrence or at diagnosis with cisplatin and etoposide: 11 of 12 patients responded, with 7 complete responses and 5 partial responses [192]. Preirradiation or neoadjuvant chemotherapy for newly diagnosed patients is currently being evaluated in multicenter trials in England, Germany, France, and the U.S. Therapeutic trials offer reduced radiotherapy to patients achieving complete response to chemotherapy [193].

Teratomas of older children that are completely mature may have an excellent prognosis if completely resected, with a five-year survival of 64% in one series [194]. The mortality in most cases was associated with surgical complications. In comparison, patients with immature teratoma had a five-year survival of 26% [194,195]. However, over 50% of these patients with immature teratoma had elevation of AFP or HCG, suggesting the presence of malignant components that were not detected on biopsy.

The majority of CNS tumors are mixed germ cell tumors, and all components may not be evident in a small biopsy. Monitoring of HCG and of AFP is particularly important in these cases. In a recent study of 50 patients with germinomas of the brain, those patients with normal HCG and AFP were all alive, but those patients with elevated HCG or AFP had only a 40% survival [187].

6.3.5. Genetic studies of central nervous system germ cell tumors. Cytogenetic analysis of central nervous system teratomas involving adolescents have show a high frequency of sex chromosomal abnormalities, most commonly increased copies of the X chromosome [196,197]. The i(12p) characteristic of adolescent testicular germ cell tumors has also been seen in some, but not all, pineal germinomas, but it has not been seen in pineal teratomas [198,199].

6.4. Hematologic malignancies

The association between germ cell tumors and hematologic malignancy is well established but uncommon. The vast majority of germ cell tumors that subsequently develop hematologic malignancies are malignant mediastinal germ cell tumors in males [200–207]. The associated hematologic abnormalities have included erythroleukemia, malignant histiocytosis, acute nonlymphocytic leukemia, myelodysplasia, and systemic mast cell disease. Three ovarian germ cell tumors have been reported in association with hematologic abnormalities; two of these were in 46, XY phenotypic females. The median interval between the diagnosis of the germ cell tumor and that of the hematologic malignancy is six months, much shorter than the 25–60-month interval commonly seen in chemotherapy-related hematologic malignancies. It has been proposed that the germ cell tumor may provide the stem line of the hematologic malignancy.

This hypothesis is supported by the presence of the i(12p) in both the germ cell tumor and hematopoetic malignancy in several cases [207,208].

References

1. Malogolowkin M, Mahour G, Krailo M, Ortega J. 1990. Germ cell tumors in infants and childhood: a 45-year experience. Pediatr Pathol 10:231–241.
2. Strohmeyer T, Reese D, Press M, Ackermann R, Hartmann M, Slamon D. 1995. Expression of the c-kit proto-oncogene and its ligand stem cell factor (SCF) in normal and malignant human testicular tissue. J Urol 153:511–515.
3. Besmer P, Manova K, Duttlinger R, Huang E, Packer A, Gyssler C, Bachvarova R. 1993. The kit-ligand (steel factor) and its receptor c-kit/W: pleiotropic roles in gametogenesis and melanogenesis. Development (Suppl):125–137.
4. Coucouvanis EC, Jones PP. 1993. Changes in protooncogene expression correlated with general and sex-specific differentiation in murine primordial germ cells. Mech Dev 42:49–58.
5. Strohmeyer T, Peter S, Hartmann M, Munemitsu S, Ackermann R, Ulrich A, Slamon D. 1991. Expression of the hst-1 and c-kit protooncogenes in human testicular germ cell tumors. Cancer Res 51:1811–1816.
6. Inoue M, Kyo S, Fujita M, Enomoto T, Kondoh G. 1994. Coexpression of the c-kit receptor and the stem cell factor in gynecological tumors. Cancer Res 54:3049–3053.
7. Ohama K, Nomura K, Okamoto E, Fukuda Y, Ihara T, Fujiwara A. 1985. Origin of immature teratoma of the ovary. Am J Obstet Gynecol 152:896–900.
8. Surti U, Hoffner L, Chakravarti A, Ferrell RE. 1990. Genetics and biology of human ovarian teratomas. I. Cytogenetic analysis and mechanism of origin. Am J Hum Genet 47:635–643.
9. Inoue M, Fujita M, Azuma C, Saji F, Tanizawa O. 1992. Histogenetic analysis of ovarian germ cell tumors by DNA fingerprinting. Cancer Res 52:6823–6826.
10. Falin LI. 1969. The development of genital glands and the origin of germ cells in human embryogenesis. Acta Anat 72:195–232.
11. Jirasek J. 1976. Principles of reproductive embryology. In Simpson J (ed.), Disorders of Sexual Differentiation. Academic Press: New York, pp. 51–110.
12. Upadhyay S, Zamboni L. 1982. Ectopic germ cells: natural model for the study of germ cell sexual differentiation. Proc Natl Acad Sci USA 79:6584–6588.
13. Luciano Z, Upadhyay S. 1983. Germ cell differentiation in mouse adrenal glands. J Exp Zool 228:173–193.
14. Kaplan CG, Askin FB, Benirschke K. 1979. Cytogenetics of extragonadal tumors. Teratology 19:261–266.
15. Mann BD, Sparkes RS, Kern DH, Mortno DL. 1983. Chromosomal abnormalities of a mediastinal embryonal cell carcinoma in a patient with 47,XXY Klinefelter syndrome: evidence for the premeiotic origin of a germ cell tumor. Cancer Genet Cytogenet 8:191–196.
16. Hoffner L, Deka R, Chakravarti A. 1994. Cytogenetics and origins of pediatric germ cell tumors. Cancer Genet Cytogenet 74:54–58.
17. Owen D, Hill A, Argent S. 1975. Origin of extragonadal teratomas and endodermal sinus tumors. Nature 254:597–599.
18. Gonzalez-Crussi F. 1984. Extragonadal Teratomas. Washington, D.C.: Armed Forces Institute of Pathology.
19. Dehner LP. 1983. Gonadal and extragonadal germ cell neoplasia of childhood. Hum Pathol 14:493–511.
20. Dehner LP. 1986. Gonadal and extragonadal germ cell neoplasms. In Finegold MJ (ed.), Pathology of Neoplasia in Children and Adolescents. W.B. Saunders: Philadelphia, pp. 282–312.
21. Ulbright TM, Loehrer PJ, Roth LM, Einhorn LH, Williams SD, Clark SA. 1984. The development of non-germ cell malignancies within germ cell tumors. Cancer 54:1824–1833.

191

22. Harms D, Janig U. 1985. Immature teratomas of childhood. Pathol Res Pract 179:388–400.
23. Thurlbeck WM, Scully RE. 1960. Solid teratoma of the ovary: a clinicopathological analysis of 9 cases. Cancer 13:804–811.
24. Norris HJ, Zirkin HJ, Benson WL. 1976. Immature (malignant) teratoma of the ovary: a clinical and pathologic study of 58 cases. Cancer 37:2359–2372.
25. Wollner N, Ghavimi F, Wachtel A, Luks E, Exelby P, Woodruff J. 1991. Germ cell tumors in children: gonadal and extragonadal. Med Pediatr Oncol 19:228–239.
26. Ho DM, Liu H. 1992. Primary intracranial germ cell tumor. Cancer 70:1577–1584.
27. Bahari CM, Lurie M, Schoenfeld A, Joel-Cohen SJ. 1980. Ovarian teratoma with peritoneal gliomatosis and elevated serum alpha-fetoprotein. Am J Clin Pathol 73:603–607.
28. Esterhay R, Shapiro H, Sutterland J, McIntire R, Wiernik P. 1973. Serum alpha-fetoprotein concentration and tumor growth dissociation in a patient with ovarian teratocarcinoma. Cancer 31:835–839.
29. Hawkins E, Isaacs H, Cushing B, Rogers P. 1993. Occult malignancy in neonatal sacroccygeal teratomas. A combined POG and CCG study. Pediatr Hematol Oncol 15:406–409.
30. Zuckman MH, Williams G, Levin HS. 1988. Mitosis counting in seminoma: an exercise of questionable significance. Human Pathol 19:329–335.
31. Ulbright T, Roth L. 1987. Recent developments in the pathology of germ cell tumors. Semin Diag Pathol 4:304–319.
32. Niehans GA, Manivel JC, Copland GT, Scheithauer BW, Wick MR. 1988. Immunohistochemistry of germ cell and trophoblastic neoplasms. Cancer 62:1113–1123.
33. Manivel JC, Jessurun J, Wick MR, Dehner LP. 1987. Placental alkaline phosphatase immunoreactivity in testicular germ-cell neoplasms. Am J Surg Pathol 11:21–29.
34. Washiyama K, Sekiguchi K, Tanaka R, Yamazaki K, Kumanishi T, Oyake Y. 1987. Immunohistochemical study on AFP, HCG and PLAP in primary intracranial germ cell tumors. Prog Exp Tumor Res 30:296–306.
35. Burke AP, Mostofi FK. 1988. Placental alkaline phosphatase immunohistochemistry of intratubular malignant germ cells and associated testicular germ cell tumors. Hum Pathol 19:663–670.
36. Shinoda J, Miwa Y, Sakai N, Yamada H, Shima H, Kato K, Takahashi M, Shimakawa K. 1985. Immunohistochemical study of placental alkaline phosphatase in primary intracranial germ-cell tumors. J Neurosurg 63:733–739.
37. Kurman RJ, Norris HJ. 1976. Endodermal sinus tumor of the ovary. Cancer 38:2404–2419.
38. Ulbright TM, Roth LM, Brodhecker CA. 1986. Yolk sac differentiation in germ cell tumors. Am J Surg Pathol 10:151–164.
39. Talerman A. 1986. Germ cell tumors. In Talerman A, Roth LM (eds.), Pathology of the Testis and its Adnexa. Churchill Livingstone: New York, pp. 29–65.
40. Huddart SN, Mann JR, Gornall P, Pearson D, Barrett A, Raafat F, Barnes JM, Wallendus KR. 1990. The UK Children's Cancer Study Group: testicular malignant germ cell tumours 1979–1988. J Pediatr Surg 25:406–410.
41. Shebib S, Sabbah RS, Sackey K, Akhtar M, Aur RJA. 1989. Endodermal sinus (yolk sac) tumor in infants and children. Am J Pediatr Hematol Oncol 11:36–39.
42. Ulbright TM. 1993. Germ cell neoplasms of the testis. Am J Surg Pathol 17:1075–1091.
43. Kurman RJ, Ganjei P, Nadji M. 1984. Contributions of immunocytochemistry to the diagnosis and study of ovarian neoplasms. Int J Gynecol Pathol 3:3–26.
44. Latza U, Fossa SD, Durkop H, Eitelbach F, Diekmann KP, Loy V, Unger M, Pizzolo G, Stein H. 1995. CD30 antigen in embryonal carcinoma and embryogenesis and release of the soluble molecule. Am J Pathol 146:463–471.
45. Belchis DA, Mowry J, Davis JH. 1993. Infantile choriocarcinoma: re-examination of a potentially curable entity. Cancer 72:2028–2032.
46. Gitlin D, Perricelli A, Gitlin GM. 1972. Synthesis of alpha fetoprotein by liver, yolk sac, and gastrointestinal tract of the human conceptus. Cancer Res 32:979–982.
47. Kaplan GW, Cromie WC, Kelalis PP, Silber I, Tank ES. 1988. Prepubertal yolk sac testicular tumors — report of the testicular tumor registry. J Urol 140:1109–1112.

48. Wu JT, Book L, Sudar K. 1991. Serum alpha fetoprotein levels in normal infants. Pediatr Res 15:50–52.
49. Marina N, Fontanesi J, Kun L, Rao B, Jenkins JJ, Thompson EI, Etcubanas E. 1992. Treatment of childhood germ cell tumors. Cancer 70:2568–2575.
50. Livingston RR, Sarembock LA. 1986. Testicular tumors in children. S Afr Med J 70:168–169.
51. Kooijman CD. 1988. Immature teratomas in children. Histopathology 12:491–502.
52. Schropp KP, Lobe TE, Rao B, Mutabagani K, Kay GA, Gilchrist BF, Philippe PG, Boles ET. 1992. Sacrococcygeal teratoma: the experience of four decades. J Pediatr Surg 27:1075–1079.
53. Gonzalez-Crussi F, Winkler RF, Mirkin DL. 1978. Sacrococcygeal teratomas in infants and children: relationship of histology and prognosis in 40 cases. Arch Pathol Lab Med 102:420–425.
54. Valdiserri RO, Yunis EJ. 1981. Sacrococcygeal teratomas: a review of 68 cases. Cancer 48:217–221.
55. Altman RP, Randolph JG, Lilly JR. 1974. Sacrococcygeal teratoma: American Academy of Pediatrics Surgical Section Survey — 1973. J Pediatr Surg 9:389–398.
56. Tapper D, Lack EE. 1983. Teratomas in infancy and childhood. Ann Surg 198:398–409.
57. Cushing B, Giller H, Cohen D, et al. 1996. Surgery alone is effective treatment of resected immature teratoma in children: a pediatric intergroup report. Med Pediatr Oncol 27:221.
58. Andrews PE, Kelalis PP, Haase GM. 1992. Extrarenal Wilms' tumor: results of the National Wilms' Tumor Study. J Pediatr Surg 27:1181–1184.
59. Kapoor G, Advani SH, Nair CN, Pai SK, Kurkure PA, Nair R, Saikia TK, Vege D, Desai PB. 1995. Pediatric germ cell tumor. J Pediatr Hematol Oncol 17(4):318–324.
60. Davidoff AM, Hebra A, Bunin N, Shochat SJ, Schnaufer L. 1996. Endodermal sinus tumor in children. J Pediatr Surg 31(8):1075–1079.
61. Jordan R, Gauderer M. 1988. Cervical teratomas: an analysis. Literature review and proposed classification. J Pediatr Surg 23:583–591.
62. Dehner LP, Mills A, Talerman A, Billman GF, Krous HF, Platz CE. 1990. Germ cell neoplasms of head and neck soft tissues: a pathologic spectrum of teratomatous and endodermal sinus tumors. Hum Pathol 21:309–318.
63. Watanatittan S, Othersen J, Hughson M. 1981. Cervical teratomas in children. Prog Pediatr Surg 14:225–239.
64. Lack EE, Travis WD, Welch KJ. 1985. Retroperitoneal germ cell tumors in childhood. Cancer 56:602–608.
65. Senocak M, Kale G, Buyukpamukcu N, Hicsonmez A, Calgar M. 1990. Gastric teratoma in children including the third reported female case. J Pediatr Surg 25:681–684.
66. Coulson W. 1990. Peritoneal gliomatosis from gastric teratoma. Am J Clin Pathol 94:87–89.
67. Fraumeni JF, Li FP, Dalager N. 1973. Teratomas in children: epidemiologic features. J Natl Cancer Inst 51:1425–1430.
68. Wakely J, Krummel T, Johnson D. 1991. Yolk sac tumor of the liver. Mod Pathol 4:121–125.
69. Rueda-Pedraza ME, Heifetz SA, Seserhenn IA, Clark GB. 1987. Primary intracranial germ cell tumors in the first two decades of life. Perspect Pediatr Pathol 10:160–207.
70. Hawkins EP, Finegold MJ, Hawkins HK, Krischer JP, Starling KA, Weinberg A. 1986. Nonseminomatous malignant germ cell tumors in children. Cancer 58:2579–2584.
71. Copeland LJ, Sneig N, Ordonez NG, Hancock KC, Gershenson DM, Saul PB, Kavanagh JJ. 1985. Endodermal sinus tumor of the vagina and cervix. Cancer 55:2558–2565.
72. McHenry C, Revnolds M, Raffensperger J. 1988. Vaginal neoplasms in infancy: the combined role of chemotherapy and conservative surgical resection. J Pediatr Surg 23:842–845.
73. Green DM. 1986. Testicular tumors in infants and children. Semin Surg Oncol 2:156–162.
74. Malogolowkin MH, Ortega JA, Krailo M, Gonzalez O, Mahour GH, Landing BH, Siegel SE. 1989. Immature teratomas: identification of patients at risk for malignant recurrence. J Natl Cancer Inst 81:870–874.
75. Carney JA, Kelalis PP, Lynn HB. 1973. Bilateral teratoma of testis in an infant. J Pediatr Surg 8:49–54.

76. Kashiwagi A, Nagamori S, Toyota K, Maeno K, Koyanagi T. 1993. DNA ploidy of testicular germ cell tumors in childhood: difference from adult testicular tumors. Nippon Hinyokiki Gekkai Zasshi 84:1655–1659.

77. Silver SA, Wiley JM, Perlman EJ. 1994. DNA ploidy analysis of pediatric germ cell tumors. Mod Pathol 7:951–956.

78. Perlman EJ, Cushing B, Hawkins E, Griffin CA. 1994. Cytogenetic analysis of childhood endodermal sinus tumors: a Pediatric Oncology Group study. Ped Pathol 14:695–708.

79. Oosterhuis JW, Castedo SMMJ, de Jong B, Seruca R, Buist J, Koops HS, Leeuw JB. 1988. Karyotyping and DNA flow cytometry of an orchidoblastoma. Cancer Genet Cytogenet 36:7–11.

80. Jenderny J, Koster E, Meyer A, Borchers O, Grote W, Harms D, Janig U. 1995. Detection of chromosome aberrations in paraffin sections of seven gonadal yolk sac tumors of childhood. Hum Genet 96(6):644–650.

81. Perlman EJ, Ho D. 1997. Genetic analysis of childhood endodermal sinus tumors by comparative genomic hybridization. Mod Pathol 10:158A.

82. Gurney JG, Davis S, Severson RK, Fang J, Ross JA, Robinson LL. 1996. Trends in cancer incidence among children in the U.S. Cancer 79(3):532–541.

83. Skakkebaek NE. 1978. Carcinoma in situ of the testis: frequency and relationship to the invasive germ cell tumours in infertile men. Histopathology 2:157–170.

84. Manivel JC, Reinberg Y, Niehans GA, Fraley EE. 1989. Intratubular germ cell neoplasia in testicular teratomas and epidermoid cysts. Cancer 64:715–720.

85. Klein FA, Melamed MR, Whitmore WF. 1985. Intratubular malignant germ cells (carcinoma in situ) accompanying invasive testicular germ cell tumors. J Urol 133:413–415.

86. Giwercman A, Bruun E, Frimodt-Moller C, Skakkebaek NE. 1989. Prevalence of carcinoma in situ and other histopathological abnormalities in testes of men with a history of cryptorchidism. J Urol 142:998–1002.

87. Niehans GA, Wick MR, Manivel JC, Dehner LP. 1989. Immunohistochemistry of intratubular germ cell neoplasia. Surg Pathol 2:213–229.

88. Koide O, Iwai S, Baba K, Iri H. 1987. Identification of testicular atypical germ cells by an immunohistochemical technique for placental alkaline phosphatase. Cancer 60:1325–1330.

89. Berthelsen JG, Skakkebaek NE. 1981. Value of testicular biopsy in diagnosing carcinoma in situ testis. Scand J Urol Nephrol 15:165–168.

90. Capelouto CC, Clark PE, Ransil BJ, Loughlin KR. 1995. A review of scrotal violation in testicular cancer: Is adjuvant local therapy necessary? J Urol 153(3 Pt 2):981–985.

91. Einhorn L. 1993. Clinial trials in testicular cancer. Cancer 71(10):3182–3184.

92. Pant J, Albrecht W, Postner G, Sellner F, Angel K, Holtl W. 1996. Adjuvant chemotherapy for high-risk clinical stage I nonseminomatous testicular germ cell cancer: long-term results of a prospective trial. J Clin Oncol 14(2):441–448.

93. Motzer RJ, Sheinfeld J, Mazumdar M, Bajorin DF, Bosl GJ, Herr H, Lyn P, Vlamis V. 1995. Etoposide and cisplatin adjuvant therapy for patients with pathologic stage II germ cell tumors. J Clin Oncol 13(11):2700–2704.

94. Williams SD, Birch R, Einhorn LH, Irwin L, Greco FA, Loehrer PJ. 1987. Treatment of disseminated germ-cell tumors with cisplatin, bleomycin, and either vinblastine or etoposide. N Engl J Med 316:1435–1440.

95. Nichols CR, Saxman S, Williams SD, Loehrer PJ, Miller ME, Wright C, Einhorn LH. 1990. Primary mediastinal sonseminomatous germ cell tumors: a modern single institution experience. Cancer 65:1641–1646.

96. Peckham MJ, Husband JE, Barrett A, Hendry WF. 1982. Orchidectomy alone in testicular stage I non-seminomatous germ cell tumors. Lancet 1:678–680.

97. Stephenson WT, Poirier SM, Rubin L, Einhorn L. 1995. Evaluation of reproductive capacity in germ cell tumor patients following treatment with cisplatin, etoposide, and bleomycin. J Clin Oncol 13(9):2278–2280.

98. Puc HS, Heelan R, Mazumdar M, Herr H, Scheinfeld J, Vlamis V, Bajorin DF, Bosl G, Mencel P, Motzer RJ. 1996. Management of residual mass in advanced seminoma: results

and recommendations from the memorial Sloan-Kettering Cancer Center. J Clin Oncol 14(2):454–460.

99. Fung CY, Kalish LA, Brodsky GL, Richie JP, Garnick MB. 1988. Stage I nonseminomatous germ cell testicular tumor: prediction of metastatic potential by primary histopathology. J Clin Oncol 6:1467–1473.

100. Sturgeon JFG, Jewett MAS, Alison RE, Gospodarowicz MK, Blend R, Herman S, Richmond H, Thomas G, Duncan W, Munro A. 1992. Surveillance after orchidectomy for patients with clinical stage I nonseminomatous testis tumors. J Clin Oncol 10:564–568.

101. Dunphy CH, Ayala AG, Swanson DA, Ro JY, Logothetis C. 1988. Clinical stage I nonseminomatous and mixed germ cell tumors of the testis. Cancer 62:1201–1206.

102. Moriyama N, Daly JJ, Keating MA, Lin C-W, Prout GR. 1985. Vascular invasion as a prognosticator of metastatic disease in nonseminomatous germ cell tumors of the testis. Cancer 56:2492–2498.

103. Javadpour N, Canning DA, O'Connell KJ, Young JD. 1986. Predictors of recurrent clinical stage I nonseminomatous testicular cancer. Urology 27:508–511.

104. Wishnow KI, Johnson DE, Swanson DA, Tenney DM, Babaian RJ, Dunphy CH, Ayala AG, Ro JY, von Eschenbach AC. 1989. Identifying patients with low-risk clinical stage I nonseminomatous testicular tumors who should be treated by surveillance. Urology 39:339–343.

105. Cullen MH, Stenning SP, Parkinson MC, Fossa SD, Kaye SB, Horwich AH, Harland SJ, Williams MV, Jakes R. 1996. Short-course adjuvant chemotherapy in high-risk stage I nonseminomatous germ cell tumors of the testis: a medical research council report. J Clin Oncol 14(4):1106–1113.

106. Read G, Stenning SP, Cullen MH, Parkinson MC, Horwich AH, kaye SB, Cook PA. 1992. Medical research council prospective study of surveillance for stage I testicular teratoma. J Clin Oncol 10:1762–1768.

107. Freedman LS, Jones WG, Peckham MJ, Newlands ES, Parkinson MC, Oliver RTD, Read G, Williams CJ. 1987. Histopathology in the prediction of relapse of patients with stage I testicular teratoma treated by orchidectomy alone. Lancet 1:294–301.

108. Culine S, Theodore C, Terrier-Lacombe MJ, Droz JP. 1996. Primary chemotherapy in patients with nonseminomatous germ cell tumors of the testis and biological disease only after orchiectomy. J Urol 155(4):1296–1298.

109. Farhat F, Culine S, Theodore C, Bekradda M, Terrier-Lacombe M, Droz J. 1996. Cisplatin and ifosfamide with either vinblastine or etoposide as salvage therapy for refractory or relapsing germ cell tumor patients. Cancer 77(6):1193–1197.

110. Blanke C, Loehrer PJ, Nichols CR, Einhorn LH. 1996. A phase II trial of VP-16, ifosfamide, cisplatin, vinblastine, and bleomycin in advanced germ-cell tumors. Am J Clin Oncol 19(5):487–491.

111. Motzer RJ, Gulati SC, Tong WP, Menendez-Botet C, Lyn P, Mazumdar M, Vlamis V, Lin S, Bosl GJ. 1993. Phase I trial with pharmacokinetic analyses of high-dose carboplatin, etoposide, and cyclophosphamide with autologous bone marrow transplantation in patients with refractory germ cell tumors. Cancer Res 53(16):3730–3735.

112. Motzer RJ, Mazumdar M, Bosl GJ, Bajorin DF, Amsterdam A, Vlamis V. 1996. High-dose carboplatin, etoposide, and cyclophosphamide for patients with refractory germ cell tumors: treatment results and prognostic factors for survival and toxicity. J Clin Oncol 14(4):1098–1105.

113. Beyer J, Kramar A, Mandanas R, Linkesch W, Greinix A, Droz JP, Pico JL, Diehl A, Bokemeyer C, Schmoll HJ, Nichols CR, Einhorn LH, Siegert W. 1996. High-dose chemotherapy as salvage treatment in germ cell tumors: a multivariate analysis of prognostic variables. J Clin Oncol 14(10):2638–2645.

114. Oosterhuis JW, de Jong B, Cornelisse CJ, Molenaar IM, Meiring A, Idenburg V, Koops HS, Sleijfer DT. 1986. Karyotyping and DNA flow cytometry of mature residual teratoma after intensive chemotherapy of disseminated nonseminomatous germ cell tumors of the testis: a report of two cases. Cancer Genet Cytogenet 22:149–157.

195

115. Castedo SMMJ, de Jong B, Oosterhuis JW, Idenburg VJS, Seruca R, Buist J, te Meerman GJ, Koops HS, Sleijfer DT. 1989. Chromosomal changes in mature residual residual teratomas following polychemotherapy. Cancer Res 49:672–676.

116. Kusuda L, Leidich RB, Das S. 1986. Mature teratoma of the testis metastasizing as mature teratoma. J Urol 135:1020–1022.

117. Atkin NB, Baker MC. 1992. X-chromatin, sex chromosomes, and ploidy in 37 germ cell tumors of the testis. Cancer Genet Cytogenet 59:54–56.

118. El-Naggar AK, Ro JY, McLemore D, Ayala AG, Batsakis JG. 1992. DNA ploidy in testicular germ cell neoplasms. Am J Surg Pathol 16:611–618.

119. Oosterhuis JW, Castedo SMMJ, de Jong B, Cornelisse CJ, Sleijfer DT, Dam A, Koops HS. 1989. Ploidy of primary germ cell tumors of the testes. Lab Invest 60:14–21.

120. de Jong B, Oosterhuis JW, Castedo SMMJ, Vos A, te Meerman GJ. 1990. Pathogenesis of adult testicular germ cell tumors. Cancer Genet Cytogenet 48:143–167.

121. Gibas Z, Prout GR, Sandberg AA. 1984. Malignant teratoma of the testis with an isochromosome number 12, (i12p), as the sole structural cytogenetic abnormality. J Urol 131:762–763.

122. Atkin NB, Baker MC. 1983. i(12p): Specific chromosomal marker in seminoma and malignant teratoma of the testis? Cancer Genet Cytogenet 10:199–204.

123. Bosl GJ, Dmitrovsky E, Reuter VE, Samaniego F, Rodriguez E, Geller NL, Chaganti RSK. 1989. Isochromosome of chromosome 12: clinically useful marker for male germ cell tumors. J Natl Cancer Inst 81:1874–1878.

124. Samaniego F, Rodriguez E, Houldsworth J, Murty VVVS, Ladanyi M, Lele KP, Chen Q, Dimitrovsky E, Geller NL, Reuter V, Jhanwar SC, Bosl GJ, Chaganti RSK. 1990. Cytogenetic and molecular analysis of human male germ cell tumors: chromosome 12 abnormalities and gene amplification. Genes Chromosomes Cancer 1:289–300.

125. Castedo SMMJ, de Jong B, Oosterhuis JW, Seruca R, Idenburg VIS, Dam A, te Meerman G, Koops HS. 1989. Chromosomal changes in human primary testicular nonseminomatous germ cell tumors. Cancer Res 49:5696–5701.

126. Delozier-Blanchet CD, Walt H, Engel E, Vuagnat P. 1987. Cytogenetic studies of human testicular germ cell tumors. Int J Androl 10:69–77.

127. Gibas Z, Prout GR, Pontes JE, Sandberg AA. 1986. Chromosome changes in germ cell tumors of the testis. Cancer Genet Cytogenet 19:245–252.

128. Atkin NB, Baker MC. 1985. Chromosome analysis of three seminomas. Cancer Genet Cytogenet 17:315–323.

129. Sinke RJ, Suijkerbuijk RF, de Jong B, Oosterhuis JW, van Kessell AG. 1993. Uniparental origin of i(12p) in human germ cell tumors. Genes Chromosomes Cancer 6:161–165.

130. Looijenga LHJ, Gillis JM, Van Putten WLJ, Oosterhuis JW. 1993. In situ numeric analysis of centromeric regions of chromosomes 1, 12, and 15 of seminomas, nonseminomatous germ cell tumors, and carcinoma in situ of human testis. Lab Invest 68:211–219.

131. Suijkerbuijk RF, Sinke RJ, Weghuis DEMO, Roque L, Forus A, Stellink F, Siepman A, van de Kaa C, Soares J, van Kessel AG. 1994. Amplification of chromosome subregion 12p11.2–p12.1 in a metastasis of an i(12p)-negative seminoma: relationship to tumor progression. Cancer Genet Cytogenet 78(2):145–152.

132. Korn WM, Weghuis DEMO, Suijkerbuijk RF, Schmidt U, Otto T, du Manoir S, van Kessel AG, Harstrick A, Seeber S, Becher R. 1996. Detection of chromosomal DNA gains and losses in testicular germ cell tumors by comparative genomic hybridization. Genes Chromosomes Cancer 17(2):78–87.

133. Murty VVVS, Houldsworth J, Baldwin S, Reuter V, Hunziker W, Besmer P, Bosl G, Chaganti RSK. 1992. Allelic deletions in the long arm of chromosome 12 identify sites of candidate tumor suppressor genes in male germ cell tumors. Proc Natl Acad Sci USA 89:11006–11010.

134. Norris HJ, Jensen RD. 1972. Relative frequency of ovarian neoplams in children and adolescents. Cancer 30:713–719.

196

135. Harms D, Janig U, Gobel U. 1989. Gliomatosis peritonei in childhood and adolescence: clinicopathological study of 13 cases including immunohistochemical findings. Pathol Res Pract 184:422–430.

136. Shafie M, Furay RW, Chablani LV. 1984. Ovarian teratoma with peritoneal and lymph node metastases of mature 'glial' tissue: a benign condition. J Surg Oncol 27:18–22.

137. Perrone T, Steiner M, dehner LP. 1986. Nodal gliomatosis and alpha-fetoprotein production: two unusual facets of grade I ovarian teratoma. Arch Pathol Lab Med 110:975–977.

138. Piver MS, Patton T. 1986. Ovarian cancer in children. Semin Surg Oncol 2:163–169.

139. Gershenson DM, Del Junco G, Silva EG, copeland LJ, Wharton JT. 1986. Immature teratoma of the ovary. Obstet Gynecol 68:624–629.

140. Gershenson DM, Morris M, Cangir A, Kavanagh JJ, Stringer CA, Edwards CL, Silva EG, Wharton JT. 1990. Treatment of malignant germ cell tumors of the ovary with bleomycin, etoposide, and cisplatin. J Clin Oncol 8:715–720.

141. Bonazzi C, Peccatori F, Colombo N, Lucchini V, Grazia M, Mangioni C. 1994. Pure ovarian immature teratoma, a unique and curable disease: 10 years' experience of 32 prospectively treated patients. Obstet Gynecol 84:598–604.

142. Chow SN, Yang JH, Lin YH, Chen YP, Lai JI, Chen RJ, Chen CD. 1996. Malignant ovarian germ cell tumors. Int J Gynecol Obstet 53:151–158.

143. Williams SD, Blessing JA, DiSaia PJ, Major FJ, Ball HG, Liao SY. 1994. Second-look laparotomy in ovarian germ cell tumors: the Gynecologic Oncology Group experience. Gynecol Oncol 52:287–291.

144. Gallion HH, van Nagell JR, Donaldson ES, Powell DE. 1988. Ovarian dysgerminoma: report of seven cases and review of the literature. Am J Obstet Gynecol 158:591–595.

145. Williams SD. 1991. Treatment of germ cell tumors of the ovary. Semin Oncol 18:292–296.

146. Afridi MA, Vongtama V, Tsukada Y, Piver MS. 1976. Dysgerminoma of the ovary: radiation therapy of recurrence and metastases. Am J Obstet Gynecol 126:190–194.

147. Gershenson DM, Wharton JT, Kline RC, Larson DM, Kavanagh JJ, Rutledge FN. 1986. Chemotherapeutic complete remission in patients with metastatic ovarian dysgerminoma. Cancer 58:2594–2599.

148. Javaheri G, Lifchez A, Valle J. 1983. Pregnancy following removal of and long-term chemotherapy for ovarian malignant teratoma. Obstet Gynecol 61:8S–9S.

149. Williams SD, Blessing JA, Moore DH, Homesley HD, Adcock L. 1989. Cisplatin, vinblastine, and bleomycin in advanced and recurrent ovarian germ-cell tumors. Ann Intern Med 111:22–27.

150. Peccatori F, Bonazzi C, Chiari S, Landoni F, Colombo N, Mangioni C. 1995. Surgical management of malignant ovarian germ-cell tumors: 10 years experience of 129 patients. Obstet Gynecol 86:367–372.

151. Slayton RE, Park RC, Silverger SG, Shingleton H, Creasman WT, Blessing JA. 1985. Vincristine, dactinomycin, and cyclophosphamide in the treatment of malignant germ cell tumors of the ovary. Cancer 56:243–248.

152. Culine S, Lhomme C, Michel G, Leclere J, Duvillard P, Droz J. 1996. Is there a role for second-look laparotomy in the management of malignant germ cell tumors of the ovary? Experience at Institut Gustave Roussy. J Surg Oncol 62:40–45.

153. Williams S, Blessing JA, Lian S-Y, Ball H, Hanjani P. 1994. Adjuvant therapy of ovarian germ cell tumors with cisplatin, etoposide, and bleomycin: a trial of the Gynecologic Oncology Group. J Clin Oncol 12:701–706.

154. Park IJ, Pyeatte JC, Jones HW, Woodruff JD. 1972. Gonadoblastoma in a true hermaphrodite with 46,XY genotype. Obstet Gynecol 40:466–472.

155. Scully RE. 1970. Gonadoblastoma. Cancer 25:1340–1356.

156. Olsen MM, Caldamone AA, Jackson CL, Zinn A. 1988. Gonadoblastoma in infancy: indications for early gonadectomy in 46XY gonadal dysgenesis. J Pediatr Surg 23:270–271.

157. Hart WR, Burkons DM. 1979. Germ cell neoplasms arising in gonadoblastomas. Cancer 43:669–678.

158. Page DC. 1987. Hypothesis: a Y-chromosomal gene causes gonadoblastoma in dysgenetic gonads. Development 101:151–155.

159. Parrington JM, West LF, Povey S. 1984. The origin of ovarian teratomas. J Med Genet 21:4–12.

160. Corfman PA, Richardt RM. 1975. Chromosome number and morphology of benign ovarian cystic teratomas. N Engl J Med 271:1241–1244.

161. Linder D, McCaw BK, Hecht F. 1975. Human benign ovarian teratomas. N Engl J Med 292:63–66.

162. King ME, DiGiovanni LM, Yung J, Clarke-Pearson DL. 1990. Immature teratoma of the ovary grade 3, with karyotype analysis. Int J Gynecol Pathol 9:178–184.

163. Yang-Feng TL, Katz SN, Cancang ML, Schwartz PE. 1988. Cytogenetic analaysis of ependymoma and teratoma of the ovary. Cancer Genet Cytogenet 35:83–89.

164. Gibas Z, Talerman A, Faruqi S, Carlson J, Noumoff J. 1993. Cytogenetic analysis of an immature teratoma of the ovary and its metastasis after chemotherapy-induced maturation. Int J Gynecol Pathol 12:276–280.

165. Baker BA, Figueroa L, Hawkins E, Perlman EJ. 1996. Ploidy analysis in subsets of ovarian germ cell tumors. Mod Pathol 9:88A.

166. Atkin NB, Baker MC. 1987. Abnormal chromosomes including small metacentrics in 14 ovarian cancers. Cancer Genet Cytogenet 26:355–361.

167. Speleman F, DePotter C, Dal Cin P, Mangelschots K, Ingelaere H, Laureys G, Benoit Y, Leroy J, Van Den Berghe H. 1990. i(12p) in a malignant ovarian tumor. Cancer Genet Cytogenet 45:49–53.

168. Riopel MA, Perlman EJ. 1997. Genetic analysis of ovarian germ cell tumors by comparative genomic hybridization. Mod Pathol 10:108A.

169. Hoffner L, Shen-Schwarz S, Deka R, Chakravarti A. 1992. Genetics and biology of human ovarian teratomas. III. Cytogenetics and origins of malignant ovarian germ cell tumors. Cancer Genet Cytogenet 62:58–65.

170. Hainsworth JD, Greco FA. 1992. Extragonadal germ cell tumors and unrecognized germ cell tumors. Sem Oncol 19:119–127.

171. Gerl A, Clemm C, Lamerz R, Wilmanns W. 1996. Cisplatin-based chemotherapy of primary extragonadal germ cell tumors. Cancer 77(3):526–532.

172. Saxman S, Nichols CR, Einhorn LH. 1994. Salvage chemotherapy in patients with extragonadal nonseminomatous germ cell tumors: the Indiana University experience. J Clin Oncol 12:1390–1393.

173. Oosterhuis JW, Rammeloo RHU, Cornelisse CJ. 1990. Ploidy of malignant mediastinal germ cell tumors. Hum Pathol 21:732729–732.

174. Dal Cin P, Drochmans A, Moerman P, Van Den Berghe H. 1989. Isochromosome 12p in mediastinal germ cell tumor. Cancer Genet Cytogenet 42:243–251.

175. Fujimoto Y, Monden Y, Nakahara K, Kawashima Y. 1985. Benign mediastinal teratoma associated with Klinefelter's syndrome. Jpn J Surg 15:221–224.

176. Lachman MF, Kim K, Koo B. 1986. Mediastinal teratoma associated with Klinefelter's syndrome. Arch Pathol Lab Med 110:1067–1071.

177. Daugaard G, Rorth M, von der Maase J, Skakkebaek ME. 1992. Management of extragonadal germ cell tumors and the significance of bilateral testicular biopsies. Am Oncol 3:283–289.

178. Fuller BG, Kapp DS, Cox R. 1993. Radiation therapy of pineal region tumors: 25 new cases and a review of 208 previously reported cases. Int J Radiat Oncol Biol Phys 28:229–245.

179. Baumgartner JE, Edwards MSB. 1992. Pineal tumors. Neurosurg Clin North Am 3:853–862.

180. Jennings MT, Gelman R, Hochberg F. 1985. Intracranial germ-cell tumors: natural history and pathogenesis. J Neurosurg 63:155–167.

181. Dearnaley DP, A'Hern RP, Whittaker S, Bloom HJG. 1990. Pineal and CNS germ cell tumors: Royal Marsden Hospital experience 1962–1987. Inc J Rad Oncol Biol Phys 18(4):773–781.

182. Wara W, Jenkin D, Evans A, Ertel I, Hittle R, Ortega J, Wilson C, Hammond D. 1979. Tumors of the pineal and suprasellar region: Childrens Cancer Study Group treatment results 1960–1975. Cancer 43:698–701.

183. Chan HSL, Humphreys RP, Hendrick EB, Chuang SH, Fitz CR, Becker LE. 1984. Primary intracranial choriocarcinoma: a report of two cases and a review of the literature. Neurosurgery 15(4):540–545.

184. Edwards MSB, Hudgins RJ, Wilson CB, Levin VA, Wara WM. 1988. Pineal region tumors in children. J Neurosurg 68:689–697.

185. Hoffman HJ. 1987. Pineal region tumors. Prog Exp Tumor Res 30:281–288.

186. Jooma R, Kendall B. 1983. Diagnosis and management of pineal tumors. J Neurosurg 58:654–665.

187. Balmaceda C, Finlay J, Heller G, Vlamis V, Maher P, Rosenblum M. 1993. Prognostic factors at diagnosis in patients with primary central nervous system germ cell tumors (CNS GCT): a report of an international collaborative trial of chemotherapy (abstract). Acta Neurochir 120:111.

188. Danoff BF, Cowchock FS, Marquette C, Mulgrew L, Kramer S. 1982. assessment of the long-term effects of primary radiation therapy for brain tumors in children. Cancer 49(8):1580–1586.

189. Duffner PK, Cohen ME, Thomas P. 1982. Late effects of treatment on the intelligence of children with posterior fossa tumors. Cancer 51(2):233–237.

190. Duffner PK, Cohen ME, Thomas PRM, Lansky SB. 1985. The long-term effects of cranial irradiation on the central nervous system. Cancer 56(7):1841–1846.

191. Matsutani M, Takakura K, Sano K. 1987. Primary intracranial germ cell tumors: pathology and treatment. Prog Exp Tumor Res 30:307–312.

192. Kobayashi T, Yoshida J, Sugita K, et al. 1989. Combination chemotherapy with cisplatin and etoposide for intracranial germ cell tumors. Pediatr Neurosci 14:151.

193. Allen JC. 1987. Management of primary intracranial germ cell tumors of childhood. Pediatr Neurosci 13:152–157.

194. Takakura K. 1984. Intracranial germ cell tumors. In Clinical Neurosurgery, Proceedings of the Congress of Neurological Surgeons. Williams and Wilkins: Baltimore, pp. 429–444.

195. Kageyama N, Kobayashi T, Kida Y, Yoshida J, Kato K. 1987. Intracranial germinal tumors. Prog Exp Tumor Res 30:255–267.

196. Casalone R, Righi R, Granata P, Portentoso P, Minelli E, Meroni E, Solero CL, Allegranza A. 1994. Cerebral germ cell tumor and XXY karyotype. Cancer Genet Cytogenet 74:25–29.

197. Yu IT, Griffin CA, Phillips PC, Strauss LC, Perlman EJ. 1995. Numerical sex chromosomal abnormalities in pineal teratomas by cytogenetic analysis and fluorescence in situ hybridization. Lab Invest 72:419–423.

198. Shen V, Chaparro M, Choi BH, Young R, Bernstein R. 1990. Absence of isochromosome 12p in a pineal region malignant germ cell tumor. Cancer Genet Cytogenet 50:153–160.

199. de Bruin TWA, Slater RM, Defferrari R, van Kessell AG, Suijkerbuijk RF, Jansen G, de Jong B, Oosterhuis JW. 1994. Isochromosome 12p-positive pineal germ cell tumor. Cancer Res 54:1542–1544.

200. Mihal V, Dusek J, Jarosova M, Zidova L, Pospisilova D, Indrak K, Scudla V, Krc I, Bradova E, Gregurkova J, Spidlova A. 1989. Mediastinal teratoma and acute megakaryoblastic leukemia. Neoplasma 36:739–747.

201. DeMent SH. 1990. Association between mediastinal germ cell tumors and hematologic malignancies: an update. Hum Pathol 21:699–703.

202. Mascarello JT, Cajulis TR, Billman GF, Spruce WE. 1993. Ovarian germ cell tumor evolving to myelodysplasia. Genes Chromosomes Cancer 7:227–230.

203. Koo CH, Reifel J, Kogut N, Cove JK, Rappaport H. 1992. True histiocytic malignancy associated with a malignant teratoma in a patient with 46XY gonadal dysgenesis. Am J Surg Pathol 16:175–183.

204. Chariot P, Monnet I, Gaulard P, Abd-Alsamad I, Ruffie P, De Cremoux H. 1993. Systemic

199

mastocytosis following mediastinal germ cell tumor: an association confirmed. Hum Pathol 24:111–112.

205. Chariot P, Monnet I, LeLong F, Chleq C, Droz J, De Cremoux H. 1991. Systemic mast cell disease associated with primary mediastinal germ cell tumor. Am J Surg Pathol 90:381–385.

206. Nichols CR, Roth BJ, Heerema N, Griep J, Tricot G. 1990. Hematologic neoplasia associated with primary mediastinal germ-cell tumors. N Engl J Med 322:1425–1429.

207. Ladanyi M, Samaniego F, Reuter VE, Motzer RJ, Jhanwar SC, Bosl GL, Chaganti RSK. 1990. Cytogenetic and immunohistochemical evidence for the germ cell origin of a subset of acute leukemias associated with mediastinal germ cell tumors. J Natl Cancer Inst 82:221–227.

208. Chaganti RSK, Ladanyi M, Samaniego F, Offit K, Reuter VE, Jhanwar SC, Bosl GJ. 1989. Leukemic differentiation of a mediastinal germ cell tumor. Genes Chromosomes Cancer 1:83–87.

209. Zaloudek C, Kurman RJ. 1983. Recent advances in the pathology of ovarian cancer. Clin Obstet Gynecol 10:155–185.

7. Hepatic malignancies in childhood and adolescence (hepatoblastoma, hepatocellular carcinoma, and embryonal sarcoma)

Edwin C. Douglass

1. Introduction

Primary malignant liver tumors are uncommon in pediatric patients. Hepatoblastoma, hepatocellular carcinoma, and embryonal sarcoma are the primary entities that challenge the pediatric oncologist. Although these tumors are potentially curable, the efficacy of treatment is highly dependent on anatomic location and responsiveness to chemotherapy.

2. Hepatoblastoma

Hepatoblastoma is the most common malignant hepatic tumor of childhood, with a median age of presentation of 1 year. The majority of tumors present before 2 years of age, but some may be diagnosed in older children and even in adolescents. The annual incidence rate is approximately one per million children.

2.1. Genetic factors

The two most important genetic conditions associated with the development of hepatoblastoma are familial adenomatous polyposis (FAP) and Beckwith–Wiedemann syndrome (BWS). The incidence of hepatoblastoma in FAP kindreds in increased by a factor of 200 to 800 times that of the general population [1–3]. The incidence of hepatoblastoma is also increased in BWS and in its variants, such as hemihypertrophy. Loss of heterozygosity at chromosome 11p15, the region of BWS, has been observed in sporadic hepatoblastoma [4]. Loss of genetic imprinting with retention of paternal alleles has also been observed at this locus [5,6].

Cytogenetic studies have demonstrated that trisomies of chromosomes 2q and 20 are common in hepatoblastoma. Double minutes have also been observed [7,8]. A recurring translocation, t(1;4)(q12;q34), has been reported in four cases of hepatoblastoma [9]. A unique translocation, t(10:22), also has been reported in a case of small cell (anaplastic) hepatoblastoma [10].

D.O. Walterhouse and S.L. Cohn (eds), DIAGNOSTIC AND THERAPEUTIC ADVANCES IN PEDIATRIC ONCOLOGY. Copyright © 1997. Kluwer Academic Publishers, Boston. All rights reserved.

A single epidemiologic study of hepatoblastoma noted an association with maternal exposure to metals, paints, and oil products [11]. A significant number (approximately 10%) of children diagnosed with hepatoblastoma have a history of prematurity with prolonged stay in a neonatal intensive care unit; however, the tumorigenic factor in this association remains to be elucidated.

2.2. Pathology

2.2.1. Classification. The two primary epithelial cell types seen in hepatoblastoma are described as *fetal* and *embryonal*. Fetal cells are slightly smaller than normal hepatocytes and form slender cords separated by sinusoids. Embryonal cells have a high nuclear:cytoplasmic ratio and exhibit a higher cell density with more frequent mitoses than fetal cells. Both types may be mixed in the same tumor. Hepatoblastomas may be *epithelial*, with purely fetal or embryonal histology or an admixture of the two. Alternatively, they may exhibit *mixed* histology, with epithelial components combined with mesenchymal elements. These mesenchymal elements typically take the form of collections of spindle cells, and osteoid may also be present. Rare histologic patterns also found in hepatoblastoma include the *macrotrabecular* variant seen in epithelial tumors and the *small cell* (anaplastic) pattern, which resembles neuroblastoma [12]. Table 1 lists the classification schema proposed by Conran et al. [13], with the distribution seen in their series of 105 cases. This classification adds a category of mixed hepatoblastoma with *teratoid* features, where elements from all three germ layers can be distinguished in the tumor.

2.2.2. Pathology and prognosis. A number of authors have tried to discern a relationship between pathologic subtypes of hepatoblastoma and prognosis [13–15]. However, there has yet to be a clear demonstration of prognostic import to histopathology in the majority of cases of hepatoblastoma. It has been demonstrated that tumors with purely fetal histology that have been entirely removed have an excellent prognosis [16]. The rare small cell (anaplastic) variant of hepatoblastoma, usually accompanied by low serum alpha-

Table 1. Histologic classification hepatoblastoma [13]

Epithelial type	
Fetal pattern	28%
Embryonal pattern	17%
Macrotrabecular pattern	3%
Small cell pattern	3%
Mixed epithelial/mesenchymal	
Mixed pattern	31%
Mixed pattern/teratoid features	9%
Hepatoblastoma not otherwise specified	9%

fetoprotein levels, appears to confer a particularly poor prognosis and has been resistant to most forms of treatment [17].

2.3. Diagnostic workup

Hepatoblastoma is the most common liver tumor in childhood, particularly in children younger than 5 years of age. Other lesions that could be considered in the child presenting with a primary liver tumor include hepatocellular carcinoma, embryonal sarcoma of the liver, and vascular malformations (primarily hemangioendothelioma), as well as more uncommon malignancies in this location, such as angiosarcoma, embryonal rhabdomyosarcoma, and neuroblastoma.

The serum alpha-fetoprotein level is markedly elevated in patients with hepatoblastoma, except in cases of the small cell variant, where minimal or no elevation may be seen. It should be noted that alpha-fetoprotein is *normally* elevated at birth, particularly in premature infants, and declines to normal adult levels over the first year of life (table 2).

Hepatoblastoma infrequently presents with precocious puberty in males. This phenomenon is associated with β-HCG-excreting tumors.

Diagnostic imaging studies should include computerized tomography (CT) or magnetic resonance imaging (MRI) of the liver. CT scans cannot be relied upon to accurately predict tumor resectability [18]; MRI may be more useful, particularly as a preoperative evaluation. A CT scan of the chest should be performed, since this site is the most common location for metastatic disease. Although bone metastases may occur rarely in hepatoblastoma, bone scans at diagnosis are not useful and may be misleading because of the occurrence of osteopenia associated with hepatoblastoma [19]. This osteopenia will regress after treatment of the tumor.

2.4. Staging

Postsurgical disease extent has been the primary criterion used in the staging of hepatoblastoma in most North American clinical studies (table 3). Such a staging system is dependent on the surgical expertise and familiarity of the

Table 2. Normal serum alpha-fetoprotein of infants at various ages [59]

Age	Mean ± S.D. (ng/mL)
Premature	134,734 ± 41,444
Newborn	48,406 ± 34,713
1 mo.	2654 ± 3080
2 mo.	323 ± 278
4 mo.	74 ± 56

Table 3. Postsurgical staging of hepatoblastoma

Stage I — completely resected tumor
Stage II — microscopic residual posttumor resection (tumor at margins of resected specimen)
Stage III — partially resected or unresected specimen confined to liver, or tumor spill during operative procedure
Stage IV — distant metastatic disease

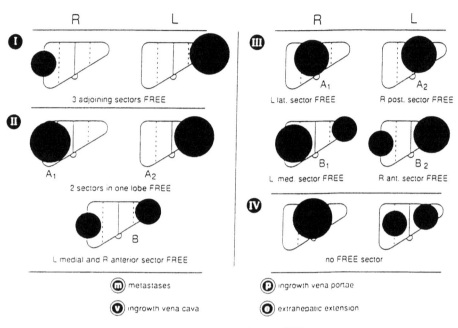

Figure 1. Pretreatment Staging System for Hepatoblastoma [20].

individual surgeon with reference to resection of liver tumors. Criteria for pretreatment staging have been proposed (figure 1) and may be most useful for comparison of patients in multi-institutional studies [20].

2.5. Treatment

The following discussion of treatment of hepatoblastoma will be divided into three topics: early case reports/small clinical series, clinical trials, and management of resistant/recurrent disease. Orthotopic liver transplant, an increasingly important modality in the management of this disease, will be discussed later in the chapter, since this topic relates to all the malignant liver tumors of childhood.

2.5.1. Early case reports. Responses of childhood 'hepatomas' were noted even in the early clinical trials of doxorubicin [21]. Reports by Andrassy [22] and Weinblatt [23] indicated the effectiveness of doxorubicin in combination chemotherapy given preoperatively to children with hepatoblastoma. Cisplatin emerged as an important agent in the treatment of hepatoblastoma, with reports of its therapeutic efficacy both in combination with doxorubicin [24] and combined with vincristine and 5-fluorouracil [25,26]. Even when used as a single agent, cisplatin, used in a high dose of $150\,mg/m^2$, produced marked preoperative tumor responses in seven patients with advanced disease [27].

2.5.2. Clinical trials. The first two multi-institutional studies of hepatoblastoma were reported by Evans in 1982 [28]. All children with malignant liver tumors, both hepatoblastoma and hepatocellular carcinoma, were eligible for these studies, and the two histologic types were combined in the analyses of survival. In study 1 (1972–1976), children with stage I tumors received no further treatment, and those with residual or metastatic disease received vincristine, actinomycin-D, and cyclophosphamide together with radiation therapy to areas of disease. Metastatic disease occurred in 7 of the 11 children with stage I tumors. Only 7 of the 40 patients entered survived; there were no survivors who did not have either complete resection or minor residual disease that received radiotherapy. No responses occurred to chemotherapy alone. Study 2 (1972–1978) employed a more aggressive chemotherapy combination of vincristine, cyclophosphamide, doxorubicin, and 5-fluorouracil. All patients (including those with stage I disease) received chemotherapy, while those with residual or metastatic disease continued to receive radiation therapy. This study demonstrated a marked survival improvement in patients with stage I disease: 20 of 24 patients survived with the addition of adjuvant chemotherapy. Responses to chemotherapy were noted in 12 of 37 patients with measurable disease (stages III and IV); however, their overall survival remained poor, with only two patients surviving after resection of residual disease. A third study ran from 1981–1984 and added cisplatin and bleomycin to the four-drug regimen of study 2. No analysis of the data from this study has been published; however, the outcome was similar enough to the previous studies to include patients in an analysis of histology and prognosis in hepatoblastoma [16].

From the mid-1980s, both the Pediatric Oncology Group (POG) and the Children's Cancer Group (CCG) developed treatment protocols based primarily on the use of cisplatin. The CCG demonstrated that a regimen of cisplatin and continuous-infusion doxorubicin achieved a measurable tumor response in 25 of 33 children (75%) with initially unresectable hepatoblastoma. This response allowed gross tumor excision in 20 of the 25 patients, and 19 of these 29 remained free of disease following treatment [29]. The POG employed cisplatin combined with vincristine and 5-fluorouracil in a pilot study for patients with all stages of hepatoblastoma. Patients with tumor excised initially (stages I and II) had a 90% disease-free survival following four courses of adjuvant chemotherapy. In patients with advanced disease (stages III and IV), 36 of 39 achieved a partial response to chemotherapy (92%), and 24 of 31 stage III patients had a complete excision of tumor after chemotherapy. Patients with stage IV disease fared poorly, with only 1 of 8 experiencing a long-term disease-free survival [30].

The cisplatin/doxorubicin regimen and the cisplatin/vincristine/5-fluorouracil regimen were subsequently compared in a randomized intergroup protocol (CCG 8881/POG 8945) that ran from 1989 through 1992 and registered 173 eligible patients with hepatoblastoma. There was no difference in survival between the two regimens. Patients with stages I and II disease continued to do well, with 95% event-free survival (EFS) of patients with stage I/II disease, 60% EFS of patients with stage III disease, and 25% EFS of patients with stage IV disease. Toxicity was more pronounced in patients receiving the cisplatin/doxorubicin regimen, particularly cardiotoxicity and severe neutropenia, and it was concluded that the cisplatin/vincristine/5-fluorouracil regimen should be considered the preferable treatment [31,32].

The International Society for Pediatric Oncology (SIOP) has also evaluated the use of cisplatin and doxorubicin used preoperatively in all patients presenting with primary liver tumors and elevated AFP levels. They report a response rate of 86% in patients with hepatoblastoma [33].

The German cooperative Pediatric Liver Tumor Study evaluated the use of a combination of ifosfamide, doxorubicin, and cisplatin in 37 patients with advanced or metastatic hepatoblastoma. Thirty-five of the 37 patients responded to the chemotherapy, with a disease-free survival rate of 73% (23 patients) at a median of 36 months follow-up [34]. No patients with lymph node involvement or metastatic disease were long-term survivors, and a rising AFP level during therapy was a predictor of poor survival.

2.5.3. Management of resistant/recurrent disease. The management of resistant and/or recurrent disease in hepatoblastoma remains unsatisfactory; however, it is possible, on an individual basis, for patients to benefit and even enjoy long-term disease-free survival after failing primary treatment. The child with rising AFP levels after achieving a complete remission represents a particularly perplexing and not uncommon clinical situation. Such children may be reasonably managed by continued close follow-up with imaging of the chest and abdomen until the tumor source of the rising AFP level is apparent. Recurrent disease confined to the lungs may be managed by metastatectomy alone or with concurrent chemotherapy with a feasible chance of cure [35–37]. Recurrent disease in the remaining liver or abdomen carries a much worse prognosis and warrants the use of aggressive treatment regimens if a cure is sought.

Resistant disease confined to the liver after primary chemotherapy represents another common clinical situation in the management of hepatoblastoma. There is some evidence of the benefit of radiotherapy in selected cases [30,38], and intratumoral chemoembolization has also been used, but it is here that orthotopic liver transplantation offers the greatest possibility cure (see section 4 below).

Patients whose tumors are resistant to chemotherapy with standard platinum-containing regimens may benefit from treatment with increased dose intensity of cisplatin. In the POG 9345 study, 12 hepatoblastoma patients who continued to have unresectable or metastatic disease following chemotherapy with carboplatin ($700\,mg/m^2$), vincristine, and 5FU received cisplatin ($40\,mg/ m^2/d \times 5$ days) with VP-16; 9 of 12 achieved further tumor shrinkage, and this therapy allowed complete tumor resection in three of these patients.

3. Hepatocellular carcinoma

In contrast to hepatoblastoma, hepatocellular carcinoma is seen more frequently in children over 5 years of age, although it may occur in infants [12]. An abdominal mass, sometimes associated with pain, is the usual presenting feature. A number of underlying conditions, all characterized by hepatocellular damage, may be associated with hepatocellular carcinoma, including biliary atresia, Fanconi's anemia, type 1 glycogen storage disease, and hereditary tyrosinemia. Hepatocellular carcinoma has also been reported in neurofibromatosis type 1, fetal alcohol syndrome, and ataxia-telangiectasia [12]. Hepatocellular carcinomas have occurred as second malignant neoplasms in patients who received abdominal irradiation as treatment for Wilms' tumor [39].

Several institutional series of hepatocellular carcinoma in childhood have noted the very high mortality rate associated with this malignancy (<90%) [39–41]. In a review of cases combined from early Pediatric Intergroup Studies, Haas reported only one survivor out of 28 patients. Although the fibrolamellar variant of hepatocellular carcinoma has been reported as carrying an improved prognosis, this outcome was not confirmed by the Intergroup series [16]. In the latest Pediatric Intergroup Study, children and adolescents with hepatocellular carcinoma were randomized to receive therapy with either cisplatin/vincristine/5-fluorouracil or cisplatin/doxorubicin. While 7 of 7 patients whose tumors were initially completely resected survive free of disease, only 4 of 38 patients with more advanced disease at diagnosis survive. Although this study suggests a good prognosis for those patients whose disease can be resected, both chemotherapy regimens proved inadequate for the treatment of patients with advanced disease [42].

There are a number of treatment modalities that have been used in the treatment of hepatocellular carcinoma. These include (in addition to surgery and numerous chemotherapeutic regimens) cryosurgery, embolization, chemoembolization, isolated hepatic perfusion, percutaneous intratumoral alcohol injection, radiation therapy, and radioimmunotherapy. None has had a significant impact on patient outcome [41,43]. However, individual patients may benefit from one or more of these modalities. A reasonable approach to unresectable nonmetastatic hepatocellular carcinoma may include standard chemotherapy such as ICE (ifosfamide, carboplatin, etoposide) or chemoembolization with combinations such as cisplatin, doxorubicin, and mitomycin. If tumor shrinkage is achieved, resection should be attempted. If the tumor remains unresectable, orthotopic liver transplantation may be considered (see section 4 below). Patients with metastatic hepatocellular carcinoma at diagnosis have a very poor prognosis, but chemotherapy may still provide some palliative benefit.

4. Transplantation for hepatic malignancy

The cure of primary hepatic malignancy in childhood depends ultimately on surgical extirpation of the tumor. While chemotherapy may provide tumor shrinkage adequate for subsequent resection in the majority of cases of hepatoblastoma, a significant minority (10%–25%) of children remain who have tumors that can only be removed by complete hepatectomy and orthotopic liver transplant. There is much more experience with liver transplantation in adults with hepatocellular carcinoma, where the chance of significant survival after transplant has been reported to be from 25% to 50% [44–46]. Because of its rarity, experience with transplantation from hepatoblastoma is more limited; however, several reviews have reported a 50%–75% long-term survival for children with hepatoblastoma treated with liver transplantation [47–49]. The more favorable chances of survival with hepatoblastoma are most likely due to its greater chemotherapeutic responsiveness compared to hepatocellular carcinoma. Informative literature on the outcome of liver transplantation in children with hepatocellular carcinoma is also limited, but the survival of these children seems to parallel that of adults [49]. Hepatocellular carcinoma is an occasional finding in the livers of children who receive an orthotopic transplant for chronic liver disease but does not seem to affect the chances for survival of these children [50].

Liver transplantation is a reasonable therapeutic strategy for the child with unresectable hepatoblastoma that has shown some response to chemotherapy. The chances for recurrence of tumor after transplant in these children is small, due in part to the effectiveness of chemotherapy in preventing the appearance of metastatic disease. The child with unresectable hepatocellular carcinoma (which usually shows little response to chemotherapy) may not be as likely to be cured by liver transplantation; however, long-term survival has been reported.

5. Embryonal sarcoma of the liver

Embryonal sarcoma of the liver is an undifferentiated sarcomatous neoplasm. It is the third most common hepatic malignancy in childhood, with an incidence of occurrence slightly less than hepatocellular carcinoma. It presents typically in late childhood (6–10 years) as a rapidly growing abdominal mass that may be associated with pain [51]. Immunohistochemical and ultrastructural attempts have not clearly defined its histogenesis [52–54].

Older series have noted a very poor prognosis conferred by this tumor [51]; however, recent reports have demonstrated the efficacy of combined modality therapy with chemotherapy followed by surgical resection of residual disease. Earlier chemotherapy reports indicated that 'sarcoma therapy' with vincristine, actinomycin, cyclophosphamide, and doxorubicin could produce tumor responses [55,56]. More recent reports indicate that cisplatin and ifosfamide may be even more effective [56,57]. Some patients enjoy long-term survival after surgical resection without adjuvant chemotherapy [54,58]. Children presenting with unresectable tumors should receive chemotherapy, e.g., vincristine, ifosfamide, and doxorubicin, followed by attempted surgical resection.

6. Summary

Hepatoblastoma is the most common malignant liver tumor of childhood. Clinical trials have demonstrated its responsiveness to chemotherapy, especially with platinum-based chemotherapeutic agents. In patients with completely resected tumors, recurrent disease is effectively controlled by adjuvant chemotherapy. In patients with initially unresectable tumors, chemotherapy can induce tumor shrinkage sufficient to allow complete extirpation of tumor and also to prevent recurrent disease. The child with tumor resistant to primary therapy or with recurrent disease presents a special problem requiring individualized and innovative therapies, including consideration of orthotopic liver transplant.

Hepatocellular carcinoma in children and adolescents carries a much poorer prognosis compared to hepatoblastoma. Complete resection of tumor offers the only hope of cure, but these tumors are unfortunately resistant or partially resistant to conventional doses of chemotherapy. A number of innovative treatment strategies have been employed, but optimal treatment remains elusive. Transplant for tumor localized to the liver may offer the only hope of cure.

Embryonal (undifferentiated) sarcoma of the liver is a rare tumor that has not been studied prospectively in any clinical trial. Small published series indicate that it can be responsive to chemotherapy, and cure may be possible.

References

1. Iwama T, Mishima Y. 1994. Mortality in young first-degree relatives of patients with familial adenomatous polyposis. Cancer 73:2065–2068.

2. Li FP, Thurber WA, Seddon J, et al. 1987. Hepatoblastoma in families with polyposis coli. JAMA 257:2475–2477.

3. Garber JE, Li FP, Kingston JE, et al. 1988. Hepatoblastoma and familial adenomatous polyposis. J Natl Cancer Inst 80:1626–1628.

4. Simms LA, Reeve AE, Smith PJ. 1995. Genetic mosaicism at the insulin locus in liver associated with childhood hepatoblastoma. Genes Chromosomes Cancer 13:72–73.

5. Rainier S, Dobry CJ, Feinberg AP. 1995. Loss of imprinting in hepatoblastoma. Cancer Res 55:1836–1838.

6. Albrecht S, von Schweinitz D, Waha A, et al. 1994. Loss of maternal alleles on chromosome arm 11p in hepatoblastoma. Cancer Res 54:5041–5044.

7. Mascarello JT, Jones MC, Kadota RP, et al. 1990. Hepatoblastoma characterized by trisomy 20 and double minutes. Cancer Genet Cytogenet 47:243–247.

8. Fletcher JA, Kozakewich HP, Pavelka K, et al. 1991. Consistent cytogenetic aberrations in hepatoblastoma: a common pathway of genetic alterations in embryonal liver and skeletal muscle malignancies? Genes Chromosomes Cancer 3:34–43.

9. Schneider NR, Cooley LD, Finegold MJ, et al. In press. Report of the first recurring chromosome translocation in hepatoblastoma: der(4)t(1;4)(q12;q34). Genes Chromosomes Cancer. 19:291–294, 1977.

10. Hansen K, Bagtas J, Mark HF, et al. 1992. Undifferentiated small cell hepatoblastoma with aunique chromosomal translocation: a case report. Pediatr Pathol 12:457–462.

11. Buckley JD, Sather H, Ruccione K, et al. 1989. A case–control study of risk factors for hepatoblastoma. Cancer 64:1169–1176.

12. Weinberg AG, Finegold MJ. 1983. Primary hepatic tumors of childhood. Hum Pathol 14:512–537.

13. Conran RM, Hitchcock CL, Waclawiw MA, et al. 1992. Hepatoblastoma: the prognostic significance of histologic type. Pediatr Pathol 12:167–183.

14. Dehner LP, Manivel JC. 1988. Hepatoblastoma: an analysis of the relationship between morphologic subtypes and prognosis. Am J Pediatr Hematol Oncol 10:310–307.

15. von Schweinitz D, Wischmeyer P, Leuschner I, et al. 1994. Clinico-pathological criteria with prognostic relevance in hepatoblastoma. Eur J Cancer 30A:1052–1058.

16. Haas JE, Muczynski KA, Krailo M, et al. 1989. Histopathology and prognosis in childhood hepatoblastoma and hepatocarcinoma. Cancer 64:1082–1095.

17. Lack EE, Neave C, Vawter GF. 1982. Hepatoblastoma: a clinical and pathologic study of 54 cases. Am J Surg Pathol 6:693–705.

18. King SJ, Babyn PS, Greenberg ML, et al. 1992. Value of CT in determining the resectability of hepatoblastoma before and after chemotherapy. Am J Roentgen 160:793–798.

19. Archer D, Babyn P, Gilday D, et al. 1993. Potentially misleading bone scan findigns in patients with hepatoblastoma. Clin Nucl Med 18:1026–1031.

20. Mackinlay GA, Pritchard J. 1992. A common language for childhood liver tumours. Pediatr Surg Int 7:325–326.

21. Tan C, Rosen G, Ghavimi F, et al. 1975. Adriamycin (NSC-123127) in pediatric malignancies. Cancer Chemother Rep 6:259–266.

22. Andrassy RJ, Brennan LP, Siegel MM, et al. 1980. Preoperative chemotherapy for hepatoblastoma in children: report of six cases. J Pediatr Surg 15:517–522.

23. Weinblatt ME, Siegel SE, Siegel MM, et al. 1982. Preoperative chemotherapy for unresectable primary hepatic malignancies in children. Cancer 50:11061–11064.

24. Quinn JJ, Altman AJ, Robinson HT, et al. 1985. Adriamycin and cisplatin for hepatoblastoma. Cancer 56:1926–1929.

25. Douglass EC, Green AA, Wrenn E, et al. 1985. Effective cisplatin (DDP) based chemotherapy in the treatment of hepatoblastoma. Med Pediatr Oncol 13:187–190.

26. Douglass EC, Green AA, Priest JR, et al. 1987. Effective therapy for metastatic/unresectable hepatoblastoma (HB) (abstract). Proc Am Soc Clin Oncol 6:214.

27. Black CT, Cangir A, Choroszy M, et al. 1991. Marked response to preoperative high-dose cisplatinum in children with unresectable hepatoblastoma. J Pediatr Surg 26:1070–1073.

28. Evans A, Land VJ, Newton WA, et al. 1982. Combination chemotherapy (vincristine, adriamycin, cyclophosphamide, and 5-fluorouracil) in the treatment of children with malignant hepatoma. Cancer 50:821–826.

29. Ortega JA, Krailo MD, Haas JE, et al. 1991. Effective treatment of unresectable or metastatic hepatoblastoma with cisplatin and continuous infusion doxorubicin chemotherapy: a report from the Children's Cancer Study Group. J Clin Oncol 9:2167–2176.

30. Douglass EC, Reynolds M, Finegold M, et al. 1993. Cisplatin, vincristine, and fluorouracil therapy for hepatoblastoma: a Pediatric Oncology Group Study. J Clin Oncol 11:96–99.

31. Ortega JA, Douglass E, Feusner J, et al. 1994. A randomized trial of cisplatin/vincristine/5-fluorouracil vs. cisplatin/doxorubicin i.v. continuous infusion for the treatment of hepatoblastoma. Results from the Pediatric Intergroup Hepatoma Study (CCG-8881/POG 9845) (abstract). Proc Am Soc Clin Oncol 13:416.

32. Ortega JA, Douglass EC, Feusner J, et al. In press. A randomized of trial of cisplatin/vincristine/5-fluorouracil vs. cisplatin/adriamycin I.V. continuous infusion for the treatment of hepatoblastoma: a report from the Pediatric Liver Tumor Intergroup (CCG 8881/POG 8945). J Clin Oncol.

33. Perilongo G, Plaschkes J, Brown J, et al. 1996. Response of hepatoblastoma to pre-operative chemotherapy with cisplatin and doxorubicin (PLADO) in the International Society of Paediatric Oncology Liver tumor Study (abstract). Proc Am Soc Clin Oncol 14:444.

34. von Schweinitz D, Hecker H, Harms D, et al. 1995. Complete resection before development of drug resistance is essential for survival from advanced hepatoblastoma: a report from the German Cooperative Pediatric Liver tumor Study HB-89. J Pediatr Surg 30:845–852.

35. Feusner JH, Krailo MD, Haas JE, et al. 1993. Treatment of pulmonary metastases of initial stage I hepatoblastoma in childhood: report from the Children's Cancer Group. Cancer 71:859–864.

36. Black CT, Luck SR, Musemeche CA, et al. 1991. Aggressive excision of pulmonary metastases is warranted in the management of childhood hepatic tumors. J Pediatr Surg 26:1082–1085.

37. Passmore SJ, Noblett HR, Wisheart JD, et al. 1995. Prolonged survival following multiple thoracotomies for metastatic hepatoblastoma. Med Pediatr Oncol 24:58–60.

38. Habrand J-L, Nehme D, Kalifa C, et al. 1992. Is there a place for radiation therapy in the management of hepatoblastomas and hepatocellular carcinomas in children? (Abstract.) Int J Radiat Oncol Biol Phys 23:525–531.

39. Kovalic JJ, Thomas PRM, Beckwith JB, et al. 1991. Hepatocellular carcinoma as second malignant neoplasms in successfully treated Wilms' tumor patients. Cancer 67:342–344.

40. Lack EE, Neave C, Vawter GF. 1983. Hepatocellular carcinoma: review of 32 cases in childhood and adolescence. Cancer 52:1510–1515.

41. Farmer DG, Busuttil RW. 1994. The role of multimodal therapy in the treatment of hepatocellular carcinoma. Cancer 73:2669–2670.

42. Douglass E, Ortega J, Feusner J, et al. 1994. Hepatocellular carcinoma in children and adolescents: Results from the Pediatric Integroup Hepatoma Study (CCG 8881/POG 8945) (abstract). Proc Am Soc Clin Oncol 13:420.

43. Venook AP. 1994. Treatment of hepatocellular carcinoma: too many options? J Clin Oncol 12:1323–1334.

44. Ringe B, Wittekind C, Bechstein WO, et al. 1989. The role of liver transplantation in hepatobiliary malignancy. Ann Surg 209:88–98.

45. Olthoff KM, Millis JM, Rosove MH, et al. 1990. Is liver transplantation justified for the treatment of hepatic malignancies? Arch Surg 125:1261–1268.

46. Iwatsuki S, Starzl TE, Sheahan DG, et al. 1991. Hepatic resection versus transplantation for hepatocellular carcinoma. Ann Surg 214:221–229.

47. Penn I. 1991. Hepatic transplantation for primary and metastatic cancers of the liver. Surgery 110:726–734.

48. Koneru B, Flye MW, Busuttil RW, et al. 1991. Liver transplantation for hepatoblastoma: the American experience. Ann Surg 213:118–121.

211

49. Tagge EP, Tagge DU, Reyes J, et al. 1992. Resection including transplantation, for hepatoblastoma and hepatocellular carcinoma: impact on survival. J Pediatr Surg 27:292–297.
50. Esquivel CO, Gutierrez C, Cox KL, et al. 1994. Hepatocellular carcinoma and liver cell dysplasia in children with chronic liver disease. J Pediatr Surg 11:1465–1469.
51. Stocker JT, Ishak KG. 1978. Undifferentiated (embryonal) sarcoma of the liver: report of 31 cases. Cancer 42:336–348.
52. Parham DM, Kelly DR, Donnelly WH, et al. 1991. The immunohistochemical and ultrastructural spectrum of hepatic sarcomas of childhood: evidence for a common histogenesis. Mod Pathol 4:648–653.
53. de Chadarevian J-P, Pawel BR, Faerber EN, et al. 1994. Undifferentiated (embryonal) sarcoma arising in conjunction with mesenchymal hamartoma of the liver. Mod Pathol 7:490–493.
54. Leuschner I, Schmidt D, Harms D. 1990. Undifferentiated sarcoma of the liver in childhood. Hum Pathol 21:68–76.
55. Horowitz ME, Etcubanas E, Webber BL, et al. 1987. Hepatic undifferentiated (embryonal) sarcoma and rhabdomyosarcoma in children: results of therapy. Cancer 59:396–402.
56. Babin-Boilletot A, Flamant F, Lacombe-Terrier M-J, et al. 1993. Primitive malignant nonepithelial hepatic tumors in children. Med Pediatr Oncol 21:634–639.
57. Urban CE, Mache CJ, Schwinger W, et al. 1993. Undifferentiated (embryonal) sarcoma of the liver in childhood: successful combined-modality therapy in four patients. Cancer 72:2511–2516.
58. Walker NI, Horn MJ, Strong RW, et al. 1992. Undifferentiated (embryonal) sarcoma of the liver. Pathologic findings and long-term survival after complete surgical resection. Cancer 69:52–59.
59. Wu JT, Book L, Sudar K. 1981. Serum alpha fetoprotein levels in normal infants. Pediatr Res 15:50–52.

212

III

Sarcomas

8. Osteosarcoma

Jeffrey S. Dome and Cindy L. Schwartz

1. Introduction

Only three decades ago, osteosarcoma was considered incurable; treatment options were greeted with great skepticism and pessimism [1]. The recognition of the efficacy of adjuvant chemotherapy has allowed 70% of patients with osteosarcoma to be cured of their disease. With the advances in our understanding of the biology of osteosarcoma, we are poised to improve this cure rate even further. This chapter highlights the latest information on the biology and treatment of osteosarcoma.

2. Epidemiology and etiology

Osteosarcoma is the most common primary malignancy of bone in childhood and adolescence. There is a bimodal pattern of incidence, with the first peak occurring in the second decade of life and the second, much smaller, peak occurring around age 70 (see figure 1). Osteosarcoma is rare in early childhood, with only a few documented cases in patients less than 3 years of age [2–4]. In the pediatric population, bone tumors compose 5% of malignancies in children aged 0–14 years; 52% of these are osteosarcoma and 40% are Ewing's sarcoma [5]. Osteosarcoma thus composes 2.6% of pediatric malignancies in the United States, with an age-specific incidence rate of 3.3 per million children under age 15 [6]. Although not generally included in statistics of childhood cancer, adolescents account for the highest frequency of osteosarcomas diagnosed [7].

The incidence of osteosarcoma is slightly higher in males, with a male:female ratio of about 1.4:1 [7–9]. The median age of onset is 17 years in females and 20 years in males [7]. There is some international variation in incidence of osteosarcoma, as well as racial differences within the United States [8–10]. The latest Surveillance, Epidemiology, and End Results (SEER) data indicate an incidence rate in black children that is 15% higher than in white children [6].

The etiology of osteosarcoma is unknown, although rapid bone growth,

D.O. Walterhouse and S.L. Cohn (eds), DIAGNOSTIC AND THERAPEUTIC ADVANCES IN PEDIATRIC ONCOLOGY. Copyright © 1997. Kluwer Academic Publishers, Boston. All rights reserved.

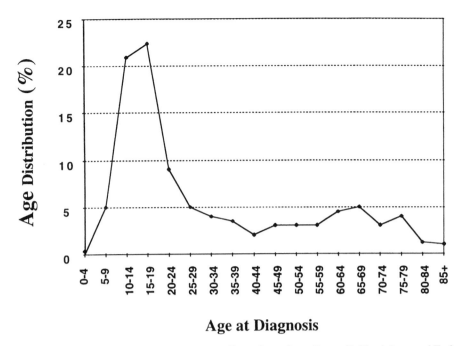

Age at Diagnosis

Figure 1. Epidemiology of osteosarcoma according to latest Surveillance, Epidemiology, and End Results (SEER) data, 1973–1987 [7].

both physiologic and pathologic, was one of the first associated factors identified [11]. Osteosarcoma, with its peak incidence during the pubertal growth spurt, occurs at the time of maximal expansion of bone. The most frequently affected sites are the metaphyses of long bones, the location of growth [12]. Children with osteosarcoma have been reported to be significantly taller than controls [13], and giant breeds of dogs are at greater risk of developing osteosarcoma than smaller dogs [14]. Conditions characterized by excessive cellular proliferation such as fibrous dysplasia, Paget's disease, bone infarcts, osteomyelitis, and unresolved calluses are also associated with the development of osteosarcoma. It is speculated that rapidly dividing cells have an increased susceptibility to carcinogenic agents or genetic mutations.

Various environmental agents have been postulated as causative factors for osteosarcoma, but only ionizing radiation has a well-documented effect. Jaw tumors were first reported in the 1920s in luminizers, women who painted watch dials with paint containing radium and other radioactive substances [15]. Since then, radiation exposure, both accidental and therapeutic, has been demonstrated in numerous studies to predispose to bone sarcomas. In a report of late effects of pediatric primary cancer treatment, the risk of developing secondary osteosarcoma correlated with radiation dose. Childhood cancer

216

survivors who received 1000–2999 rads of radiation therapy had a sixfold increased risk of developing secondary bone cancer, rising to 38-fold at doses of more than 6000 rads [16]. The average latency period to secondary osteosarcoma is in the 9–11 year range [17]. Notably, while most secondary osteosarcomas occur within the initial radiation field, there is an increased risk even outside radiation portals and in patients treated with chemotherapy alone. The increased risk may be explained by the genetic predisposition of some patients, particularly those with hereditary retinoblastoma and the Li–Fraumeni syndrome, towards developing osteosarcoma. It is also possible that prior treatment with alkylating agents can increase the risk of bone sarcomas [16].

While other environmental agents have been implicated in the development of osteosarcoma, their role in the causation of this disease has not been well substantiated. The National Toxicology Program released a study several years ago suggesting fluoride as an etiologic agent of osteosarcoma in male rats [18]. However, subsequent epidemiological studies found no relationship between fluoride levels in drinking water and osteosarcoma [19]. Herbicides, fertilizers, and pesticides have also been associated with osteosarcoma [20,21], but reports are conflicting and definitive evidence is lacking.

Viruses as causative agents of human osteosarcoma have been thoroughly investigated, but only circumstantial evidence linking the two has surfaced. By inoculating animals with a variety of sarcoma viruses, researchers have been able to elicit osteosarcomas in mice and rats [22–24]. Osteosarcomas have also been induced in hamsters injected with extracts from human osteosarcomas, suggesting the presence of an infectious agent within the extract [25]. In the same report, viral particles were seen by electron microscopy within the tumor tissue. Immunological studies have detected specific antibody to a common sarcoma antigen in sera from 100% of patients with osteosarcoma, 85% of their family members, and 29% of normal blood donors [26]. The high percentage of family members carrying the antibody suggests the possibility of a virus or other infectious agent. Further, cytotoxic lymphocytes directed against osteosarcoma cells have been found in rats and humans [24,27]. Despite this evidence, a specific human virus has never been demonstrated to play a role in the genesis of osteosarcoma.

3. Cytogenetics

The cytogenetics of osteosarcoma indicate that this tumor is characterized by extreme chromosomal irregularity. Unlike other tumors that may have classic alterations in karyotype, osteosarcoma cells are frequently aneuploid and contain a disparate array of chromosome aberrations. Only the parosteal variant of osteosarcoma is associated with a predictable cytogenetic abnormality, namely, the ring chromosome [28,29]. The percentage of osteosarcomas with cytogenetic abnormalities varies according to he detection technique

217

used. In series using classic chromosome banding techniques, 50%–80% of tumor samples had karyotype aberrations [29–31]. Using the technique of comparative genomic hybridization (CGH), more than 91% of tumor samples had cytogenetic changes [32]. The high degree of karyotypic irregularity reflects a combination of clonal and nonclonal alterations, the latter presumably a result of chromosome instability. Higher-grade tumors tend to have more of both types of alterations [33].

It has been difficult to pinpoint which chromosomal loci are important in the pathogenesis of osteosarcoma because of the multitude of changes seen. Nevertheless, a few loci have nonrandomly been observed to be involved in deletions or rearrangements. Two important hot spots occur at chromosomes 13q14 and 17p13, which contain the retinoblastoma (Rb) and p53 tumor suppressor genes, respectively. Other frequent deletion sites, detected by allelotyping, are located on 3q and 18q [34]. Karyotyping and flow cytometry reveal that osteosarcomas can range from being near-diploid to pentaploid, with the majority of tumors containing both hypodiploid and hyperdiploid clones of cells [35,36].

4. Molecular biology

The recent boom in the field of molecular oncology has greatly expanded our understanding of the events that initiate cancer. The study of osteosarcoma has been particularly exciting due to the variety of molecular biological phenomena characterized in this tumor. This section summarizes the oncogenes of both the tumor suppressor and dominant-acting varieties, that have been associated with osteosarcoma.

4.1. Tumor suppressor genes

Tumor suppressor genes, also called *recessive oncogenes*, are genes that exert an inhibitory effect on growth. Tumor suppressor genes cause malignant change through loss of function rather than overexpression. Hereditary retinoblastoma and the Li–Fraumeni syndrome, both associated with high rates of osteosarcoma, are caused by deletions or mutations in their respective tumor suppressor genes, Rb and p53. There is now abundant evidence that these two genes play a role in the genesis of osteosarcoma.

The discovery of the retinoblastoma gene, Rb, had its beginnings when Knudson proposed a two-hit model for retinoblastoma development based on the observation that the hereditary from of this disease occurs at a younger age than the sporadic form [37]. According to the model, mutations in two genes are necessary in order to develop this ocular tumor. Patients with a genetic predisposition carry one mutation from birth and thus require only one additional alteration to express the disease. When this hypothesis was proposed, the nature and location of the purported genes was a mystery. Later, a region conferring susceptibility to retinoblastoma was localized to chromosome 13q14 and the gene for retinoblastoma was cloned [38–40]. It is now clear that Rb encodes a phosphoprotein that serves as a critical checkpoint for entry into the cell cycle. Absent or dysfunctional Rb protein enables cells to progress through cell division unregulated, predisposing to the genesis of malignancy.

The first suggestion of a relationship between the Rb gene and osteosarcoma was epidemiologic. The actuarial risk of developing a second sarcoma, predominantly osteosarcoma, in hereditary retinoblastoma survivors has been estimated to be 6%–50% at 20 years and 38%–90% at 30 years [41–44]. This finding suggests that the two tumors may share a common genetic etiology. This observation was later substantiated in the laboratory. Concurrent with the reports on retinoblastoma, cytogeneticists detected karyotypic anomalies at chromosome 13q14 in osteosarcoma [45], and molecular analyses confirmed mutations in the Rb gene [46–48]. In two large series of osteosarcoma specimens, approximately 40% had structural abnormalities of the Rb gene, 63% had loss of heterozygosity (LOH) at the Rb locus, and 54% had absent Rb protein expression [49,50]. Functionally, when copies of the Rb gene were introduced into Rb-negative osteosarcoma cell lines, restoration of expression of the gene resulted in a change in cell morphology, inhibition of growth, and suppression of tumor formation in nude mice [51].

While the Rb gene is associated with osteosarcoma, not all osteosarcomas harbor Rb mutations, nor do all patients with hereditary Rb mutations develop osteosarcomas, implicating the involvement of other genes. Studies on osteosarcoma specimens have revealed a high frequency of LOH on chromosome 17, the locus that contains the gene for p53 [49,52].

The p53 gene, like Rb, encodes a nuclear phosphoprotein that acts as a tumor suppressor. The exact mechanisms of p53 action continue to be studied, but it appears that it regulates the transition from the G1 to the S phase of the cell cycle [53]. DNA-damaging agents, such as radiation and carcinogens, induce an increased expression of p53 protein, allowing cells time to repair damaged DNA. If such repair does not successfully occur, p53 may promote cell death through apoptosis [54–56]. Absent or dysfunctional protein, as well as inactivation by binding to viral proteins or cytoplasmic sequestration, are mechanisms by which p53 may contribute to oncogenesis. The p53 gene is the most frequently altered gene in sporadically occurring human cancer [53].

Numerous lines of evidence implicate absent or defective p53 as a causative factor in osteosarcoma. Transgenic mice carrying a mutated p53 gene develop osteosarcomas, [57] and osteosarcoma cell lines have gene rearrangements and deletions in p53 [58–61]. With high-resolution techniques, 42% of human osteosarcoma specimens examined harbored either a gross or subtle p53 mutation [62]. Multifocal tumors had a higher likelihood of containing such a mutation [63].

Osteosarcoma is included in the spectrum of cancers of the Li–Fraumeni syndrome, a familial predisposition to cancer associated with germline p53 mutations [64]. Among children with osteosarcoma, 3%–4% have germline p53 mutations, even without a family history of Li–Fraumeni syndrome [65,66]. With further scrutiny, the families of these children sometimes meet the criteria for Li–Fraumeni syndrome [67]. It is therefore imperative to take a careful family history in osteosarcoma patients, and some clinicians advocate testing all patients for p53 mutations.

Mechanisms other than genomic alteration may cause inactivation of the p53 gene. The human homologue of the murine double-minute 2 gene (MDM2) encodes a protein that binds p53 and inactivates it [68]. Up to 27% of osteosarcomas overexpress the MDM2 gene [68–70]. Overexpression of MDM2 is much more prevalent in metastatic or recurrent tumors, suggesting that this finding may be a marker of, and possibly a contributor to, progression of disease.

There is now early evidence that the cyclins and cyclin-dependant kinases (CDKs), critical regulators of the cell cycle, may be altered in osteosarcoma [71]. The complexity of cell cycle control suggests that initiation of tumorigenesis may be the result of disturbances of any number of genes.

4.2. Dominant-acting oncogenes

Simply described, proto-oncogenes are a general class of genes that promote cell growth. These genes are present in normal cells and are critical to the regulation of cellular processes such as progression through the cell cycle. When these genes are altered such that they promote growth excessively, they are termed *oncogenes*. Oncogenes have been incriminated in osteosarcoma development, though their role is less substantiated than that of the tumor suppressor genes. Many oncogenes, including c-abl, c-raf, c-ras, c-met, c-mos and c-sis, have been investigated, but the best-described oncogenes associated with osteosarcoma are c-myc and c-fos.

The myc family of oncogenes encodes proteins that serve as transcription factors in the regulation of cell growth, apoptosis, and transformation. Overall, myc expression promotes growth and inhibits differentiation. The complex means by which myc exerts its actions and its regulatory elements have recently been reviewed [72,73]. Aberrant myc expression has been reported in a variety of pediatric tumors, most notably neuroblastoma (n-myc) and Burkitt's lymphoma (c-myc). Evidence also implicates this oncogene in osteosarcoma development. An analysis of six osteosarcoma cell lines revealed 5–20-fold amplification [74]. Radiation-induced murine osteosarcomas had c-myc amplification in 12 of 53 (23%) tumors, with decreased differentiation markers in those tumors with the highest amplification [75]. Analyses of human tumors also reveal myc amplification [76,77], though only 7% were affected in the largest series reported [78]. Notably, this does not exclude the overexpression of myc protein, through transcriptional, translational, or post-translational mechanisms.

The fos and jun oncogenes encode proteins that compose the activator

Table 1. Genes implicated in osteosarcoma development

Gene	Chromosome	Class	Documented mechanism of alteration
p53	17p13	Tumor suppressor	Deletion, mutation, rearrangement
Rb	13q14	Tumor suppressor	Deletion, mutation, rearrangement
MDM2	12q13–14	Oncogene	Gene amplification
Myc	8q24	Oncogene	Gene amplification
fos	14q21	Oncogene	↑ RNA/protein expression

protein-1(AP-1) complex of transcription factors. These factors may play a role in the signal transduction pathway from the cell membrane to the nucleus. The fos and jun proteins are inducible by various external stimuli and form heterodimers that bind DNA and transactivate growth-related genes [79,80]. The association of the fos oncogene with bone tumors was first made when the FBJ sarcoma virus (containing v-fos) induced osteosarcomas when injected into mice [22,81,82]. Knockout mice lacking this gene develop osteopetrosis, whereas transgenic mice overexpressing this gene develop osteosarcoma [83–86]. The role of fos in human osteosarcoma is less clear. Fos gene amplification and RNA overexpression were observed only in a small minority of human osteosarcoma cell lines [87,74]. In situ hybridization revealed detectable fos RNA expression in 33% of human osteosarcomas but not in normal cells [88]. Fos protein expression, assayed by immunohistochemistry, was elevated in approximately 60% of human tumors [89]. While it is premature to draw definitive conclusions regarding a causative role for c-fos in osteosarcoma, the evidence is very suggestive.

In summary, oncogenes and tumor suppressor genes are altered in a significant proportion of osteosarcomas (see table 1). In some cases, multiple genes are aberrant in the same tumor. It is fair to hypothesize that osteosarcoma follows a multihit model of tumorigenesis, with alterations of critical combinations of genes precipitating tumor development. The implications of specific mutations for the prognosis of osteosarcoma are actively being investigated.

5. Pathology

By definition, osteosarcoma is a tumor of malignant connective tissue that produces osteoid. Since this tumor arises from a mesenchymal stem cell, various types of differentiation may be seen. Osteosarcomas may have fibroblastic, chondroblastic, or osteoblastic components, but the common thread is that they all produce osteoid. Fibrosarcomas and osteochondromas may look very similar histologically to osteosarcoma, but they lack the bone production. Raymond et al. suggest lumping osteosarcomas into two categories, conventional and variant [90]. The *conventional osteosarcomas*, which constitute the majority of osteosarcomas in children and adolescents, behave in a stereotypically aggressive manner, and fine histologic distinctions are usually of academic interest only. The *variants*, however, may have distinct clinical courses and therefore must be recognized.

The World Health Organization recently published a revised malignant osteosarcoma classification schema in which the tumors are grouped according to whether they arise in the center or surface of bone [91]. The central, or intramedullary, tumors include osteosarcomas of the conventional, telangiectatic, well-differentiated and small cell varieties. The conventional osteosarcomas, in turn, are divided into osteoblastic, chondroblastic, and fibroblastic subtypes. All the central osteosarcomas are aggressive with the exception of the well-differentiated intramedullary subtype. The surface, or peripheral, osteosarcomas include the parosteal (juxtacortical), periosteal, and high-grade surface variants. The parosteal osteosarcomas are very low grade and rarely metastasize, although they may contain areas of dedifferentiated tumor. The periosteal osteosarcomas are somewhat differentiated and are intermediate in their metastatic potential. The high-grade surface tumors are aggressive and behave similarly to conventional osteosarcoma. The histologic features of these subtypes are summarized in table 2.

A few types of osteosarcoma warrant special mention because they have different clinical behaviors [9]. Osteosarcoma of the jaw is seen mainly in patients beyond the second decade and is associated with chondroblastic differentiation with small amounts of osteoid. It has an indolent course and metastasizes less frequently than classic osteosarcoma. Paget's disease-associated osteosarcoma occurs in patients beyond the fifth decade of life and carries a poor prognosis. Postradiation osteosarcoma has a long latency period between radiation and disease onset (average 9–11 years). As a result, it occurs only rarely in childhood, usually in the setting of hereditary retinoblastoma. Like Paget's-associated osteosarcoma, postradiation osteosarcoma has a poor response to chemotherapy. Post-radiation extraosseous osteosarcoma has also been described. A small percentage of osteosarcomas are multifocal (5%), involving different areas of bone at diagnosis. It is unclear whether multifocal tumors represent metastases or multiple primary malignancies.

Although the current histologic categorization of osteosarcomas has proven useful, pathologists are attempting to better define subclasses for this neoplasm. Immunohistochemical assays using antibodies against collagen subtypes have been developed to identify osteoid, since this matrix material characteristically contains collagen types I and V and lacks collagen types II, III, IV, and VI [92]. This test has helped to properly diagnose cases with scant amounts of osteoid, which may be confused with Ewing's sarcoma, fibrosarcoma, malignant fibrous histiocytoma, or poorly differentiated chondrosarcoma [93]. Markers against collagen also help distinguish between different classes of conventional osteosarcoma, although the clinical utility of this remains to be determined. Immunohistochemical studies using antibodies against the noncollagenous proteins osteonectin and osteocalcin, presumed osteoblastic markers, initially showed promise to distinguish osteoblastic tu-

Table 2. Pathologic classification of malignant osteosarcomas

Pathologic subtype	%[a]	Peak age affected	Histologic features
Central tumors (medullary)			
• Conventional osteosarcoma	87	2nd	
Osteoblastic (50%)		decade	Tumor cells with nuclear and mitotic atypia; osteoid or bony trabeculae interspersed among tumor cells; may have extensive sclerosis
Fibroblastic (25%)			Tumor cells are spindle shaped and may be in a herringbone pattern; osteoid production focal
Chondroblastic (25%)			Cells lie in lacunae and form chondroid lobules
• Telangiectatic osteosarcoma	3	2nd decade	Septa surrounded by malignant cells separated by spaces; may have few pleomorphic cells in bloody background; benign giant cells present
• Intraosseous well differentiated (low grade)	1.2	3rd decade	Well-differentiated spindle cells with little cytological atypia; interlacing pattern permeates surrounding structures
• Small cell (round cell)	1.3	2nd decade	Small cells resembling those of Ewing's sarcoma, but osteoid matrix is produced
Surface tumors (peripheral)			
• Parosteal (juxtacortical)	4	3rd decade	Slightly atypical spindle cells between normal-appearing bony trabeculae
• Periosteal	1.5	2nd decade	Resembles a moderately differentiated chondroblastic osteosarcoma
• High-grade surface	0.7	2nd decade	Highly anaplastic osteosarcoma originating on surface of bone

[a] Percentages reflect data from the Mayo Clinic series of 1718 osteosarcoma patients [9] applied to the WHO classification system [91].

mors from those with fibroblastic or chondroblastic differentiation [94]. Additional date did not support such specificity [95].

6. Clinical presentation and patterns of spread

The most common sites of osteosarcoma occurrence in children and adolescents are the femur (44%), tibia (17%), and humerus (15%) [8,9] (figure 2). Other bones may be involved, particularly in older individuals where osteosarcoma is frequently seen in the axial skeleton. Pain, either sudden or insidious, is the most frequent presenting symptom. Patients may recall a traumatic event to the tender area, but this is often coincidental; the trauma merely draws attention to the involved site. It is possible, however, to have a

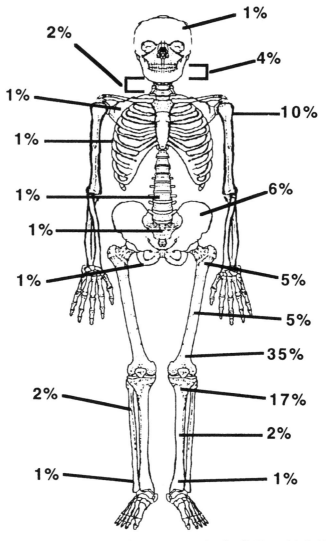

Figure 2. Distribution of osteosarcoma (adapted from Mirra [194]). The unlabeled bones constitute less than 1% of osteosarcoma cases. This series includes middle-aged and elderly patients; if
only children and adolescents were considered, there would be even fewer cases in the axial
skeleton.

pathological fracture through a tumor-infiltrated bone. Swelling is another
sign of osteosarcoma, which may be minimal at first but becomes progressively
more significant over time. The skin overlying the tumor may be taut and
shiny, and superficial venous congestion may be seen. Osteosarcoma presentation with local signs and symptoms is the rule; it is distinctly uncommon to
have constitutional symptoms.

Approximately 15%–20% of patients with newly diagnosed osteosarcoma have metastases detectable on imaging studies [96]. This disease spreads hematogenously, with an impressive predilection towards the lungs. Distant bone is the next most common metastatic site, affecting 2%–4% of patients. It is unclear whether this entity represents multifocal tumor arising synchronously or metastasis from the primary tumor. Authors have cited lack of pulmonary metastases in these patients as evidence for multifocal disease, but others have refuted this claim [97]. Other reported, but infrequent, locations of spread include the lymph nodes, liver, kidney, brain, soft tissue, and heart [8].

7. Clinical evaluation and diagnostic studies

The evaluation of suspected osteosarcoma begins with a detailed history and physical examination focusing on the typical presenting features of local pain and swelling. Metastases are rarely detected on initial history and physical, except in very advanced disease.

7.1. Radiologic evaluation

The radiologic evaluation of osteosarcoma involves multiple imaging modalities. Conventional radiography remains the most valuable initial tool in the detection of osteosarcoma. In most cases, typical radiographic features illustrate the aggressive osteoid-forming nature of this disease. Lesions may be lytic (30%) , sclerotic (45%), or mixed (25%) [98]. They may be confined to the medulla but often destroy the cortex and elevate soft tissue. Osteoid produced by tumor cells appears cloudlike with ill-defined margins. Periosteal reaction, commonly appearing as triangular-shaped elevations (Codman's triangles), frequently occurs in osteosarcoma but is not specific to this disease. The major drawback of plain films is their relative insensitivity in delineating extent of tumor involvement in bone.

The advent of magnetic resonance imaging (MRI) has greatly enhanced our ability to document tumor location and anatomic relationships. MRI is exceptionally well suited for imaging bone tumors and has become the modality of choice for imaging osteosarcoma. T1-weighted sequences demonstrate the interface between tumor and bone marrow and T2-weighted sequences distinguish between tumor and muscle. MRI defines spatial relationships accurately, since it can image in any plane. It facilitates surgical planning because it defines tumors size, distance from the joint line, evidence of extension into the joint, and evidence of neurovascular involvement. Tumor boundary definition by MRI corresponds to that of pathologic evaluation within millimeters [99] (see figure 3). Computed tomography (CT), largely supplanted by MRI, continues to be effective in certain anatomic sites such as the pelvis and shoulder girdle [100].

225

Imaging modalities have been used to predict osteosarcoma responsiveness to chemotherapy. The contrast agent gadolinium-diethylenetriaminepentaacetic acid (Gd-DTPA), used in conjuction with MRI, highlights the tumor's vascularity; decreasing vascularity signifies tumor necrosis [101]. Angiography also measures vascularity, but has not consistently correlated with degree of necrosis. Color Doppler flow imaging has been proposed as a good predictor of tumor death [102]. Magnetic resonance spectroscopy (MRS) is a potential tool to assess tumor metabolism. ^{31}P spectoscopy measures the concentration of phosphorylated compounds (phosphomonoester, phosphodiester, inorganic phosphate, phosphocreatine, and adenosine triphosphate) in

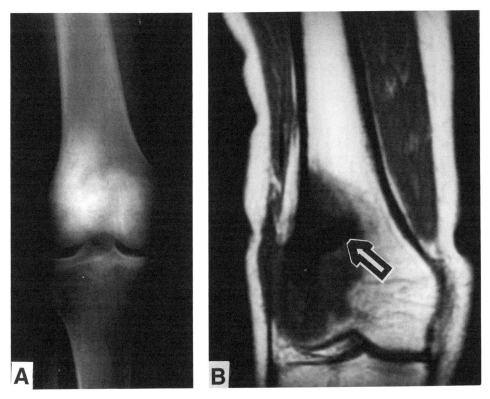

Figure 3. (**a**) PA view of plain film of the distal femur of an adolescent patient with osteosarcoma. An intramedullary ill-defined sclerotic lesion is seen. (**b,c**) Corresponding MRI images: (**b**) Coronal T1-weighted image shows low signal intensity in the distal femur with minimal cortical breakthrough, which may be secondary to the biopsy site (arrow). No involvement of the joint is seen. (**c**) Coronal inversion recovery image shows heterogenous foci of decreased and increased signal intensity, signifying areas of osteoid formation and bone marrow edema, respectively. The bone marrow is likely infiltrated with tumor cells. (Courtesy of Dr. Loralie Ma, Johns Hopkins Hospital.)

226

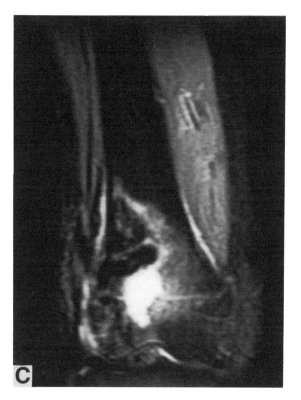

Figure 3. (continued)

soft tissue [100,103]. Malignant bone tumors have spectral characteristics distinct from those of normal tissue that change during chemotherapy. These changes have not correlated with degree of necrosis, however. Nuclear scans, such as thallium-201, have also been used to monitor response to therapy; decreased uptake correlates with degree of necrosis [104]. Some investigators advocate performing nuclear medicine scans to guide therapy even before definitive resection or amputation [105].

Workup for metastases involves imaging the lungs and bone, the two most common sites of spread. CT scans most reliably detect pulmonary spread. In cases of questionable pulmonary nodules, positron-emission tomography (PET) scanning, which indicates metabolically active tissue, may distinguish metastases from benign tissue [106]. Bone scintigraphy, using methylene diphosphonate labeled with technetium-99 m, is the most sensitive and cost-effective means for detecting skip lesions and distant bone metastases [100]. This modality is also effective in detecting spread to lung, lymph nodes, and soft tissue [107]. In initial staging, MRI should also be performed on the entire length of the affected bone to help detect skip metastases.

227

7.2. Biopsy

The histologic diagnosis of osteosarcoma may be accomplished by needle or open-surgical biopsy. While needle biopsies are less invasive, they are prone to sampling error and do not yield sufficient tissue for biological studies. Open-surgical biopsies are not trivial, since poor technique may lead to tumor seeding along the biopsy tract and subsequent local recurrence. Moreover, the biopsy site must be carefully placed in order to be included within the definitive resection planes. If biopsy placement is suboptimal, limb salvage may be precluded [108]. A study by the MD Anderson Cancer Center group reported that only 6 of 26 osteosarcomas referred by outside institutions had well-placed biopsies [109]. Fortunately, more patients are now being referred to surgeons who will perform the definitive resection for the initial biopsy.

7.3. Additional evaluation

Additional evaluation of the patient with osteosarcoma primarily assesses the baseline function of organs affected by treatment. Cardiac function, potentially compromised by doxorubicin, is best evaluated with echocardiogram or MUGA scan and ECG. Renal function, affected by cisplatin, ifosfamide, and methotrexate, is estimated by urinalysis, BUN, and creatinine. Glomerular filtration rate should be determined by 12- or 24-hour urine collection for creatinine clearance or by radioisotope elimination. Renal tubular function is assessed with electrolyte, calcium, phosphorous, and magnesium determinations. Audiologic examination is advised before administration of the ototoxic agent cisplatin.

Lactate dehydrogenase (LDH) and alkaline phosphatase levels may be prognostic indicators for osteosarcoma. High levels of both enzymes have been associated with poor outcome [110]. While these factors are not used to stratify patients into treatment groups, serial measurements may be indicative of response to therapy. The recommended workup for a patient with newly diagnosed osteosarcoma is summarized in table 3.

7.4. Differential diagnosis

The differential diagnosis of osteosarcoma includes other lesions of bone, benign and malignant. The most frequent consideration is Ewing's sarcoma. In contrast to osteosarcoma, Ewing's sarcoma occurs in flat bones or the diaphyses of long bones and typically appears as a purely lytic lesion on plain film. Another distinguishing feature of Ewing's sarcoma is the predominance of the soft tissue component of the mass. Other malignant neoplasms to consider are leukemias, lymphomas, and bone metastases from other tumor types. Benign lesions such as osteoid osteoma, osteoblastoma, enchondroma, osteochondroma, chondroblastoma, aneurysmal bone cysts, and avascular ne-

Table 3. Recommended evaluation of a patient with newly diagnosed osteosarcoma

I.   History and physical examination
II. Radiologic evaluation
• Plain films of affected bone
• MRI scan of affected bone
• PA and lateral chest x-ray
• CT scan of chest with 1.0cm intervals
• Radionuclide bone scan
III. Biopsy of primary tumor
IV. Laboratory evaluation
• Complete blood count (CBC) with differential
• Electrolytes, calcium, phosphorous, magnesium
• Blood urea nitrogen, creatinine
• Lactate dehydrogenase (LDH), alkaline phosphatase
• Liver function tests
• Varicella titers
V. Cardiac evaluation
• Echocardiogram or MUGA scan
• Electrocardiogram
VI. Renal evaluation
• Urinalysis
• Glomerular filtration rate
12- or 24-hour urine collection for creatinine clearance
or radioisotope GFR
VII. Audiogram

crosis also masquerade as osteosarcoma [111]. Osteomyelitis may also be considered in the differential diagnosis, although it more closely resembles Ewing's sarcoma on x-ray and in clinical presentation. Biopsy is essential in making the final diagnosis.

8. Prognostic factors

A plethora of prognostic factors for osteosarcoma have been identified, but in the context of variable study designs and changing treatment strategies, reports regarding their value have been contradictory. Prior to the era of neoadjuvant chemotherapy, the mainstays of prognosis were age, sex, tumor size, and location. Many studies showed age before or in the early part of the second decade, male gender, large tumors (>15cm), and location in the axial skeleton as poor prognostic indicators. While some of these prognostic factors were predictive in univariate analyses, none was consistently proven as an independent prognosticator in multivariate analyses [112]. Other suggested predictors of poor outcome have included tumor spread at diagnosis, high alkaline phosphatase levels [110,113], incomplete tumor resection, and short duration of symptoms [114,115]. A new generation of prognostic factors, such as histologic response to chemotherapy, expression of P-glycoprotein, and molecular biological changes, has now emerged (table 4).

229

Table 4. Prognostic indicators in osteosarcoma

Indicator	Prognostic implication	Comments	Recent references
Stage	Metastasis or multifocal disease → unfavorable	Even with surgical resection and modern chemotherapy, metastatic disease still portends poor long-term survival	
Response to chemotherapy	≥90% necrosis → favorable <90% necrosis → unfavorable	Other than presence of metastases, the most valuable prognostic indicator today	[110,112,117–120]
P-glycoprotein expresson	High expression → unfavorable	Promising new factor that also has therapeutic implications. Tests of expression need to be standardized	[120,127–129]
DNA ploidy	Near diploid clones → favorable		[35]
Tumor size	Large tumor (>15 cm) → unfavorable	Conflicting data on value of this marker. A recent study using sophisticated tumor volume measurements found size as an independent predictor of outcome. Cannot be dismissed yet	[186]
Tumor site	Axial skeleton → least favorable Proximal femur → unfavorable Proximal tibia → favorable	Empirically, one would think that tumors in areas difficult to resect would do worse, but data on this are conflicting	[110,112]
Histologic subtype	Parosteal variant → favorable	With the exception of rare low-grade osteosarcomas, the difference between outcome of conventional osteosarcomas is not significant	[9,115]
Duration of symptoms	Short duraton <2–6 months → unfavorable	Shown to be of importance before adjuvant chemotherapy. May not hold up any longer	[114,115]
Alkaline phosphatase /LDH levels	High levels → unfavorable	Unclear whether these markers are independent predictors with respect to tumor size	[110,120]
Gender	Male gender → unfavorable	Conflicting data. Not found to be an independent predictor of outcome	[112]
Age	Age < second decade → unfavorable	Has not stood up as an independent variable	[112]

8.1. Histologic response to chemotherapy

In the mid-1970s, with the advent of neoadjuvant chemotherapy prior to definitive surgical resection, a new prognostic possibility was described. Tumors could be assessed histologically for percent necrosis following chemotherapy [116] (see figure 4). Multiple clinical trials have since confirmed the predictive value of histologic response to treatment, with modern era event-free survival rates of 70%–90% in responsive tumors and 40%–60% in unresponsive tumors [110,112,117–120]. Most studies define a favorable response as 90% tumor necrosis or greater. The agreement between studies on the value of this prognostic indicator is remarkable; other than metastasis at presentation, histologic response to chemotherapy is regarded the best predictor of osteosarcoma outcome to date.

8.2. P-glycoprotein expression

A potential new prognostic indicator for osteosarcoma is the expression of P-glycoprotein (P-gp), which confers the multidrug resistance (MDR) phenotype. P-gp is a 170-kDa integral membrane protein encoded by the human mdr1 gene located on chromosome 7q21 [121,122]. It functions as an ATP-dependent efflux pump that prevents intracellular accumulation of anthracyclines, vinka alkaloids, epidophyllotoxins, taxanes, and actinomycin D, resulting in multidrug resistance [123]. P-gp has been documented in a number of adult cancers as well as in rhabdomyosarcoma, neuroblastoma, acute lymphoblastic leukemia, and retinoblastoma [124]. Specific normal cells also manufacture this protein, which is thought to be involved in the secretion of toxic metabolites and the maintenance of the blood–brain barrier.

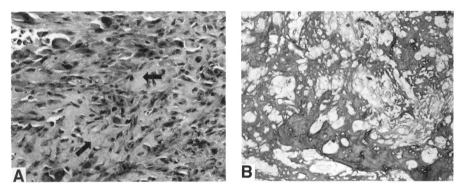

Figure 4. (**a**) Osteosarcoma showing cytologically malignant cells interspersed among osteoid (arrows) (hematoxylin and eosin ×400). (**b**) The same osteosarcoma following chemotherapy and total excision. Extensive residual osteoid and stromal fibrosis is present without viable tumor cells (hematoxylin and eosin ×125). (Courtesy of Dr. Elizabeth Perlman, Johns Hopkins Hospital.)

231

Schwartz et al. first demonstrated that the expression of P-gp may have prognostic implications for osteosarcoma [125]. Since gene amplification of mdr1 in human tumors has not been observed, assays for multidrug resistance have accordingly been directed at the RNA or protein level. Overexpression of mdr1 gene products is seen in 23%–86% of primary osteosarcomas, depending upon the technique used. Reverse transcriptase/polymerase chain reaction (RT-PCR), which measures levels of mRNA transcript, is the most sensitive method to measure mdr1 expression. Immunohistochemistry is more widely used, however, because it directly detects P-gp and can elucidate the cellular expression pattern of this protein. Each technique has its drawbacks [126], and it has been challenging to compare studies that utilize different methods of detection [127,128]. Regardless of technique, higher levels of expression are associated with metastatic osteosarcomas and a trend towards worse outcome [127,129]. In the largest study to date, Baldini et al. reported a significantly lower actuarial relapse-free survival rate in patients expressing high P-gp in their original tumors (42%) compared to those with low or absent expression (80%) [120]. The prognostic value of P-gp in this study was independent of other factors and more predictive than extent of necrosis after chemotherapy. The MDR phenotype thus shows promise as a strong prognostic factor in osteosarcoma, although standardization of assays will be needed to expand this approach.

8.3. Other molecular and cytogenetic indicators

Oncogenes and tumor suppressor genes are rapidly being characterized in osteosarcoma. It is possible that specific genetic alterations carry prognostic significance. Preliminary evidence suggests unfavorable prognosis with LOH at the p53 locus on chromosome 17 [34] and with MDM2 gene amplification [69]. A recent report suggests that Rb indirectly regulates the transcription of genes for enzymes such as dihydrofolate reductase. Alteration of the Rb gene could thus lead to resistance to methotrexate, which is commonly used in osteosarcoma treatment [130]. Genetic markers conferring a good prognosis in osteosarcoma include a near-diploid DNA content. Even in the presence of hyperdiploid cell clones, which most osteosarcomas have, the presence of at least 20% diploid cells has been linked to favorable outcome [35]. With better correlations, these observations may be applied to therapeutic approaches.

9. Treatment

Within the last 20 years, the survival rate for localized osteosarcoma has risen from 20% to 70%, largely a result of adjuvant therapy and a multidisciplinary approach to treatment. This section describes the different modalities of therapy used to treat osteosarcoma, with particular attention paid to modern treatment strategies.

9.1. Surgery

Surgery was the first available therapy for osteosarcoma and remains a cornerstone of treatment today. The traditional surgical approach to a patient with osteosarcoma is amputation of the affected bone. This procedure can reliably remove all tumor tissue, leaving clear margins. The local recurrence rate following amputation is less than 5%. Functionality following this procedure depends on the ability to fit a prosthesis. Function following a below-knee amputation is excellent, while a hemipelvectomy causes significant impairment. For above-knee amputations, it is sometimes possible to perform a tibial turnback, or rotationplasty. This involves resecting the distal femur but leaving an intact neurovascular bundle to the tibia in place. The tibia is then rotated so that the foot is inverted and fixated to the remaining femur, resulting in a functional joint (i.e., the ankle) to replace the knee. A prosthesis may then be placed with good results.

With improved control of microscopic residual disease by chemotherapy, limb-salvage procedures, which involve en bloc resection of tumor with the placement of an internal prosthesis, were developed. Today, about 60%–80% of osteosarcomas are amenable to limb-salvage operations [108]. Reconstructions use allografts, customized artificial endoprosthetic devices, or a combination of the two. The method of choice depends upon the preference and experience of the surgeon. Limb-salvage procedures may fail due to infection, nonunion, and fracture. Relative contraindications include major neurovascular involvement, pathologic fractures, and a contaminated, inappropriately placed, or infected biopsy site. Skeletal immaturity may preclude patients from limb-salvage procedures since limb-length discrepancy may be profound. Telescopic prostheses are available for selected patients. Although overall survival is not compromised by limb-salvage surgery [110], several studies reported that local failure rate was significantly higher in resected tumors than amputated tumors (9.2% to 10.5% versus 1.9% to 2.5%) [131–133]. The risk of local relapse was apparent in those with narrow surgical margins and poor response to chemotherapy. Definitive studies have not been performed.

Surgery also plays an important role in the treatment of pulmonary metastases. Although the outcome for patients with pulmonary metastases has traditionally been poor, surgical resection of both primary and metastatic disease combined with chemotherapy has increased disease-free survival rates to 25%–40%. After relapse, resection of metastases may significantly extend the survival time.

9.2. Chemotherapy

Before the era of chemotherapy, 80% of patients with localized osteosarcoma would develop pulmonary metastases within 6–9 months of amputation. In the 1970s, it was recognized that high-dose methotrexate [134], doxorubicin [135], and cisplatin [136] had activity against osteosarcoma. Compared to historical controls, disease-free survival rates rose with the introduction of these agents into adjuvant treatment regimens [137]. In 1978, the Mayo Clinic reported improved survival without chemotherapy, which was attributed to improved surgical techniques or a change in the natural history of osteosarcoma [138–141]. As a result, adjuvant chemotherapy was not the definitive standard of care until prospective randomized trials firmly established the benefit of chemotherapy [142,143]. In retrospect, the earlier study may have been affected by referral patterns or other unrecognized factors resulting in a group of patients with better prognostic features.

In the mid-1970s, the Memorial Sloan Kettering Cancer Center (MSKCC) pioneered the use of preoperative chemotherapy with response-based chemotherapy after definitive surgical resection [116]. Potential theoretical advantages of this approach included the more immediate treatment of pulmonary micrometastases and the facilitation of surgical resection by cytoreduction and encapsulation of tumor. Additionally, assessing tumor response to chemotherapy provided treatment-guiding information; poor histologic responders had their postoperative chemotherapy regimens altered. This approach proved beneficial for good histologic responders, yielding cure rates greater than 70%; however, poor responders, despite tailored chemotherapy, had cure rates of only 40%–50%. Subsequent protocols in he early 1980s demonstrated that intensifying preoperative chemotherapy increases the percentage of patients achieving good histologic response and raises the overall survival rate, but exposes all patients to enhanced toxicity. Despite intensification of therapy, cure rates of poor responders remain low [118]. Table 5 shows the results of several large multiagent osteosarcoma trials. It should be noted that since intensity and duration of therapy affect outcome, accurate comparison of trials by agents alone is limited.

Recent treatment protocols have incorporated new approaches to improve outcome. Ifosfamide and etoposide have been added to the armamentarium of efficaceous anti-osteosarcoma agents [144,145], and newer compounds such as topotecan are being investigated. The use of colony-stimulating factors to hasten recovery from neutropenia has enabled intensification of chemotherapy regimens. Pharmacokinetic studies are being undertaken to optimize the dosing and administration of already familiar drugs, most notably methotrexate, since outcome may be dependent upon peak levels [146].

It may prove feasible to identify patients with an adverse biological risk factor at diagnosis and modify treatment accordingly. The Pediatric Oncology Group (POG)/Children's Cancer Group (CCG) intergroup study is analyzing all diagnostic tumor specimens for P-glycoprotein expression. Those patients expressing this protein may have better outcome if treated with agents not removed by the P-gp pump (e.g., cisplatin, methotrexate, ifosfamide). An alternative approach is to use competitive inhibitors of P-gp to overcome multidrug resistance. Verapamil was the first such drug used in clinical trials, but because high levels were necessary to overcome the MDR phenotype, the therapeutic index was easily exceeded. Newer studies have employed CSA or

Table 5. Representative major osteosarcoma trials

Study	Pre-op chemo	Post-op chemo	# patients	% good responders	RFS (%)	Mean follow-up (yrs)	Comment	Ref.
UCLA (1981–1984)	None	DOX; BCD; HDMTX vs. Observation	59	N.A.	55 vs. 20	2	Established benefit of adjuvant therapy for osteosarcoma	[143]
MIOS/POG 8107 (1982–1986)	None	DOX; BCD; HDMTX; CDDP vs. Observation	113	N.A.	61 vs. 11	8	Established benefit of adjuvant therapy for osteosarcoma	[142,187]
MSKCC T7 (1976–1978)	BCD; HDMTX; VCR; DOX	Same as preop	75	58	Overall: 76	10+	Impressive results except for poor histologic responders	[110]
T10 (1978–1981)	BCD; HDMTX; DOX	G: same as preop P: DOX; BCD; CDDP	153	34	Overall: 73	8+	Backbone of many subsequent studies. Results irreproducible by other groups	[110,188]
GPO COSS 80 (1979–1982)	HDMTX; DOX; BCD vs. HDMTX; DOX; CDDP	Same as preop +/– IFN	101	52	Overall: 63 Good: 84 Poor: 52	8	BCD and CDDP arms similar; IFN did not make difference	[148,189]

Table 5 (continued)

Study	Pre-op chemo	Post-op chemo	# patients	% good responders	RFS (%)	Mean follow-up (yrs)	Comment	Ref.
COSS 82 (1982–1984)	HDMTX; BCD vs. HDMTX; DOX/ CDDP	G: same as preop P: DOX; CDDP vs. G: same as preop P: BCD; CDDP; IFOS	118	26 vs. 60	Overall: 44 Good: 73 Poor 41 Overall: 66 Good: 79 Poor: 52	5+	CDDP/DOX is more efficaceous than BCD. Maximizing # of good responders increases overall RFS	[118,189]
COSS 86 (1986–1988)	HDMTX; DOX; i.a. or i.v. CDDP; IFOS	Same as preop	153	68	81	<5	i.a. vs. i.v. CDDP equivalent	[189,190]
CCG-782 (1983–1986)	HDMTX; VCR; BCD	BCD; VCR; HDMTX; DOX; +CDDP for poor responders	232	27	Overall: 58 Good: 88 Poor: 57	4	Poor responders not salvagable with CDDP/DOX postoperatively	[191,192]
Rizzoli Institute (1986–1989)	DOX/ CDDP; HDMTX	G: same as preop P: same as preop + IFOS/VP-16	164	78	Overall: 66 Good: 87 Poor: 58	4.5	Best reported histologic response to chemotherapy	[113]
MD Anderson (1980–1982)	DOX; i.a. CDDP	G: same as preop +/– DTIC in lieu of CDDP P: HDMTX	37	59	Overall: 50 Good: 86 Poor: 13	5		[141]

Study (years)	Induction	Postop	N	%	Outcome	Yrs	Comments	Ref
(1983–1988)	i.a. CDDP	G: DOX; CDDP +/– DTIC in lieu of CDDP; P: HDMTX; DOX; BCD; DTIC	60	68	Overall: 60 Good: 72 Poor: 33	5		[141]
EOI 80831 (1983–1986)	CDDP/DOX; HDMTX vs. CDDP/DOX	Same as preop	198	41 vs. 22	Overall: 41 vs. Overall: 57	3	Worse outcome in 3-drug arm attributed to lower dose intensity of CDDP/DOX	[193]
Mayo Clinic Pilot I	DOX; IFOS; HDMTX × 14 wks	G: same as preop P: same as preop with CDDP added	81	72	Overall: 75	3	Backbone of current POG/CCG study	[168]
Pilot II	DOX; IFOS; HDMTX; CDDP × 14 wks	Same as above	72		Overall: 97	2	Published only in abstract form	[168]

Abbreviations: RFS, relapse-free survival; G, good responder (≥90% necrosis); P, poor responder (<90% necrosis); DOX, doxorubicin; CDDP, cisplatin; HDMTX, high-dose methotrexate; IFOS, ifosfamide; BCD, bleomycin, cyclophosphamide, actinomycin-D; VCR, vincristine; CBDCA, carboplatin; IFN, interferon; MTP-PE, muramyl tripeptide-phosphatidyl ethanolamine; GCSF, granulocyte colony-stimulating factor; MSKCC, Memorial Sloan Kettering Cancer Center; GPO, German Pediatric Oncology Group; COSS, Cooperative Osteosarcoma Study; POG, Pediatric Oncology Group; EOI, European Osteosarcoma Intergroup; CCG, Children's Cancer Study Group; MIOS, Multi-Institutional Osteosarcoma Study; SWOG, Southwest Oncology Group.

237

its analogues as a means of P-gp blockade, since levels that completely inhibit the pump are achievable in human serum with minimal toxicity. A pilot study noted responses to CSA with doxorubicin and cisplatin in patients treated for recurrent osteosarcoma [125,147]. A phase II study of this approach is ongoing in the POG (C. Schwartz, personal communication).

9.3. Biological response modifiers

Even with the most intensive treatment regimens, 20%–30% of patients will relapse. Since further manipulations of standard chemotherapeutic agents may provide only minimal increases in survival, innovative biological response modifiers are being explored as adjuvants to therapy. Interferon (IFN), a cytokine that inhibits growth of osteosarcoma cells and partially reverses the malignant phenotype in vitro, was the first such agent to be studied. Human trials found no in vivo benefit [148].

An antitumor effect may be inducible with muramyl tripeptide phosphatidyl ethanolamine (MTP-PE), a synthetic lipophilic analogue of the mycobacterial cell wall component muramyl dipeptide. MTP-PE potentiates the immune system by activating monocytes and macrophages. Human monocytes phagocytize a liposomal form of this compound very efficiently and subsequently kill tumor, but not normal, cells [149]. In a murine model, 8%–10% of liposomal MTP-PE injected intravenously localized to the lungs and caused regression of pulmonary melanoma metastases [150,151]. In a subsequent prospective study, dogs with spontaneously developed osteosarcoma survived longer if given MTP-PE versus observation alone [152]. Phase I human trials demonstrated good tolerance of this drug, with side effects limited to chills, fever, headaches, myalgias, and fatigue [153]. A phase II study revealed that, compared to resection alone, patients with chemoresistant metastatic pulmonary osteosarcoma treated with MTP-PE showed a statistically significant prolongation of time to relapse (4.5 months vesus 9 months) [154]. MTP-PE is currently being studied in phase III trials in the setting of minimal residual disease after extirpative surgery. Extension of therapy for 12 weeks beyond the chemotherapy will minimize any potential limitation of monocyte response by cytotoxic therapy.

Another class of biological response modifiers under evaluation are growth hormone (GH) antagonists. GH stimulates the transcription of insulin-like growth factor I (IGF-1), an autocrine stimulator of osteosarcoma cells in vitro. Without GH, tumor growth may be inhibited. Murine osteosarcoma has reduced metastatic potential in hypophysectomized mice [156], and GH hormone antagonists can mimic hypophysectomy [157,158]. Clinical trials may begin in the near future.

Angiogenesis inhibitors prevent the vascularization necessary for growth and metastasis of cancer. The identification of the chemical factors that mediate angiogenesis has opened new prospects for the treatment of solid tumors [159]. Several analyses of angiogenesis inhibitors have used osteosarcoma cells in animal models. When osteosarcoma cells were inoculated into mice and the angiogenesis inhibitor TNP-470 (or a control) was subsequently administered for three weeks, the number and vascularity of pulmonary metastases was significantly decreased in the TNP-470-treated group [160]. Similar results were observed in a rat model [161]. TNP-470 has been approved by the FDA for phase I trials, but results have not been reported in patients with osteosarcoma.

9.4. Radiation therapy

Osteosarcoma is generally classified as radioresistant. In clinical trials 30–40 years ago, responses to radiation doses of 80 Gy were transient, and residual tumor cells remained in amputation specimens. Enhancement of tumor response with radiosensitizers such as bromodeoxyuridine resulted in unacceptably high soft tissue damage [162]. Various studies had limited success adding radiation therapy to chemotherapy for overt pulmonary metastases, but these were not randomized, and it is difficult to tease out the actual effect of the radiation [46,166,167]. A prophylactic role for radiation therapy in preventing lung metastases has been investigated but has not proven effective in clinical trials [165]. At the cellular level, the radioresistance of osteosarcoma is predictable. Osteosarcoma cell lines show a heightened ability to repair DNA in response to radiation damage. In addition, many osteosarcomas harbor p53 mutations, which may confer a radioresistant phenotype by allowing cells to divide despite DNA damage [163,164]. With the success of preoperative chemotherapy and limb-sparing surgery, the only recognized role for radiation in the treatment of osteosarcoma is palliative.

10. Metastasis and recurrence

10.1. Metastasis at presentation

Approximately 15%–20% of patients diagnosed with osteosarcoma present with metastatic disease, usually in the lungs. Between 1975 and 1984, even with adjuvant chemotherapy and resection of metastases, only 11% of patients with metastases at presentation survived [96]. Notably, patients with chemotherapy-induced complete response who did not undergo metastatectomy had a 100% relapse rate. This confirmed other reports attesting to the necessity of complete surgical resection of metastatic osteosarcoma. A more recent report showed a two-year disease-free survival rate of 46% in patients treated with ifosfamide, high-dose methotrexate, doxorubicin, and aggressive surgery [168]. Considering these promising data, patients with metastases should be candidates for aggressive chemotherapy with subsequent primary tumor resections and metastatectomies. Even those who are not cured in the long run may experience significantly prolonged survival. Current trials for metastatic disease at diagnosis are evaluating new agents such as topotecan and etoposide/ifosfamide combinations.

10.2. Recurrent disease

Most recurrences of osteosarcoma occur in the lungs (80%), followed by distant bone (15%) and local bone (5%) [169]. Approximately 20% of patients develop metastases in multiple locations [170,171]. Less common sites of relapse include the brain, epidural space, liver, mediastinum, diaphragm, and soft tissue. The recognition of nonpulmonary metastases has increased with the advent of adjuvant chemotherapy [170]. This increase may be due to the greater efficacy of intravenous chemotherapy in the lungs compared to other locations. Alternatively, patients may be living longer, allowing previously unobserved patterns of metastasis to surface. The median time to development of metastases is now 20 months, compared to seven months historically [172]. Relapses beyond five years from diagnosis are rare, although they have been reported as late as 13 years after diagnosis.

As for primary disease, treatment for recurrent disease is multimodal. When surgery and chemotherapy are employed, five-year survival rates following recurrence are 25%–40%. Surgery plays a crucial role in the management of recurrence. Studies over the past 15 years have repeatedly confirmed the benefit of resecting pulmonary metastases, both in terms of overall survival rate and duration of survival [173–178]. In some cases, multiple thoracotomies are necessary to effect a long-term cure. In a review of long-term survivors of osteosarcoma metastases, Pastorino notes that the average number of thoracotomies performed on each patient ranges between 2 and 3, with the number of resected lesions ranging from 3 to 9 [179]. Chemotherapy also has its place in the treatment of relapsed disease. The choice of agents must be tailored to the tumor's initial response to particular drugs. Since high-dose chemotherapy with autologous bone marrow rescue has been performed on only limited numbers of osteosarcoma patients, its role in the treatment of recurrent disease is unclear [171].

Prognostic factors for survival following relapse have been assessed in multiple studies. Survival after pulmonary relapse is better than that after local or distant bone recurrence. For those patients with pulmonary metastases, complete surgical resection is the best predictor of good outcome [171]. Other favorable indicators include unilateral pulmonary disease, fewer than three pulmonary nodules, and a long disease-free interval [171,174,176,180]. The extent of necrosis of pulmonary metastases following chemotherapy does not appear to affect prognosis [180].

11. Late complications

Enhanced survival of children with osteosarcoma after intensive chemotherapy has resulted in a large cohort of patients who are at significant risk for late sequelae. While some complications of therapy are overt and easily recognized, such as the musculoskeletal complications after amputation or limb salvage, others may be subclinical. Since most osteosarcomas recur within five years, subsequent patient evaluations should concentrate on potential therapy-induced effects.

The most significant late effect of osteosarcoma treatment is doxorubicin-related cardiotoxicity. With cumulative exposure, anthracyclines cause ventricular wall thinning, increased wall stress, and elevated afterload. Most patients are clinically asymptomatic, but increasing numbers are developing frank congestive heart failure or ventricular arrhythmias. This outcome is particularly problematic in osteosarcoma patients, where cumulative doxorubicin dose as well as dose fraction, both associated with cardiotoxicity, are higher than in most other malignancies. Goorin reported cardiac effects in approximately 75% of survivors of osteosarcoma. It was once thought that the cardiac effects of anthracyclines stabilized with time, but more recent information suggests that cardiac decompensation may arise 15 or more years post-treatment [181]. Factors contributing to such decompensation include pregnancy and weight lifting. If echocardiographic changes are present after completion of therapy, the risk for developing clinical heart disease is 70%, versus 12% when changes are absent. Monitoring for anthracycline-induced cardiac damage should include history and physical exam, echocardiogram to measure fractional shortening and afterload [182], and electrocardiogram to measure QTc interval, since prolongation may be indicative of anthracycline-induced myocardial damage [183]. Holter monitoring should be performed in those with any evidence of myocardial injury. Such studies should be performed every other year in all survivors of osteosarcoma, with annual follow-up in patients with abnormal results. Treatment for anthracycline-associated congestive heart failure includes pharmacotherapy with afterload-reducing and inotropic agents and heart transplantation for those with severe end-stage disease.

Osteosarcoma survivors treated with cisplatin are susceptible to ototoxicity. Hearing loss is first noted in the high-frequency range, often in association with tinnitus and vertigo. More profound hearing loss is commonplace. Audiograms should be performed every 3–5 years unless clinical evidence of hearing loss arises. It is not yet clear whether there will be late emergence of ototoxicity after cisplatin. There has been no evidence of improvement in hearing over time [184].

Long-term glomerular and renal tubular damage may be precipitated by the agents cisplatin and ifosfamide. This toxicity generally occurs during or soon after therapy, but it may be persistent. Glomerular dysfunction results in elevated levels of serum creatinine, azotemia, and decreased glomerular filtration rate (GFR). Cisplatin-induced tubular dysfunction causes prominent urinary wasting of cations, particularly magnesium, as well as calcium and potassium. Ifosfamide may cause phosphaturia, glycosuria, amino aciduria, and inability to acidify the urine (Fanconi syndrome). Treatment of nephrotoxicity is supportive; electrolytes should be monitored and replaced as necessary.

Fertility may be compromised in patients receiving alkylating agents such as cyclophosphamide and ifosfamide. In both males and females, the likelihood of sterility is dose related; adolescent males may become sterile after $4\,g/m^2$ of cyclophosphamide (almost invariably after $10\,g/m^2$), while female teens can tolerate doses of more than $20\,g/m^2$ without infertility. Women treated with alkylating agents are at risk for the development of early menopause [185]. Sperm collection in adolescent males should be considered prior to initiating therapy.

Late mechanical complications of limb-salvage procedures include fracture, loosening of the prosthesis, and limb-length discrepancy. Revision of the prosthesis or amputation are commonly necessary. Occasionally, growth in the contralateral growth plate must be surgically impaired to avoid limb-length discrepancy. Long-term studies of function after limb-sparing surgery are ongoing. While few patients choose amputation over limb salvage, the limitations on activities may be more profound with the latter. Musculoskeletal sequelae of limb amputation include phantom pains and pressure sores from ill-fitted prostheses.

Treatment-induced second malignancies after osteosarcoma are relatively rare due to the limited use of alkylating agents and radiotherapy. However, since osteosarcoma patients have an increased risk of carrying a mutated p53 gene in the germline (Li–Fraumeni syndrome), they may be genetically predisposed to other malignancies such as breast cancer. Careful attention to familial cancer history is necessary throughout follow-up.

12. Conclusions and future directions

The progress made in treatment of osteosarcoma during the past three decades has been remarkable. Surgical techniques have been refined so that the majority of patients can now undergo limb-salvage operations rather than amputation. Effective chemotherapy combinations have been identified that allow 70% of patients to be cured of their disease. In order to take these successes to new heights, however, we must look towards novel forms of anticancer therapy. The recent boom in our understanding of the biology of osteosarcoma has enabled us to develop agents that target malignant cells via mechanisms more specific than simple disruption of DNA. Examples of novel treatments already in use include the immunomodulator MTP-PE and the multidrug resistance reversing agent cyclosporine A. As we continue to unravel the molecular mechanisms underlying osteosarcoma, we will identify even more potential therapeutic targets.

References

1. Link MP, Eilber F. 1993. Osteosarcoma. In Pizzo PA, Poplack DG (eds.), Principles and Practice of Pediatric Oncology. Philadelphia: Lippincott, pp. 841–866.

2. Siegal G, Dahlin D, Sim F. 1975. Osteoblastic osteogenic sarcoma in a 35-month old girl: report of a case. Am J Pathol 63:336–890.

3. Levy M, Jaffe N. 1982. Osteosarcoma in early childhood. Pediatrics 70(2):302–303.

4. Luiz C, Al Kharusi W, Sethu A, Buhl L, Al Lamki Z. 1992. Osteosarcoma in a 26-month old girl. Cancer 70(4):894–896.

5. Miller R, Yound J, Novakovic B. 1995. Childhood cancer. Cancer 75(Suppl 1):395–405.

6. Gurney J, Severson R, Davis S, Robison L. 1995. Incidence of cancer in children in the United States. Cancer 75(8):2186–2195.

7. Dorfman H, Czerniak B. 1995. Bone cancers. Cancer 75(Suppl 1):203–210.

8. Huvos A. 1991. Bone Tumors: Diagnosis, Treatment and Prognosis. Philadelphia: W.B. Saunders.

9. Unni K. 1996. Dahlin's Bone Tumors — General Aspects and Data on 11,087 Cases. Philadelphia, New York: Lippincott-Raven.

10. Parkin D, Stiller C, Nectoux J. 1993. International variations in the incidence of childhood bone tumours. Int J Cancer 53:371–376.

11. Johnson L. 1953. Bull NY Acad Med 29:164–171.

12. Price C. 1958. Primary bone-forming tumours and their relationship to skeletal growth. J Bone Joint Surg 40B(3):574–593.

13. Fraumeni J. 1967. Stature and malignant tumors of bone in childhood and adolescence. Cancer 20(6):967–973.

14. Tjalma R. 1966. Canine bone sarcoma: estimation of relative risk as a function of body size. J Natl Cancer Inst 36(6):1137–1150.

15. Loutit J. 1970. Malignancy from radium. Br J Cancer 24(2):195–207.

16. Tucker M, D'angio G, Boice J, et al. 1987. Bone sarcomas linked to radiotherapy and chemotherapy in children. N Engl J Med 317(10):588–593.

17. Newton W, Meadows A, Shimada H, Bunin G, Vawter G. 1991. Bone sarcomas as second malignant neoplasms following childhood cancer. Cancer 67(1):193–201.

18. Toxicology and carcinogenesis studies of sodium fluoride (CAS No. 7681-49-4) in F344/N Rats and B6C3F Mice (Drinking water studies). 1990. NIH publication 91-2848.

19. Gelberg K, Fitzgerald E, Hwand S, Dubrow R. 1995. Fluoride exposure and childhood osteosarcoma: a case–control study. Am J Public Health 85(12):1678–1683.

20. Schwartzbaum J, George S, Pratt C, Davis B. 1991. An exploratory study of environmental and medical factors potentially related to childhood cancer. Med Pediatr Oncol 19:115–121.

21. Moss M, Kanarek M, Anderson H, Hanrahan L, Remington P. 1995. Osteosarcoma, seasonality and environmental factors in Wisconsin, 1979–1989. Arch Environ Health 50(3):235–241.

22. Finkel MP, Biskis BO, Jinkins PB. 1966. Virus induction of osteosarcomas in mice. Science 151(711):698–701.

23. Czitrom A, Pritzker K, Langer F, Gross A, Luk S. 1976. Virus-induced osteosarcoma in rats. J Bone Joint Surg 58-A(3):303–308.

24. Friedlander G, Mitchell M. 1976. A virally induced osteosarcoma in rats. J Bone Joint Surg 58-A(3):295–302.

25. Finkel M, Biskis B, Farrell C. 1968. Osteosarcomas appearing in syrian hamsters after treatment with extracts of human osteosarcomas. Proc Natl Acad Sci USA 60:1223–1230.

26. Morton D, Malmgren R. 1968. Human osteosarcomas: immunologic evidence suggesting an associated infectious agent. Science 162:1279–1281.

27. Yu AHW, Jaffe N, Parkman R. 1977. Concomitant presence of tumor-specific cytotoxic and inhibitor lymphocytes in patients with osteogenic sarcoma. N Engl J Med 297:121–127.

28. Sinovic J, Bridge J, Neff J. 1992. Ring chromosome in parosteal osteosarcoma — clinical and diagnostic significance. Cancer Genet Cytogenet 62:50–52.

29. Mertens F, Mandahl N, Orndal C, et al. 1993. Cytogenetic findings in 33 osteosarcomas. Int J Cancer 55:44–50.

30. Hoogerwerf W, Hawkins A, Perlman E, Griffin C. 1994. Chromosome analysis of nine osteosarcomas. Genes Chromosomes Cancer 9:88–92.

31. Ozisik Y, Meloni A, Peier A, Altungoz O, Spanier S, Zalupski M, Leong S, Sandberg A. 1994. Cytogenetic findings in 19 malignant bone tumors. Cancer 74(8):2268–2275.
32. Tarkkanen M, Karhu R, Kallioniemi A, et al. 1995. Gains and losses of DNA sequences in osteosarcomas by comparative genomic hybridization. Cancer Res 55:1334–1338.
33. Fletcher J, Gebhardt M, Kozakewich H. 1994. Cytogenetic aberrations in osteosarcomas. Cancer Genet Cytogenet 77:81–88.
34. Yamaguchi T, Togushida J, Yamamoro T, et al. 1992. Allelotype analysis in osteosarcomas: frequent allele loss on 3q, 13q, 17p, and 18q. Cancer Res 52:2419–2423.
35. Look A, Douglass E, Meyer W. 1988. Clinical importance of near diploid tumor stem lines in patients with osteosarcoma of an extremity. N Engl J Med 318(24):1567–1572.
36. Bauer HCF. 1993. Current status of DNA cytometry in osteosarcoma. In Humphrey GB (ed.), Osteosarcoma in Adolescents and Young Adults: New Developments and Controversies. Boston: Kluwer, pp. 159–169.
37. Knudson AG Jr. 1971. Mutation and cancer: statistical study of retinoblastoma. Proc Natl Acad Sci USA 68(4):820–823.
38. Friend SH, Bernards R, Rogelj S, Weinberg RA, Rapaport JM, Albert DM, Dryja TP. 1986. A human DNA segment with properties of the gene that predisposes to retinoblastoma and osteosarcoma. Nature 323(6089):643–646.
39. Fung YK, Murphree AL, T'Ang A, Qian J, Hinrichs SH, Benedict WF. 1987. Structural evidence for the authenticity of the human retinoblastoma gene. Science 236(4809):1657–1661.
40. Lee WH, Bookstein R, Hong F, Young LJ, Shew JY, Lee EY. 1987. Human retinoblastoma susceptibility gene: cloning, identification, and sequence. Science 235(4794):1394–1399.
41. Abramson DH, Ellsworth RM, Zimmerman LE. 1976. Nonocular cancer in retinoblastoma survivors. Trans Am Acad Ophthalmol Otolaryngol 81(3 Pt 1):454–457.
42. Abramson DH, Ellsworth RM, Kitchin FD, Tung G. 1984. Second nonocular tumors in retinoblastoma survivors. Are they radiation-induced? Ophthalmology 91(11):1351–1355.
43. Draper GJ, Sanders BM, Kingston JE. 1986. Second primary neoplasms in patients with retinoblastoma. Br J Cancer 53(5):661–671.
44. Smith LM, Donaldson SS, Egbert PR, Link MP, Bagshaw MA. 1989. Aggressive management of second primary tumors in survivors of hereditary retinoblastoma. Int J Radiat Oncol Biol Phys 17(3):499–505.
45. Gilman P, Wang N, Fan S, Reede J, Khan A, Leventhal B. 1985. Familial osteosarcoma associated with 13; 14 chromosomal rearrangement. Cancer Genet Cytogenet 17:123–132.
46. Weichselbaum R, Cassady J, Jaffe N, Filler R. 1977. Preliminary results of aggressive multimodality therapy for metastatic osteosarcoma. Cancer 40:78–83.
47. Benedict W, Fung Y, Murphree A. 1988. The gene responsible for the development of retinoblastoma and osteosarcoma. Cancer 62:1691–1694.
48. Reissmann P, Simon M, Lee W, Slamon D. 1989. Studies of the retinoblastoma gene in human sarcomas. Oncogene 4:839–843.
49. Toguchida J, Ishizaki K, Sasaki M, Ikenaga M, Sugimoto M, Kotoura Y, Yamamuro T. 1988. Chromosomal reorganization for the expression of recessive mutation of retinoblastoma susceptibility gene in the development of osteosarcoma. Cancer Res 48:3939–3943.
50. Wadayama B, Toguchida J, Shimizu T, Ishizaki K, Sasaki M, Kotoura Y, Tamamuro T. 1994. Mutation spectrum of the retinoblastoma gene in osteosarcomas. Cancer Res 54:3042–3048.
51. Huang H, Yee J, Shew J, et al. 1988. Suppression of the neoplastic phenotype by replacement of the RB gene in human cancer cells. Science 242:1563–1566.
52. Toguchida J, Ishizaki K, Nakamura Y, Sasaki M, Ikenaga M, Kato M, Sugimoto M, Kotoura Y, Yamamuro T. 1989. Assignment of common allele loss in osteosarcoma to the subregion 17p13. Cancer Res 49:6247–6251.
53. Chang F, Syrjanen S, Syrjanen K. 1995. Implications of the p53 tumor-suppressor gene in clinical oncology. J Clin Oncol 13(4):1009–1022.
54. Lane DP. 1993. A death in the life of p53. Nature 362:786–787.
55. Marx J. 1993. How p53 suppresses cell growth. Science 262:1644–1645.

56. Yonish-Rouach E, Grunwald D, Wilder S, et al. 1993. p53-mediated cell death: relationship to cell cycle control. Mol Cell Biol 13:1415–1423.

57. Lavigueur A, Maltby V, Mock D, Rossant J, Pawson T, Bernstein A. 1989. High incidence of lung, bone, and lymphoid tumors in transgenic mice overexpressing mutant alleles of the p53 oncogene. Mol Cell Biol 9(9):3982–3991.

58. Masuda H, Miller C, Koeffler H, Battifora H, Cline M. 1987. Rearrangement of the p53 gene in human osteogenic sarcomas. Proc Natl Acad Sci USA 84:7716–7719.

59. Romano JW, Ehrhart JC, Duthu A, Kim CM, Appella E, May P. 1989. Identification and characterization of a p53 gene mutation in a human osteosarcoma cell line. Oncogene 4(12):1483–1488.

60. Miller CW, Aslo A, Tsay C, Slamon D, Ishizaki K, Toguchida J, Yamamuro T, Lampkin B, Koeffler HP. 1990. Frequency and structure of p53 rearrangements in human osteosarcoma. Cancer Res 50(24):7950–7954.

61. Chandar N, Billig B, McMaster J, Novak J. 1992. Inactivation of p53 gene in human and murine osteosarcoma cells. Br J Cancer 65(2):208–214.

62. Toguchida J, Yamaguchi T, Ritchie B, et al. 1992. Mutation spectrum of the p53 gene in bone and soft tissue sarcomas. Cancer Res 52:6194–6199.

63. Ivarone A, Matthay K, Steinkirchner T, Israel M. 1992. Germ-line and somatic p53 gene mutations in multifocal osteogenic sarcoma. Proc Natl Acad Sci USA 89:4207–4209.

64. Malkin D, Li F, Strong L, et al. 1990. Germ line p53 mutations in a familial syndrome of breast cancer, sarcomas, and other neoplasms. Science 250:1233–1238.

65. Toguchida J, Yamaguchi T, Dayton S, et al. 1992. Prevalence and spectrum of germline mutations of the P53 gene among patients with sarcoma. N Engl J Med 326(20):1301–1308.

66. Mcintyre J, Smith-Sorensen B, Friend S, et al. 1994. Germline mutations of the p53 tumor suppressor gene in children with osteosarcoma. J Clin Oncol 12(5):925–930.

67. Porter D, Holden S, Steel C, Cohen B, Wallace M, Reid R. 1992. A significant proportion of patients with osteosarcoma may belong to Li–Fraumeni cancer families. J Bone Joint Surg Br 74-B(6):883–886.

68. Oliner J, Kinzler K, Meltzer P, George K, Vogelstein B. 1992. Amplification of a gene encoding a p53-associated protein in human sarcomas. Nature 358:80–83.

69. Ladanyi M, Cha C, Lewis R, Jhanwar S, Huvos A, Healey J. 1993. MDM2 gene amplification in metastatic osteosarcoma. Cancer Res 52:16–18.

70. Florenes V, Maelandsmo G, Forus A, Andreassen A, Myklebost O, Fodstad O. 1994. MDM2 gene amplification and transcript levels in human sarcomas: relationship to TP53 gene status. J Natl Cancer Inst 86(17):1297–1302.

71. Miller C, Aslo A, Campbell M, Kawamata N, Lampkin B, Koeffler H. 1996. Alterations of the p15, p16, and p18 genes in osteosarcoma. Cancer Genet Cytogenet 86:136–142.

72. DePinho RA, Schreiber-Agus N, Alt FW. 1991. Myc family oncogenes in the development of normal and neoplastic cells. Adv Cancer Res 57:1–46.

73. Henriksson M, Luscher B. 1996. The myc family of oncogenes. Adv Cancer Res 68:109–182.

74. Isfort R, Cody D, Lovell G, Doersen C. 1995. Analysis of oncogenes, tumor suppressor genes, autocrine growth-factor production, and differentiation state of human osteosarcoma cell lines. Mol Carcinogenesis 14:170–178.

75. Sturm S, Strauss P, Adolph S, Hameister H, Erfle V. 1990. Amplification and rearrangement of c-myc in radiation-induced murine osteosarcomas. Cancer Res 50:4146–4153.

76. Masuda H, Battifora H, Yokota J, Meltzer S, Cline MJ. 1987. Specificity of proto-oncogene amplification in human malignant diseases. Mol Biol Med 4(4):213–227.

77. Ikeda S, Sumii H, Akiyama K, Watanabe S, Ito S, Inoue H, Takechi H, Tanabe G, Oda T. 1989. Amplification of both c-myc and c-raf-1 oncogenes in human osteosarcoma. Jpn J Cancer Res 80:6–9.

78. Ladanyi M, Park C, Lewis R, Jhanwar S, Healey J, Huvos A. 1993. Sporadic amplification of the myc gene in human osteosarcomas. Diagn Mol Pathol 2(3):163–167.

79. Angel P, Karin M. 1991. The role of jun, fos and the AP-1 complex in cell-proliferation and transformation. Biochim Biophys Acta 1072(2–3):129–157.

245

80. Radler-Pohl A, Gebel S, Sachsenmaier C, et al. 1993. The activation and activity control of AP-1 (fos/jun). Ann N Y Acad Sci 684:127–148.

81. Ward JM, Young DM. 1976. Histogenesis and morphology of periosteal sarcomas induced by FBJ virus in NIH Swiss mice. Cancer Res 36(11 Pt 1):3985–3992.

82. Curran T, Peters G, Van Beveren C, Teich NM, Verma IM. 1982. FBJ murine osteosarcoma virus: identification and molecular cloning of biologically active proviral DNA. J Virol 44(2):674–682.

83. Ruther U, Garber C, Komitowski D, Muller R, Wagner EF. 1987. Deregulated c-fos expression interferes with normal bone development in transgenic mice. Nature 325(6103):412–416.

84. Ruther U, Komitowski D, Schubert FR, Wagner EF. 1989. c-fos expression induces bone tumors in transgenic mice. Oncogene 4(7):861–865.

85. Wang ZQ, Ovitt C, Grigoriadis AE, Mohle-Steinlein U, Ruther U, Wagner EF. 1992. Bone and haematopoietic defects in mice lacking c-fos. Nature 360(6406):741–745.

86. Wang Z, Liang J, Schellander K, Wagner E, Grigoriadis A. 1995. c-fos-induced osteosarcoma formation in transgenic mice: cooperativity with c-jun and the role of endogenous c-fos. Cancer Res 55:6244–6251.

87. Schon A, Michiels L, Janowski M, Merregaert J, Erfle V. 1986. Expression of protooncogenes in murine osteosarcomas. Int J Cancer 38:67–74.

88. Wang H, Rodgers W, Chmell M, Svitek C, Schwartz H. 1995. Osteosarcoma oncogene expression detected by in situ hybridization. J Orthoped Res 13:671–678.

89. Wu JX, Carpenter PM, Gresens C, Keh R, Niman H, Morris JW, Mercola D. 1990. The proto-oncogene c-fos is over-expressed in the majority of human osteosarcomas. Oncogene 5(7):989–1000.

90. Raymond A, Simms W, Ayala A. 1995. Osteosarcoma-specimen management following primary chemotherapy. Hematol Oncol Clin North Am 9(4):841–867.

91. Schajowicz F, Sissons H, Sobin L. 1995. The World Health Organization's histologic classification of bone tumors. Cancer 75(5):1208–1214.

92. Ueda Y, Nakanishi I. 1989. Immunohistochemical and biochemical studies on the collagenous proteins of human osteosarcoma. Virchows Arch (B) 58:79–88.

93. Grundmann E, Ueda Y, Schneider-Stock R, Roessner A. 1995. New aspects of cell biology in osteosarcoma. Pathol Res Pract 191:563–570.

94. Jundt G, Schultz A, Berghauser KH, Fisher LW, Gehron-Robey P, Termine JD. 1989. Immunocytochemical identification of osteogenic bone tumors by osteonectin antibodies. Virchows Arch (A) 414:345–353.

95. Bosse A, Vollmer E, Bocker W, Roessner A, Wuisman P, Jones D, Fisher LW. 1990. The impact of osteonectin for differential diagnosis of bone tumors. An immunohistochemical approach. Pathol Res Pract 186(5):651–657.

96. Meyers P, Heller G, Healey J, Huvos A, Applewhite A, Sun M, LaQuaglia M. 1993. Osteogenic sarcoma with clinically detectable metastasis at initial presentation. J Clin Oncol 11(3):449–453.

97. Parham D, Pratt C, Parvey L, Webber B, Champion J. 1985. Childhood multifocal osteosarcoma: clinicopathologic and radiologic correlates. Cancer 55(11):2653–2658.

98. Kesselring FO, Penn W. 1982. Radiological aspects of "classic" primary osteosarcoma: value of some radiological investigations: a review. Diagn Imaging 51(2):78–92.

99. Gillespy T, Manfrini M, Ruggieri P, Spanier SS, Pettersson H, Springfield DS. 1988. Staging of intraosseous extent of osteosarcoma: correlation of preoperative CT and MR imaging with pathologic macroslides. Radiology 167(3):765–767.

100. Murphy WA. 1991. Imaging bone tumors in the 1990's. Cancer 67(4):1169–1176.

101. Fletcher BD, Hanna SL, Fairclough DL, Gronemeyer SA. 1992. Pediatric musculoskeletal tumors: use of dynamic contrast-enhanced MR imaging to monitor response to chemotherapy. Radiology 184:243–248.

102. Van der Woude HJ, Bloom JL, Schipper J, et al. 1994. Changes in tumor perfusion induced by chemotherapy in bone sarcomas: color doppler flow imaging compared with contrast-enhanced MR imaging and 3-phase bone scintigraphy. Radiology 191:421–431.

246

103. Mooyaart EL, Kamman RL, Boeve WJ. 1993. In vivo ^{31}P nuclear magnetic resonance spectroscopy of osteosarcoma. In Humphrey GB (ed.), Osteosarcoma in Adolescents and Young Adults: New Developments and Controversies. Boston: Kluwer, pp. 19–24.

104. Rosen G, Loren G, Ramanna L. 1991. Osteogenic sarcoma: early evaluation of preoperative chemotherapy with thallium-201 scintigraphy. Proc Am Soc Clin Oncol: 97.

105. Rosen G. 1993. An opinion supporting the role of high-dose methotrexate in the treatment of osteosarcoma. In Humphrey GB (eds.), Osteosarcoma in Adolescents and Young Adults: New Developments and Controversie. Boston: Kluwer, pp. 49–54.

106. Tse N, Hoh C, Hawkins R, Phelps M, Glaspy J. 1994. Positron emission tomography diagnosis of pulmonary metastases in osteogenic sarcoma. Am J Clin Oncol 17:22–25.

107. Hoefnagel CA, Bruning PF, Cohen P, Marcuse HR, van der Schoot JB. 1981. Detection of lung metastases from osteosarcoma by scintigraphy using 99mTc-methylene diphosphonate. Diagn Imaging 50(5):277–284.

108. Aboulafia A, Malawer M. 1993. Surgical management of pelvic and extremity osteosarcoma. Cancer 71:3358–3366.

109. Murray J, Jessup K, Romsdahl M, et al. 1985. Limb-salvage surgery in osteosarcoma: early experience at MD Anderson Hospital and Tumor Institute. Cancer Treatment Symp 3:131–137.

110. Meyers P, Heller G, Healey J, Huvos A, Lane J, Marcove R, Applewhite A, Vlamis V, Rosen G. 1992. Chemotherapy for nonmetastatic osteogenic sarcoma: the Memorial Sloan-Kettering experience. J Clin Oncol 10(1):5–15.

111. Rosenberg ZS, Lev S, Schmahmann S, Steiner GC, Beltran J, Present D. 1995. Osteosarcoma: subtle, rate, and misleading plain film features. Am J Radiol 165:1209–1214.

112. Davis A, Bell R, Goodwin P. 1994. Prognostic factors in osteosarcoma: a critical review. J Clin Oncol 12(2):423–431.

113. Bacci G, Picci P, Ferrari S, Oralndi M, Ruggieri P, Casadei R, Ferraro A, Biagini R, Battistini A. 1993. Prognostic significance of serum alkaline phosphatase measurements in patients with osteosarcoma treated with adjuvant or neoadjuvant chemotherapy. Cancer 71(4):1224–1230.

114. Bentzen S, Poulsen H, Kaai S, Jensen O, Johansen H, Mouridsen H, Daugaard S, Arnoldi C. 1988. Prognostic factors in osteosarcoma. Cancer 62(1):194–202.

115. Taylor W, Ivins J, Unni K, Beabout J, Gelenzer H, Black L. 1989. Prognostic variables in osteosarcoma: a multi-institutional study. J Natl Cancer Inst 81(1):21–30.

116. Rosen G, Murphy M, Huvos A, Gutierrez M, Marcove R. 1976. Chemotherapy, en bloc resection, and prosthetic bone replacement in the treatment of osteogenic sarcoma. Cancer 37(1):1–11.

117. Raymond A, Chawla S, Carrasco C. 1987. Osteosarcoma chemotherapy effect: a prognostic factor. Semin Diagn Pathol 4:212–236.

118. Winkler K, Beron G, Delling G. 1988. Neoadjuvant chemotherapy of osteosarcoma: results of a randomized cooperative trial (COSS-82) with salvage chemotherapy based on histological tumor response. J Clin Oncol 6:329–337.

119. Glasser D, Lane J, Huvos A, Marcove R, Rosen G. 1992. Survival, prognosis, and therapeutic response in osteogenic sarcoma. Cancer 69(3):698–708.

120. Baldini N, Scotlandi K, Barbanti-Brodano G, et al. 1995. Expression of P-glycoprotein in high-grade osteosarcomas in relation to clinical outcome [see comments]. N Engl J Med 333(21):1380–1385.

121. Roninson IB, Chin JE, Choi KG, Gros P, Housman DE, Fojo A, Shen DW, Gottesman MM, Pastan I. 1986. Isolation of human mdr DNA sequences amplified in multidrug-resistant KB carcinoma cells. Proc Natl Acad Sci USA 83(12):4538–4542.

122. Callen DF, Baker E, Simmers RN, Soshadri R, Roninson IB. 1987. Localization of the human multiple drug resistance gene, MDR1, to 7q21.1. Hum Genet 77(2):142–144.

123. Endicott JA, Ling V. 1989. The biochemistry of P-glycoprotein-mediated multidrug resistance. Annu Rev Biochem 58:137–171.

124. Goldstein LJ, Galski H, Fojo A, et al. 1989. Expression of a multidrug resistance gene in human cancers. J Natl Cancer Inst 81(2):116–124.
125. Schwartz C, Rosier R, Willis J, Hicks D. 1992. P-glycoprotein (P-gp) expression in osteosarcoma and clinical outcome (meeting abstract). Proc Am Soc Clin Oncol 11:A948.
126. Chan H, DeBoer G, Haddad G, Gallie B, Ling V. 1995. Multidrug resistance in pediatric malignancies. Hematol Oncol Clin North Am 9(2):275–318.
127. Wunder JS, Bell RS, Wold L, Andrulis IL. 1993. Expression of the multidrug resistance gene in osteosarcoma: a pilot study. J Orthoped Res 11(3):396–403.
128. Serra M, Scotlandi K, Manara MC, Maurici D, Benini S, Sarti M, Campanacci M, Baldini N. 1995. Analysis of P-glycoprotein expression in osteosarcoma. Eur J Cancer 31A(12):1998–2002.
129. Stein U, Wunderlich V, Haensch W, Schmidt-Peter P. 1993. Expression of the mdr1 gene in bone and soft tissue sarcomas of adult patients. Eur J Cancer 29A(14):1979–1981.
130. Li W, Fan J, Hochhauser D, et al. 1995. Lack of functional retinoblastoma protein mediates increased resistance to antimetabolites in human sarcoma cell lines. Proc Natl Acad Sci USA 91:10436–10440.
131. Winkler K, Bieling P, Bielack S. 1992. Die chemotherapie des osteosarkoms. Z Othosp 138:285–289.
132. Fuchs N, Winkler K. 1993. Osteosarcoma. Curr Opinion Oncol 5:667–671.
133. Picci P, Sangiorgi L, Rougraff B, Neff J, Casadei R, Campanacci M. 1994. Relationship of chemotherapy-induced necrosis and surgical margins to local recurrence in osteosarcoma. J Clin Oncol 12(12):2699–2705.
134. Jaffe N, Frei E, Taggis D, Bishop Y. 1974. Adjuvant methotrexate and citrovorum factor treatment of osteogenic sarcoma. N Engl J Med 291:994–997.
135. Cortes EP, Holland JF, Wang JJ, Sinks LF, Blom J, Senn H, Bank A, Glidewell O. 1974. Amputation and adriamycin in primary osteosarcoma. N Engl J Med 291:998–1000.
136. Baum E, Greenberg L, Gaynon P, Krivit W, Hammond D. 1978. Use of cis-platinum diammine dichloride (CPDD) in osteogenic sarcoma (OS) in children. Proc Am Assoc Cancer Res 19:385.
137. Grem JL, King SA, Wittes RE, Leyland-Jones B. 1988. The role of methotrexate in osteosarcoma. J Natl Cancer Inst 80:626–656.
138. Taylor WF, Ivins JC, Dahlin DC, Edmonson JH, Pritchard DJ. 1978. Trends and variability in survival from osteosarcoma. Mayo Clin Proc 53(11):695–700.
139. Edmonson JH, Green SJ, Ivins JC, Gilchrist GS, Cregan ET, Pritchard DJ, Smithson WA, Dahlin DC, Taylor WF. 1980. Methotrexate as adjuvant treatment for primary osteosarcoma (letter). N Engl J Med 303(11):642–643.
140. Taylor WF, Ivins JC, Pritchard DJ, Dahlin DC, Gilchrist GS, Edmonson JH. 1985. Trends and variability in survival among patients with osteosarcoma: a 7-year update. Mayo Clin Proc 60(2):91–104.
141. Jaffe N, Patel S, Benjamin R. 1995. Chemotherapy in osteosarcoma: basis for application and antagonism to implementation; early controversies surrounding its implementation. Hematol Oncol Clin North Am 9(4):825–839.
142. Link M, Goorin A, Miser A, et al. 1986. The effect of adjuvant chemotherapy on relapse-free survival in patients with osteosarcoma of the extremity. N Engl J Med 314(25):1600–1606.
143. Eilber F, Giuliano A, Eckardt J, Patterson K, Moseley S, Goodnight J. 1987. Adjuvant chemotherapy for osteosarcoma: a randomized prospective trial. J Clin Oncol 5(1):21–26.
144. Marti C, Kroner T, Remagen W, Berchtold W, Cserhati M, Varini M. 1985. High dose ifosfamide in advanced osteosarcoma. Cancer Treat Rep 69(1):115–117.
145. Cassano WF, Graham-Pole J, Dickson N. 1991. Etoposide, cyclophosphamide, cisplatin, and doxorubicin as neoadjuvant chemotherapy for osteosarcoma. Cancer 68(9):1899–1902.
146. Graf N, Winkler K, Betlemovic M, Fuchs N, Bode U. 1994. Methotrexate pharmacokinetics and prognosis in osteosarcoma. J Clin Oncol 12(7):1443–1451.
147. Rosier RN, Teot LA, Hicks DG, Schwartz C, O'keefe RJ, Puzas JE. 1995. Multiple drug resistance in osteosarcoma. Iowa Orthopaed J 15:66–73.

248

148. Winkler K, Beron G, Kotz R, et al. 1984. Neoadjuvant chemotherapy for osteogenic sarcoma: results of a coorperative German/Austrian study. J Clin Oncol 2(6):617–624.

149. Kleinerman E, Erickson K, Schroit A, et al. 1983. Activation of tumoricidal properties in human blood monocytes by liposomes containing lipophilic muramyl tripeptide. Cancer Res 43:2010–2014.

150. Fidler I, Sone S, Fogler W, et al. 1981. Eradication of spontaneous metastases and activation of alveolar macrophages by intravenous injection of liposomes containing muramyl dipeptide. Proc Natl Acad Sci USA 58:1680–1684.

151. Fidler I, Barnes Z, Fogler W, et al. 1982. Involvement of macrophages in the eradication of established metastases following intravenous injection of liposomes containing macrophage activators. Cancer Res 42:496–501.

152. MacEwen E, Kurzman I, Rosenthal R, et al. 1989. Therapy of osteosarcoma in dogs with intravenous injection of liposome encapsulated muramyl tripeptide. J Natl Cancer Inst 81:935–937.

153. Murray J, Kleinerman E, Cunningham J, et al. 1989. Phase I trial of liposomal muramyl tripeptidephosphatidylethanolamine in cancer patients. J Clin Oncol 7:1915–1925.

154. Kleinerman E, Gano J, Johnston D, Benjamin R, Jaffe N. 1995. Efficacy of liposomal muramyl tripepetide (CGP 19835A) in the treatment of relapsed osteosarcoma. Am J Clin Oncol 18(2):93–99.

155. Kleinerman E, Snyder J, Jaffe N. 1991. Influence of chemotherapy administration on monocyte activation by liposomal muramyl tripeptide phophatidylethanolamine in children with osteosarcoma. J Clin Oncol 9(2):259–267.

156. Pollak M, Sem AW, Richard M, Tetenes E, Bell R. 1992. Inhibition of metastatic behavior of murine osteosarcoma by hypophysectomy. J Natl Cancer Inst 84:966–971.

157. Chavez-Kappel C, Velez-Yanguas M, Hirschfeld S, Helman L. 1994. Human osteosarcoma cell lines are dependent on Insulin-like growth factor I for in vitro growth. Cancer Res 54:2803–2807.

158. Pinski J, Schally AV, Groot K, Halmos G, Szepeshazi K, Zarandi M, Armatis P. 1995. Inhibition of growth of human osteosarcomas by antagonists of growth hormone-releasing hormone. J Natl Cancer Inst 87(23):1787–1794.

159. Folkman J. 1995. Clinical applications of research on angiogenesis. N Engl J Med 333(26):1157–1163.

160. Mori S, Ueda T, Kuratsu S, Hosono N, Izawa K, Uchida A. 1995. Suppression of pulmonary metastasis by angiogenesis inhibitor TNP-470 in murine osteosarcoma. Int J Cancer 61(1):148–152.

161. Morishita T, Mii Y, Miyauchi Y, et al. 1995. Efficacy of the angiogenesis inhibitor O-(chloroacetyl-carbamoyl)fumagillol (AGM-1470) on osteosarcoma growth and lung metastasis in rats. Jpn J Clin Oncol 25(2):25–31.

162. Martinez A, Goffinet D, Donaldson S, Bagshaw M, Kaplan H. 1985. Intra-arterial infusion of radiosensitizer (BUdR) combined with hypofractionated irradiation and chemotherapy for primary treatment of osteogenic sarcoma. J Radiat Oncol Biol Phys 11(1):123–128.

163. Kastan MB, Onyekwere O, Sidransky D, Vogelstein B, Craig RW. 1991. Participation of p53 protein in the cellular response to DNA damage. Cancer Res 51(23 Pt 1):6304–6311.

164. Kuerbitz SJ, Plunkett BS, Walsh WV, Kastan MB. 1992. Wild-type p53 is a cell cycle checkpoint determinant following irradiation. Proc Natl Acad Sci USA 89(16):7491–7495.

165. Rab G, Ivins J, Childs D, Cupps R, Pritchard D. 1976. Elective whole lung irradiation in the treatment of osteogenic sarcoma. Cancer 38:939–942.

166. Jaffe N, Paed D, Farber S, et al. 1973. Favorable response of metastatic osteogenic sarcoma to pulse high dose methotrexate with citrovorum rescue and radiation therapy. Cancer 31(6):1367–1373.

167. Rosen G, Tefft M, Martinez A, Cham W, Murphy M. 1975. Combination chemotherapy and radiation therapy in the treatment of metastatic osteogenic sarcoma. Cancer 35(3):622–630.

168. Miser J, Arndt C, Smithson W, et al. 1994. Treatment of high grade osteosarcoma with

ifosfamide, mesna, adriamycin, high dose methotrexate with or without cisplatin. Results of two pilot trials. Proc ASCO 13:421.

169. Goorin A, Shuster J, Baker A, Horowitz M, Meyer W, Link M. 1991. Changing pattern of pulmonary metastases with adjuvant chemotherapy in patients with osteosarcoma: results from the Multiinstitutional Osteosarcoma Study. J Clin Oncol 9(4):600-605.

170. Giuliano A, Feig S, Eilber F. 1984. Changing metastatic patterns of osteosarcoma. Cancer 54:2160–2164.

171. Tabone M, Kalifa C, Rodary C, Raquin M, Couanet D, Lemerle J. 1994. Osteosarcoma recurrences in pediatric patients previously treated with intensive chemotherapy. J Clin Oncol 12(12):2614–2620.

172. Jaffe N, Smith E, Abelson H, Frei E. 1983. Osteogenic sarcoma: alterations in the pattern of pulmonary metastases with adjuvant chemotherapy. J Clin Oncol 1(4):251–254.

173. Rosenberg S, Flye M, Conkle D, Geipp C, Levine A, Simon R. 1979. Treatment of osteogenic sarcoma: aggressive resection of pulmonary metastases. Cancer Treatment Rep 63(5):753–756.

174. Putnam J, Roth J, Wesley M, Johnston M, Rosenberg S. 1983. Survival following aggressive resection of pulmonary metastases from osteogenic sarcoma: analysis of prognostic factors. Ann Thorac Surg 36(5):516–523.

175. Goorin A, Delorey M, Lack E, et al. 1984. Prognostic significance of complete surgical resection of pulmonary metastases in patients with osteogenic sarcoma: analysis of 32 patients. J Clin Oncol 2(5):425–431.

176. Meyer W, Schell M, Kumar A, et al. 1987. Thoracotomy for pulmonary metastatic osteosarcoma: an analysis of prognostic indicators of survival. Cancer 59:374–379.

177. Belli L, Scholl S, Livartowski A, et al. 1989. Resection of pulmonary metastases in osteosarcoma: a retrospective analysis of 44 patients. Cancer 63:2546–2550.

178. Pastorino U, Gasparini M, Tavecchio L, et al. 1991. The contribution of salvage surgery to the management of childhood osteosarcoma. J Clin Oncol 9(8):1357–1362.

179. Pastorino U, Gasparini M, Azzarelli A, Tavecchio L, Racasi G. 1993. Salvage surgery for childhood osteosarcoma. In Humphrey G (ed.), Osteosarcoma in Adolescents and Young Adults: New Developments and Controversies. Boston: Kluwer Academic.

180. Ward W, Mikaelian K, Dorey F, Mirra J, Sassoon A, Holmes E, Eilber F, Eckardt J. 1994. Pulmonary metastases of stage IIB extremity osteosarcoma and subsequent pulmonary metastases. J Clin Oncol 12(9):1849–1858.

181. Steinherz LJ, Steinherz PG, Tan C. 1995. Cardiac failure and dysrhythmias 6–19 years after anthracycline therapy: a series of 15 patients. Med Pediatr Oncol 24(6):352–361.

182. Steinherz LJ, Graham T, Hurwitz R, Sondheimer HM, Schwartz RG, Shaffer EM, Sandor G, Benson L, Williams R. 1992. Guidelines for cardiac monitoring of children during and after anthracycline therapy: report of the Cardiology Committee of the Childrens Cancer Study Group. Pediatrics 89(5 Pt 1):942–949.

183. Schwartz CL, Hobbie WL, Truesdell S, Constine LC, Clark EB. 1993. Corrected QT interval prolongation in anthracycline-treated survivors of childhood cancer. J Clin Oncol 11(10):1906–1910.

184. Schwartz CL, Hobbie WL, Ruble K, Hinkle A, Constine LS. 1996. Long term nephrotoxicity and ototoxicity after cisplatin (CDDP) therapy. Proc 4th Int Conf on Long Term Complications of Treatment of Children and Adolescents for Cancer, Buffalo, NY.

185. Nicholson HS, Byrne J. 1993. Fertility and pregnancy after treatment for cancer during childhood or adolescence. Cancer 71(Suppl 10):3392–3399.

186. Bieling P, Rehan N, Winkler P, et al. 1996. Tumor size and prognosis in aggressively treated osteosarcoma. J Clin Oncol 14(3):848–858.

187. Link M. 1993. Results of the MIOS. In Humprey G (ed.), Osteosarcoma in Adolescents and Young Adults: New Developments and Controversies. Boston: Kluwer.

188. Rosen G, Caparros B, Huvos AG, et al. 1982. Preoperative therapy for osteogenic sarcoma: selection of postoperative adjuvant chemotherapy based on the response of the primary tumor to preoperative chemotherapy. Cancer 49(6):1221–1230.

189. Winkler K, Bielack S, Delling G, Jurgens H, Kotz R, Salzer-Kuntschik M. 1993. Treatment of osteosarcoma: experience of the Cooperative Osteosarcoma Study Group (COSS). In Humphrey G (ed.), Cancer Treatment and Research: Osteosarcoma in Adolescents and Young Adults: New Developments and Controversies. Boston: Kluwer.

190. Winkler K, Bielack S, Delling G, et al. 1990. Effect of intraarterial versus intravenous cisplatin in addition to systemic doxorubicin, high-dose methotrexate, and ifosfamide on histologic tumor response in osteosarcoma (Study COSS-86). Cancer 66(8):1703–1710.

191. Provisor A, Nachman J, Krailo M, Ettinger L, Hammond D. 1987. Treatment of non-metastatic osteogenic sarcoma of the extremities with pre-and post-operative chemotherapy. Proc ASCO 6:217.

192. Miser JS, Krailo M. 1993. The Children's Cancer Group Studies. In Humphrey G (ed.), Osteosarcoma in Adolescents and Young Adults: New Developments and Controversies. Boston: Kluwer.

193. Bramwell VHC, Burger M, Sneath R, et al. 1992. A comparison of two short intensive adjuvant chemotherapy regimens in operable osteosarcoma of limbs in children and young adults: the first study of the European Osteosarcoma Intergroup. J Clin Oncol 10(10):1579–1591.

194. Mirra JM. 1989. Bone Tumors: Clinical, Radiologic, and Pathologic Correlations. Philadelphia: Lea & Febiger.

9. The Ewing's sarcoma family of tumors: Ewing's sarcoma and peripheral primitive neuroectodermal tumor of bone and soft tissue

Linda Granowetter and Daniel C. West

1. Introduction

In 1921 James Ewing described a radiosensitive tumor of the forearm composed of small round cells that he believed to be of endothelial origin [1]. These small round cell tumors of bone came to be known as *Ewing's sarcomas*. Soft tissue variants are called *extraosseous* Ewing's sarcoma [2,3] and the Askin tumor [4]. Bone and soft tissue tumors, which are quite similar to Ewing's sarcoma under the light microscope but which have notable neural differentiation, have been denoted *peripheral primitive neuroectodermal tumors* (PNETs) or *peripheral neuroepithelioma*. The distinction between Ewing's sarcoma of bone and soft tissue and other small round blue cell tumors of childhood was essentially a diagnosis of exclusion until current immunohistochemical and molecular genetic techniques gave us tools to better delineate these tumors. These tumors are defined by a common molecular marker, the (11;22)(q24;q12) translocation, or its variants. It is now thought that these tumors are all related and compose a spectrum of neuroepithelial tumors ranging from the least differentiated (Ewing's sarcoma) to the most differentiated variants (PNET). It has been suggested that these tumors be considered a family of tumors called the *Ewing's sarcoma family of tumors* (ESFT). Discussions in this chapter will refer to the Ewing family of tumors, but it should be noted that much of the epidemiological and clinical data have been derived from studies restricted to histologically defined Ewing's sarcoma of bone. A complete database of the biological and clinical spectrum of this family of tumors does not yet exist because large prospective clinical trials were generally open only to patients with Ewing's sarcoma of bone; soft tissue variants and peripheral neuroepitheliomas have been treated in trials for sarcomas or other tumors. Further, as discussed below, the criteria for distinguishing PNET and Ewing's sarcoma have not been uniform over years and among pathologists. Future studies will include all members of this family of tumors, and thus, enrich the database available.

2. Epidemiology

Ewing's sarcoma of bone is a rare tumor: in the United States, there are about 2.7 cases identified each year per million children under 15 years of age [5]. If

D.O. Walterhouse and S.L. Cohn (eds), DIAGNOSTIC AND THERAPEUTIC ADVANCES IN PEDIATRIC ONCOLOGY. Copyright © 1997. Kluwer Academic Publishers, Boston. All rights reserved.

one were to include the soft tissue variants, PNET, and older patients, the incidence would be slightly amplified. Horowitz and colleagues compiled data from 17 studies, performed over 10 years, which included Ewing's sarcoma, peripheral PNET and extraosseous Ewing's sarcoma, and found that among 1505 reported patients 87% had Ewing's sarcoma of bone, 8% extraosseous Ewing's sarcoma, and 5% peripheral PNET [6]. Among these patients, more than half the tumors occurred in the second decade of life, close to one third in the first decade, and less than 10% in the third decade. These data are very similar to those from the Children's Cancer Group (CCG)–Pediatric Oncology Group (POG) intergroup study (1988–1992) of Ewing's sarcoma of bone and PNET, in which 30% of patients were younger than 10 years, 57% were age 10–17, and 13% were between 18 and 30 years of age [7,8]. Less commonly, ESFT occurs in patients over 30 years of age [9–11]. The spectrum of age of patients with peripheral neuroepitheliomas is said to include an increased number of younger patients. Ewing's sarcoma is rare among non-white populations [12–15]. In New York state, 22% of primary bone malignancies among white patients are Ewing's sarcoma, but only 7% of primary bone tumors diagnosed in African Americans are Ewing's sarcoma [12].

Clear predisposing factors to Ewing tumors have not been identified. A recent report [16] from Canada linked an increased risk of death from bone cancer (osteosarcoma, Ewing's sarcoma, and chondrosarcoma) to elevated levels of radium in the drinking water of recorded birthplace, but this finding has not been confirmed in other reports. In an analysis from England, low birth weight was associated with Ewing's sarcoma [17]. A report for the National Cancer Institute [18] demonstrated an increased risk of stomach and neuroectodermal cancers in family members of Ewing's sarcoma patients; however, a similar (albeit smaller) study of patients ascertained from the Manchester bone tumor registry [19] found no excess of cancer in relatives. The risk of cancer in mothers of children with Ewing's sarcoma does not appear to be increased [20]. There have been reports of Ewing's sarcoma in siblings [21,22]; however, the Ewing family of tumors is not associated with the Li–Fraumeni familial cancer syndrome [23]. Although osteosarcoma following chemotherapy and radiation treatment for Ewing's sarcoma is well described, Ewing's sarcoma as a second malignancy is rare [24–27]. There is no convincing evidence that Ewing's sarcoma is associated with skeletal abnormalities, genitourinary abnormalities, or other congenital abnormalities, although case reports and associations have been reported.

3. Pathology

The Ewing's sarcoma family of tumors consists of classic Ewing's sarcoma (ES) of bone, extraosseous Ewing's sarcoma, and peripheral primitive neuro-ectodermal tumors (PNETs) of bone and soft tissue (including the so-called Askin tumor of the chest wall) [4]. These tumors are grouped together because they share the t(11;22)(q24;q12) chromosomal rearrangement and are widely believed to be of common neural histogenesis [28,29]. In fact, many pathologists and oncologists now view the distinction between ES and PNET as unimportant and consider all ES and PNETs of bone and soft tissues as Ewing tumors with varying degrees of neural differentiation [30]. As a family, Ewing tumors are part of the larger group of small round cell tumors of childhood (SRCTs), which also include rhabdomyosarcoma, neuroblastoma, and non-Hodgkin's lymphoma [28]. Differentiating between these can be difficult because they are of such similar morphology, but the distinction is important, since therapy and prognosis vary depending on subtype. The process of making a definitive diagnosis requires identification of subtle features of differentiation derived from a combination of methods, including light microscopy (LM), electron microscopy (EM), and immunohistochemistry (IC). A summary of the immunohistochemistry of Ewing tumors and other SRCTs is shown in table 1.

Classic Ewing's sarcoma, the most undifferentiated SRCT, is characterized by sheets of homogeneous small round cells with scant cytoplasm, well-defined cellular borders, absence of intercellular material, and relatively few mitotic figures (figure 1) [1,6,28,29,31]. Atypical forms of ES are common and generally demonstrate larger and more pleomorphic cells with slightly more cytoplasm and greater numbers of mitotic figures. Typically, ES shows no evidence of differentiation by LM or EM and, until recently, stained negatively for routinely available immunohistochemical markers. ES cells usually contain cytoplasmic glycogen demonstrated by PAS staining, which can be useful for differentiating ES from an osteosarcoma. However, PAS staining is of no value in differentiating ES from other SRCTs, since they are often PAS positive as well.

Peripheral PNET is a primitive neural tumor that by LM shows some evidence of neural differentiation in the form of pseudorosettes or true rosettes but lacks ganglion cell differentiation and frank neuropil [6,31,32]. Ul-

Table 1. Immunohistochemical characteristics of small round cell tumors of childhood

| Marker | Ewing tumors | | Neuroblastoma | Rhabdomyosarcoma | Lymphoma |
	Es	PNET			
S-100	−	+/−	+	+/−	−
NSE	−	+	+	+/−	−
Desmin	−	−	−	+	−
Actin	−	−	−	+	−
Vimentin	+	+/−	−	+	+/−
LCA	−	−	−	−	+
013/HBA71 (p30/32^{MIC2})	+	+	−	+/−	+/−

Symbols: +, majority of cells show positive staining; −, majority of cells show negative staining; +/−, tumor may show positive or negative staining. Abbreviations: NSE, neuron-specific enolase; LCA, leukocyte common antigen.

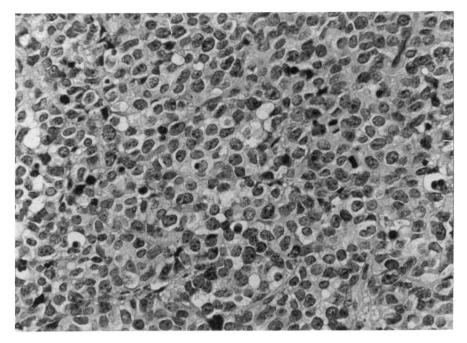

Figure 1. The light microscopy appearance of a Ewing tumor, demonstrating sheets of homogeneous small round cells with relatively scant cytoplasm and no evidence of differentiation. (Courtesy of Deborah Schofield, M.D., Department of Pathology, Children's Hospital, Boston.)

trastructural and immunostaining provide further evidence of neural differentiation, with the presence of neurites and dense core granules by EM and staining with neural immunohistochemical markers, such as S100 and NSE [6,29,32].

In the past, classic ES was often a diagnosis of exclusion, because there was no specific tumor marker available to distinguish ES from other SRCTs. Recently, ES and PNETs have been shown to express large amounts of the cell-surface glycoprotein p30/32^{MIC2}, which is encoded by the *MIC2* gene located on the pseudoautosomal portion of the X and Y chromosome [31]. Several monoclonal antibodies (HBA71, 12E7, and O13) to p30/32^{MIC2} have been developed, and numerous studies demonstrate that they are quite sensitive and reasonably specific for Ewing tumors [31,33,34]. For example, Fellinger and colleagues [34] demonstrated that 61 of 63 Ewing's sarcomas and 9 of 11 peripheral PNETs were positive for HBA71. In a larger study, Perlman et al. found that 221 of 244 (91%) Ewing family tumors stained positively for the monoclonal antibody 12E7 [31]. Unfortunately some cross-reactivity with other neoplasms, such as rhabdomyosarcomas, astrocytomas, Wilms' tumors, and T-cell lymphomas, has been observed [33,34]. Nevertheless, the non-ESFT generally demonstrates a heterogeneous and speckled staining pattern

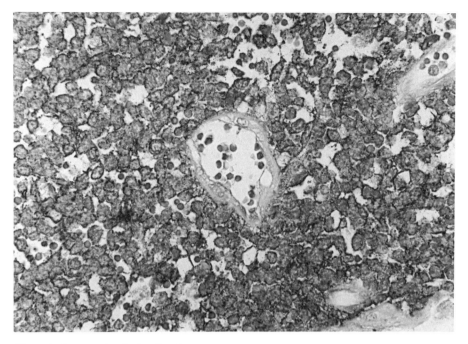

Figure 2. Immunochemical stain of a Ewing tumor with the 013 (HBA71) antibody, which recognizes the cell surface glycoprotein p30/32^{MIC2}. Note the membranous staining pattern characteristic of Ewing tumors. (Courtesy of Deborah Schofield, M.D., Department of Pathology, Children's Hospital, Boston.)

that can often be distinguished from the intense and diffuse membranous staining pattern of ESFT (figure 2) [34].

4. Histogenesis

The histogenesis of Ewing's sarcoma has been a point of debate since the tumor was first described by Dr. James Ewing in 1921 [1]. Ewing speculated that the tumor was of endothelial cell origin; however, today the bulk of ultrastructural, immunohistochemical, genetic, and experimental data suggest a neural origin [29,32]. This hypothesis is supported by several lines of evidence. First, primarily on the basis of the shared t(11;22), ES appears to be closely related to peripheral PNET, a tumor with clear ultrastructural and immunohistochemical evidence of neural differentiation [35]. Second, ES and PNET demonstrate similar patterns and levels of oncogene expression [36]. Third, a small fraction of ES (atypical ES) tumors and cell lines stain with neural markers such as S100 or NSE, and ultrastructural data have shown that rare ES tumors contain neurosecretory granules [32,36,37]. Finally, there are

257

limited experimental data demonstrating that treatment of certain ES cells lines with differentiating agents such as cAMP or retinoic acid can induce morphologic and immunohistochemical evidence of neuronal differentiation [38]. Thus, the prevailing hypothesis is that the ES family of tumors originate from a common neural precursor cell but show varying degrees of neural differentiation. In such a paradigm, ES would be considered the most undifferentiated member of the family, with atypical forms of ES being somewhat intermediate and peripheral PNET furthermost down the neural differentiation pathway [28,29].

5. Tumor genetics

The (11;22)(q24;q12) chromosomal translocation, first described in the early 1980s, is present in 85%–95% of Ewing tumors [39–43]. At the cytogenetic level, this chromosomal marker is so specific that it is often used to distinguish Ewing tumors from other SRCTs [44,45]. The DNA containing the t(11;22)(q24;q12) breakpoint has been cloned and found to involve *EWS*, a novel gene on chromosome 22, and *FLI*, the human homologue of the mouse Fli-1 gene on chromosome 11 and member of the Ets family of DNA transcription factors [46]. Transcription across the breakpoint on the derivative 22 chromosome produces a hybrid mRNA consisting of the 5′ half of *EWS* fused to the 3′ half of *FLI* (*EWS/FLI*) (figure 3) [47]. There is no evidence of transcription from the derivative 11 chromosome.

The genomic structure of *EWS* on chromosome 22 consists of 17 exons distributed over 40kb, while *FLI* is encoded by nine exons over 100kb on chromosome 11 [48,49]. Restriction enzyme mapping and reverse-transcriptase PCR studies of numerous tumors demonstrate that all breakpoints occur within introns, and transcription of mRNA across these breakpoints results in fusion of intact and in-frame exons [45,48,50]. Zucman and colleagues analyzed 54 Ewing tumors and found that the most common fusions were between exon 7 of *EWS* and either exons 6 (27 of 54) or 5 (11 of 54) of *FLI* [48]. These hybrid RNAs correspond to breakpoints within intron 7 (between exon 7 and 8) of *EWS* and either intron 5 or 4 of *FLI* (figure 3) [45,48]. *EWS* exon 7/*FLI* exon 6 and *EWS* exon 7/*FLI* exon 5 correspond to the type 1 and type 2 fusion transcripts, respectively [45,47,50,51] The type 1 rearrangement accounts for 55%–60% of cases, while type 2 occurs in approximately 25% of cases. The remaining 15%–20% of tumors have more complex and variable rearrangements; however, in all rearrangements described thus far, DNA from at least the first seven exons of *EWS* and exons 8 and 9 of *FLI* are included [45,48].

In the process of cloning the t(11;22), it was observed that some Ewing tumors demonstrated rearrangements of *EWS*, but not *FLI*. Zucman et al. showed that these tumors contain a t(21;22) involving *EWS* and *ERG*, another Ets transcription factor and closely related to *FLI*, located on chromosome 21

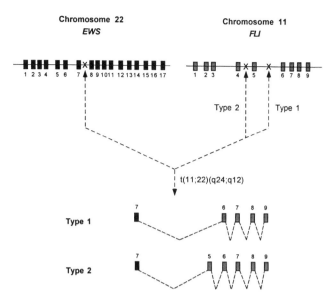

Figure 3. A schematic representation of the two most common t(11;22)(q24:q12) rearrangements in Ewing tumors. The type 1 rearrangement breaks intron 7 of *EWS* and intron 5 of *FLI*, resulting in fusion of *EWS* exons 1–7 to *FLI* exons 6–9. The type 2 rearrangement breaks *EWS* intron 7 and intron 5 of *FLI*, resulting in the fusion of *EWS* exons 1–7 to *FLI* exons 5–9. The type 1 fusion occurs in 55%–60% of cases and the type 2 in approximately 25% of cases. The remaining 15%–25% of cases have rearrangements that are more complex and variable; however, all fusions include at least exons 1–7 of *EWS* and at least exons 8–9 of *FLI*.

Table 2. Tumors associated with rearrangement of *EWS*

Tumor	Translocation	Fusion gene	References
ESFT	t(11;2)(q24;q12)	*EWS/FL1*	[46–47]
	t(21;22)(q22;q12)	*EWS/ERG*	[48]
	t(7;22)(p22;q12)	*EWS/ETV-1*	[52]
		EWS/E1A-F	[53]
Desmoplastic small round cell tumor (DSRCT)	t(11;22)(p13;q12)	*EWS/WT1*	[55–56]
Malignant melanoma of soft parts	t(12;22)(q13;q12)	*EWS/ATF-1*	[196]
Mixoid chondrosarcoma	t(9;22)(q22–31;q12)	*EWS/CHN*	[60]
Mixoid liposarcoma	t(12;22)(q13;q12)	*EWS/CHOP*	[61]

[48]. As many as 5%–10% of Ewing tumors appear to contain this alternate translocation, which produces an *EWS/ERG* fusion mRNA [45,50,51].

There are several single case reports of other rearrangements involving *EWS* in Ewing tumors (table 2). Jeon et al. described a case of ES with a t(7;22)(p22;q12) that results in the fusion of exons 1–7 of *EWS* to another Ets family member called *ETV1* (*E*TS *T*ranslocation *V*ariant) [52]. In another

259

report, an extraosseous ES was found to fuse *EWS* (again exons 1–7) with the 3' end of *E1A-F*. This gene encodes the adenovirus E1A enhancer binding protein, which contains an Ets DNA binding domain, again similar to *FLI1*, *ERG*, and *ETV1* [53]. Thus, in all *EWS* rearrangements in Ewing tumors described thus far, a hybrid RNA is produced that fuses at least exons 1–7 of *EWS* to the 3' half of an Ets transcription factor.

Additional chromosomal rearrangements not involving the *EWS* locus on chromosome 22 have also been reported. A t(1;16)(q21;q13) has been reported to occur together with the t(11;22) in a substantial fraction of tumors [54]. This translocation breakpoint has not yet been cloned.

6. EWS: other genes and other tumors

Translocations involving *EWS* are known to occur in several other tumor types outside the Ewing family of tumors. These include malignant melanoma of soft parts, myxoid chondrosarcomas, myxoid liposarcoma, and desmoplastic small round cell tumors. The cytogenetic abnormalities and the genes involved are listed in table 2. In each case, the first seven exons of *EWS* are fused to genes whose protein products are putative transcription factors. Perhaps the most interesting of these occurs in desmoplastic small round cell tumors in which the t(11;22)(p13;q12) results in the fusion of exon 7 of *EWS* with exon 8 of *WT1* [55,56]. *WT1* is a putative tumor suppressor gene mutated in a subset of Wilms' tumors. This tumor represents the only example of a translocation involving *WT1* and ultimately could have important implications regarding the role of *WT1* in tumorgenesis.

7. Biological consequences of the t(11;22)

7.1. Normal EWS and FLI

EWS is an ubiquitously expressed gene that encodes a novel protein of 656 amino acids [47]. In the amino terminal half of the protein, there is a region that shares partial homology (40%) with the large subunit of eukaryotic RNA polymerase II. The carboxy terminal half contains sequences homologous to the RNA binding domain of several proteins (figure 4). Recently, a *Drosophila* homologue of *EWS* has been cloned and termed SARFH (sarcoma-associated RNA-binding fly homologue) [57]. SARFH is expressed in the fly embryo at the earliest stages of development and in a variety of adult cell types. Antibody studies indicate that SARFH colocalizes with RNA polymerase II, implying that SARFH — and by homology, *EWS* — participate in functions common to the expression of many or most genes transcribed by RNA polymerase II. Recall that RNA polymerase II is responsible for transcription of almost all eukaryotic genes.

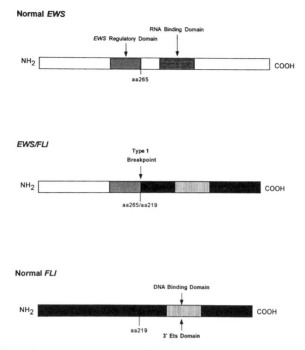

Normal *EWS*

RNA Binding Domain

EWS Regulatory Domain

NH₂ ☐ COOH

aa265

EWS/FLI

Type 1
Breakpoint

NH₂ ☐ COOH

aa265/aa219

Normal *FLI*

DNA Binding Domain

NH₂ ☐ COOH

aa219

3' Ets Domain

Figure 4. A schematic representation of the protein structure of normal or wild-type *EWS*, *FLI*, and *EWS/FLI*. *EWS* has a regulatory domain within the amino-terminal half of the protein that is being conserved in all *EWS/FLI* rearrangements. Normal *FLI* has an Ets DNA binding domain in its carboxy-terminal half that is required for transcriptional activation. *EWS/FLI* results in the replacement of the RNA binding domain of *EWS* with the DNA binding domain of *FLI*. In the type 1 rearrangement depicted here, the breakpoint occurs at amino acid 265 of *EWS* and 219 of *FLI*. This rearrangement places the *FLI DNA* binding domain under the control of the *EWS* regulatory domain.

Much more is known about *FLI* than *EWS*. *FLI* expression is somewhat more selective than *EWS*, although it is highly expressed in many adult tissues, including thymus, muscle, heart, spleen, and bone marrow [58]. *FLI* is a member of the Ets family of transcription factors, and its protein product presumably functions to regulate the expression of specific, but as yet unknown, target genes [59]. Mouse Fli-1 is involved in the induction of erythroleukemia by the Friend murine leukemia virus (F-MuLV) and serves as the integration site for F-MuLV. The apparent effect of proviral DNA integration is overexpression of normal Fli-1, rather than a rearrangement of fusion of F-MuLV with Fli-1 [60,61].

7.2. Ets family of transcription factors

The Ets family of transcription factors consists of over 30 related proteins that have been implicated in gene-specific transcriptional activation, in DNA rep-

261

lication, and more generally as participating in the general transcriptional activation complex [59]. These proteins have been shown to play an important role in a variety of cellular activities, such as developmental programs, growth control, and transformation [59]. All members of the family share common domains, termed *Ets domains*, usually located in the C-terminal region of the protein (figure 4) [59]. It is via these Ets domains that DNA binding occurs. These proteins bind specifically to promoter elements over a 10-base-pair region of DNA with a core GGA trinucleotide sequence, termed an *Ets box*. Subtle differences in flanking sequences on either side of the core sequence define an Ets box and determine which Ets protein binds to a specific promoter site.

The Ets family can be divided into five subfamilies based on similarities at the Ets domains, the position of the Ets domain within the protein, and other sequence/structural similarities. Both *FLI* and *ERG* are members of the same Ets subfamily, while *ETV1* and *E1A-F* are members of different Ets subfamilies. All are potent transcriptional activators, although the specific genes on which they act are unknown. While DNA binding is mediated through the Ets domain in the carboxy-terminal half of the *FLI* or *ERG* protein, there also is an important regulatory or modulatory domain in the amino-terminal half of the protein [62,63]. Evidence in several experimental systems suggests that most Ets proteins cooperate with other nuclear proteins and function as a part of larger protein complexes to regulate transcriptional activation. These interactions occur primarily via the amino-terminal region of the protein.

7.3. EWS/FLI hybrid

The *EWS/FLI* fusion results in the substitution of the 3' or carboxy terminal (CTD) half of *EWS* with the 3' or CTD half of *FLI* (figure 4) [47]. The effect is replacement of the RNA binding domain of *EWS* with the Ets DNA binding domain of *FLI*. Alternatively, from the perspective of the *FLI*, the result is the removal of the amino transcriptional activation and regulatory domain of *FLI* and replacement by the amino terminal half of *EWS*. This rearrangement also places the fusion gene under the transcriptional control of the ubiquitously expressed *EWS* promoter.

In the past three years, tremendous progress has been made in the understanding of the biological consequences of the t(11;22) and the *EWS/FLI* fusion gene. Several groups have shown that *EWS/FLI* mRNA is translated into a protein of approximately 68 kDa, and that this protein, like wild-type *FLI*, localizes to the nucleus [64–66]. May et al. showed that *EWS/FLI* is a potent transforming gene in NIH 3T3 cells, while *FLI* alone is not [66]. By creating large deletions in either the *EWS* or the *FLI* half of *EWS/FLI*, these authors further demonstrated that both *EWS* and *FLI* sequences are necessary for this transformation activity. These data indicate that the transforming potential of *EWS/FLI* is dependent on the presence of both *EWS* and *FLI*, and not merely due to overexpression of *FLI* under transcriptional control of the *EWS* promoter.

7.4. EWS/FLI chimeric protein

The *EWS/FLI* chimeric protein binds to DNA in a sequence-specific manner identical to wild-type *FLI*, and the 3′ Ets domain of *FLI* is necessary and sufficient for this activity [64,65,67]. In several different in vitro systems, both wild-type *FLI* and *EWS/FLI* function as sequence-specific transcriptional activators; however, *EWS/FLI* is much more potent. This transcriptional activation activity is dependent not only on DNA binding through the Ets domain of *FLI* but also on the *EWS* portion of the protein [64,65,67,68]. Deletion analysis has demonstrated that the region of *EWS* most important to its transcriptional activation activity lies within amino acids 210–265 (figure 4). In fact, it is possible to delete all of *EWS* up to amino acid 210 and still maintain this activity [65]. This region of the protein (aa210–265) is encoded by exon 7 and, as noted previously, is conserved in all *EWS* rearrangements described to date.

There are conflicting data as to whether amino acids 210–265 of *EWS* constitute a true transcriptional activation domain or whether they represent a regulatory or modulatory domain [64,65,68]. Structurally, this region is very proline and glutamine rich, and the predicted protein structure yields a turn-loop-turn/sheet-loop-sheet structure that has been seen in other transcriptional activation domains [65]. Based on these structural predictions, this region is probably involved in protein–protein interactions that modulate the transcriptional activation activity of *EWS/FLI*.

7.5. Altered transcriptional control

With the above experimental and structural data in mind, one could hypothesize that *EWS/FLI* transforms cells by altering normal transcriptional controls. Additional supporting data for this hypothesis comes from in vitro experiments comparing the ability of wild-type *FLI* and *EWS/FLI* to bind to the serum responsive element (SRE) within the *c-fos* promoter [69]. To activate the target gene in this system, wild-type *FLI* must form complexes with a second protein, serum response factor (SRF), via its amino-terminal transcriptional activation domain. Once the complex is formed, binding to the SRE within the target gene promoter occurs. *EWS/FLI* is capable of autonomously binding to DNA and initiating transcription in the absence of SRF, thus bypassing the regulatory control of this protein. Deletion of the amino-terminal half of *FLI* results in similar autonomous DNA binding, implying that an amino-terminal regulatory domain is present in wild-type *FLI* that is fundamentally altered in the *EWS/FLI* chimeric protein. These data, coupled with the observation that *EWS/FLI* is a more potent transcriptional activator than wild-type *FLI*, suggest that *EWS/FLI* may not be as limited or constrained as *FLI* [69,70]. Wild-type *FLI* may be limited to simulating only those genes with the correct Ets binding site in its promoter and in an environment that contains appropriate cofactors. On the other hand, *EWS/FLI* appears capable of activating transcription of target genes in the absence of these cofactors; thus subverting normal transcriptional controls to activate transforming genes that wild-type *FLI* cannot [70].

The genes on which *EWS/FLI* acts, the signal transduction pathways in which it induces transformation, and the proteins that regulate or fail to regulate its activity remain unknown. The only clues thus far come from Braun et al., who showed by representational difference analysis that transformation by *EWS/FLI* in NIH 3T3 cells induces expression of transformation-associated genes such as stromelysin 1 and cytokeratin 15 [71]. The significance of this finding is as yet unknown. Identification of target genes and proteins that regulate *EWS/FLI* is an area of active investigation.

8. Clinical significance

In addition to fascinating and profound biological effects, *EWS/FLI* and *EWS/ERG* provide important nucleic acid tumor markers that can be used clinically for a variety of purposes. From tumor to tumor, the t(11;22) breakpoints occur over a very broad range of genomic DNA, making detection by conventional PCR impractical. However, the *EWS/FLI* fusion RNA is easily detectable by reverse-transcriptase PCR (RT-PCR) using a single set of oligonucleotide primers. *EWS/ERG* is detectable in a similar fashion.

A PCR-based assay has many important potential applications. It has obvious diagnostic utility, especially since SRCTs can be so difficult to classify — so much so that Delattre et al. have suggested that RT-PCR evidence of *EWS/FLI* RNA be used as the primary criterion for distinguishing Ewing tumors from other SRCTs [45]. Other groups have investigated whether particular types of *EWS/FLI* fusion transcripts in a given tumor correlate with clinical parameters and/or prognosis. In a large European multicenter trial, Zoubek et al. compared the expression of different fusion transcripts to patient age, sex, primary tumor location tumor volume, and disease extension [50]. They found no significant correlation between various fusion types and these features; however, there was a suggestion that relapse-free survival for patients with localized disease tended to be longer for those with the type I fusion transcript.

The power of RT-PCR to detect as few as one tumor cell in 10^6 normal cells has obvious application in the detection and monitoring of submicroscopic disease or minimal residual disease. Our early data in the Pediatric Oncology Group, along with data from several other groups, demonstrate that it is possible to detect evidence of circulating tumor cells in the bone marrow and peripheral blood of approximately 25% of patients with nonmetastatic and 50% of patients with metastatic Ewing tumors [72,73]. One could hypothesize that this finding may be of prognostic importance in that it may be an indication of tumor burden, significant occult metastatic disease, or perhaps a reflection of particularly malignant tumor phenotype. In any case, if true, it might allow one to identify a group of poor-prognosis patients who might benefit from more intensive therapy. Alternatively, one might be able to identify a group of patients with an especially good prognosis who could be spared excessive treatment. We are currently conducting a prospective trial within the Pediatric Oncology Group, as are several groups in Europe, to test this hypothesis.

Finally, early data suggesting that Ewing tumors may provide an excellent target for gene therapy. Ouchida et al. created stable transfections with antisense *EWS/FLI* or antisense *EWS/ERG* in Ewing cell lines [74]. Expression of antisense *EWS/FLI* or *EWS/ERG* resulted in the loss of endogenous *EWS/FLI* and *EWS/ERG* protein and tumorigenicity in nude mice. Thus, perhaps Ewing tumors will become potential targets for antisense therapy in the future.

9. Extent of disease and sites at presentation

Among 530 patients with PNET or ES of bone registered on the CCG–POG intergroup Ewing's sarcoma study performed between 1988 and 1992, 76% were localized at diagnosis and 24% were metastatic. The most common primary sites, in order of occurrence, were pelvis (27%), femur (17%), rib (12%), humerus (7%), and vertebrae and fibula (5% each) [8]. Data regarding soft tissue ES and PNET are more difficult to ascertain. Among the ESFT tumors reviewed by Horowitz and colleagues [6], only 5% were defined as PNET of bone or soft tissue. Three quarters of those defined as PNET arose in the central axis; half arose in the chest or chest wall.

The distinction between extraosseous Ewing (EOE) tumors and a primary bone tumor is not always clear: soft tissue extension is exceedingly common in Ewing tumors of bone, and soft tissue tumors may invade adjacent bone. For example, in the chest wall tumors, the rib is often involved and may be the primary site or not. It is not known if bone primaries and soft tissue primaries differ in natural history and/or response to therapy. The ongoing CCG–POG intergroup study, which includes both soft tissue and apparent bone primaries, may clarify this question.

10. Clinical presentation

Almost all patients with ESFT with bone primaries report pain on presentation, more than half of patients will have a palpable mass, and about a fifth will present with fever [75]. Among patients with extraosseous tumors, a mass is more often the presenting symptom, but pain is still reported in the majority of patients. In a Mayo clinic series, 16% of patients with extremity bone tumors presented with a pathologic fracture [75]. The pain of Ewing's sarcoma may be intermittent, and a significant delay from the onset of symptoms and diagnosis is not uncommon, particularly among patients with pelvic tumors. Many patients report symptoms beginning greater than three months before diagnosis [76]. Fever, fatigue, and generalized malaise are not uncommon presenting complaints.

Given the wide range of possible primary sites of this tumor, more specific presenting complaints vary widely. However, some typical patterns of presentation are worth noting. Patients with pelvic tumors often have a prolonged history of hip or back pain, progressing to extremity weakness and/or peripheral nerve involvement, such as a sciatica-like syndrome. Back pain may be a harbinger of spinal cord compression in patients with vertebral or paraspinal tumors, and such patients require urgent investigation and initiation of treatment to prevent neurologic compromise [77]. Patients with rib or chest wall tumors may present with chest wall pain and with respiratory symptoms due to mass and/or to pleural effusion. Effusions may be sympathetic or malignant; when the fluid is examined histologically, close to half the patients will show malignant cells [78,79]. Most investigators consider ipsilateral pleural effusion to be regional rather than metastatic disease.

The most common sites of distant spread are the lungs, bone, and bone marrow. In the 1988–1992 CCG–POG intergroup study of ES and PNET of bone, among those with metastatic disease at diagnosis, the most common site was lung, followed by bone and bone marrow [7,8]. In the long-term follow-up of the first Intergroup Ewing's Sarcoma Study (IESS) for patients nonmetastatic at diagnosis, the first site of relapse was lung in 34% of patients, bone in 33%, and more than one site in 27% (most often bone and lung). Other, less common sites of first relapse were bone marrow, lymph node, soft tissue, brain, and spinal cord [76]. Among sites of bone metastasis, vertebral metastases appear to be common [76]. Liver metastases are uncommon, and isolated central nervous system metastases are rare [76,80]. Recent studies evaluating blood and bone marrow specimens for molecular evidence of micrometastases has proven that tumor cells may be found in blood or marrow in patients in whom metastasis is not clinically evident [72,73].

11. Prognostic features

Among patients with nonmetastatic disease, the primary site is an important risk factor: patients with pelvic tumors have the worst prognosis, and those with rib or distal primaries enjoy the best outlook [76,81]. In general, patients with larger tumors have a less sanguine prognosis [82,83]. An elevated lactate dehydrogenase, probably as evidence of a higher tumor burden, has been reported as a high-risk feature, as have elevated erythrocyte sedimentation rates [83–85]. It is interesting to note that in the German Cooperative Ewing's Sarcoma Study (CESS) series, tumors with greater than 100 mL volume had a significantly worse outlook in the 1981 trial, but this difference was no longer significant in the CESS 1986 trial, demonstrating that sufficient therapy can obviate some 'poor-prognosis' characteristics [86]. The absence of extraosseous extension in bone tumor primaries is considered to be a favorable sign [87]. The extent of neural differentiation has been thought to confer poor prognosis in some analyses [88,89]; however, in a large retrospective analysis of 315 patients from France, Spain, and the United States, neuroectodermal features were not associated with a poor prognosis, but 'filigree pattern and dark cells' were associated with a poorer outlook [90]. The confirmation of these findings in a large prospective series would be enlightening. Oberlin and others have reported that good histopathologic response to chemotherapy is correlated to survival [91]. Picci and colleagues report similar findings. They found statistically significant differences in five-year disease-free survival (DFS) in nonmetastatic extremity patients correlated with histologic response — 90% five-year DFS in patients with no visible tumor apparent in surgical specimens resected after chemotherapy, compared to 53% for those with microscopic nodules and 32% for those with macroscopic nodules remaining [92]. Most studies have demonstrated that older patients fare less well; the CCG–POG intergroup study (1988–1992) demonstrated a distinct advantage for nonmetastatic patients less than nine years of age when compared to the older patients treated in that trial [7,8].

Metastatic disease at diagnosis confers a poor prognosis. Long-term follow-up of patients treated from 1968 to 1980 documented two survivors among 27 patients metastatic at diagnosis [93]. The 1988–1992 POG–CCG study demonstrated a less than 20% four-year survival for patients with metastases at diagnosis, and patients with bone metastases at diagnosis did significantly worse than those with metastases restricted to the lung [7,8].

12. Diagnosis

When signs and symptoms suggest the possibility of Ewing's sarcoma, the first step towards diagnosis is appropriate imaging of the primary site. For tumors of long bones, a destructive lesion of the diaphysis is most common. Cortical bone changes and an accompanying soft tissue mass are common. Periosteal reaction, either 'onion-peel' lamellar changes or elevation of the periosteum (called *Codman's triangle*), is the most common feature noted [94]. In flat bones, a sclerotic appearance may be seen [94]. These features, however, are not pathognomonic: other possibilities in the differential diagnosis are benign lesions such as eosinophilic granuloma and osteomyelitis, which radiographically may mimic changes seen in ES. Other malignant lesions such as osteosarcoma, neuroblastoma (particularly in younger children), primary lymphoma of bone, and other sarcomas of bone should be considered. Computed tomography (CT) scans with contrast define the primary site well, particularly the extent of bone disease [95]. Magnetic resonance imaging

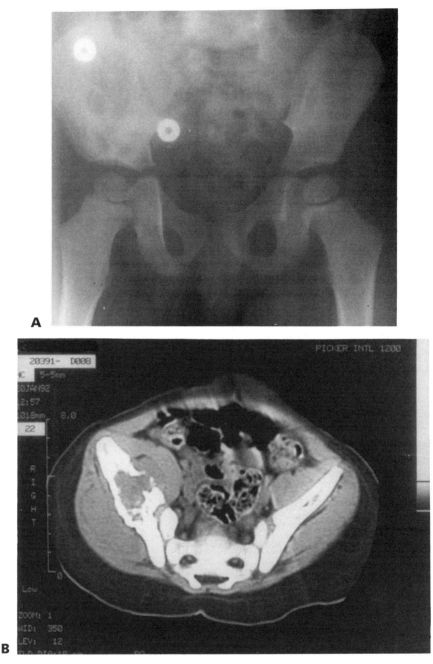

Figure 5. PNET of the ilium in a 2-year-old child before therapy and after chemotherapy and surgery. (**A**) Radiograph of the pelvis at diagnosis. Note osteolytic and blastic changes in the right ilium, with a soft tissue mass protruding into the pelvis. (**B**) Magnetic resonance imaging of the pelvis at diagnosis. Note large soft tissue mass surrounding the right iliac wing, with erosion of the right iliac crest.

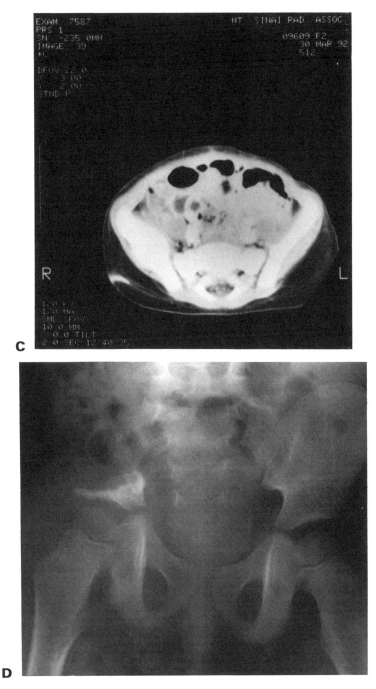

Figure 5. (**C**) Magnetic resonance imaging after chemotherapy, before resection. (**D**) Radiograph of the pelvis after chemotherapy and surgery. Right ilium has been excised except for a small rim of acetabulum holding femoral head in place.

The patient is now 6 years old, has no evidence of recurrence, and walks with a mild limp. These images were originally reproduced in Med Pediatr Oncol 21:297–294, 1993.

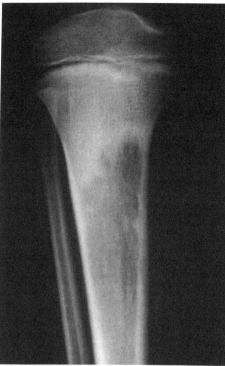

A

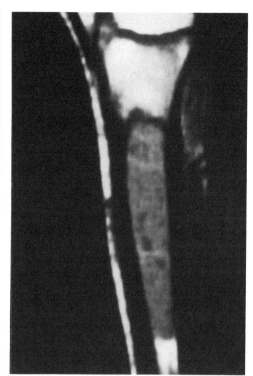

B

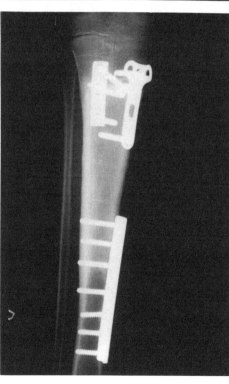

C

Figure 6. (**A**) Radiograph of ES of the proximal tibia in a 6-year-old. Note lytic changes and minimal periosteal reaction. (**B**) Magnetic resonance image of the same tumor. Note demarcation of involved bone and marrow. (**C**) Radiograph of the tibia after completion of chemotherapy and limb-sparing procedure.

The child is now 11 years old, has no evidence of recurrence, and enjoys full activity. Courtesy of Samuel Kenan, M.D. (Hospital for Joint Diseases, New York), and Karen Norton, M.D., Department of Radiology, Mount Sinai Medical Center, New York.

(MRI) is generally thought to best delineate the extent of soft tissue and marrow disease (figures 5 and 6) [96]. Technetium bone scans of the whole body will help define the primary as well as start the metastatic evaluation. Ewing family tumors are generally thallium and gallium avid; although such studies may be helpful in discerning response to therapy, they are not specific enough to be useful in differential diagnosis [97,98].

On the basis of clinical presentation and radiographs alone, there is no absolute way to distinguish among the diagnostic possibilities. Additional studies to help refine the diagnostic possibilities include a urine for VMA or HVA, which, if positive, indicates neuroblastoma. A complete blood count demonstrating blasts would be consistent with leukemia or lymphoma. If there is a clinical suspicion of neuroblastoma or lymphoma, bone marrow biopsy and aspirate may be diagnostic, sparing the patient a more invasive biopsy of the primary. If the marrow is overtly positive for cells suggestive of an ESFT, the diagnosis may be established employing cytogenetics. There are no standard examinations of the blood that are specific for ES. Commonly encountered nonspecific findings include an elevated sedimentation rate, anemia, and an elevated lactate dehydrogenase [84,85].

After the initial laboratory and imaging evaluation is complete, the diagnosis must be made by biopsy. There is no proven advantage to excisional biopsy or an attempt at complete resection at the time of diagnosis; in fact, such attempts may be counterproductive. After induction chemotherapy, surgical procedures are likely to be less morbid than attempts at complete resection at the time of diagnosis. Further, postchemotherapy surgery yields valuable information regarding the response to chemotherapy, as well as a clear sense of the need for radiation based on the assessment of surgical margins. An attempt at complete resection of chest wall tumors at the time of diagnosis may actually complicate later attempts at local control considerably [99,100]. In the past, open biopsy has been the preferred procedure so that sufficient material can be obtained for a full battery of studies, including light microscopy, electron microscopy, and chromosome and molecular studies. However, fine-needle aspiration may be sufficient for evaluation in selected cases since the advent of PCR-based molecular techniques [101]. The biopsy must be done in an institution equipped to process the material appropriately. Frozen section of the material obtained should be examined to be certain that the tissue obtained is sufficient for diagnosis because spontaneous necrosis is a near constant feature of ESFT.

Ideally, the surgeon who does the biopsy will also perform later definitive resection. At the very least, the biopsy should be performed by a surgeon familiar with both the principles of cancer surgery and reconstructive techniques so that the biopsy does not limit reconstructive options for the patient should surgery be chosen as the method of local control. Biopsy of the extraosseous extension of primary bone tumors is generally recommended to lessen the risk of subsequent pathologic fracture at the site of a bone biopsy, particularly in a weight-bearing bone. It is critical that the biopsy be performed to avoid contamination of surrounding tissue, and in a site and place that can be excised at the time of definitive local control surgery.

The surgical team planning a biopsy should keep in mind all the needs of the patient: if a malignant tumor is suspected, the family and patient should be prepared for this possibility. Consultation with the oncology team early will facilitate appropriate handling of all tissue samples. Moreover, if the patient requires general anesthesia, consideration should be given to the option of having the oncologist obtain marrow specimens for the metastatic evaluation at the same time as the biopsy procedure. Further, consideration should be given to the placing of central venous access; although it is virtually impossible to know the definitive diagnosis in the operating theater, a presumptive diagnosis of malignancy is often clear, which makes appropriate the placement of catheters and obtaining marrow under the same anesthetic.

Once the diagnosis of an ESFT is definite, a more specifically directed evaluation of the patient should ensure rapidly. The first element of the evaluation is a more careful definition of the extent of the disease. There is no uniformly accepted staging system for Ewing's sarcoma; patients are generally classified as nonmetastatic or metastatic. Many treatment programs also stratify tumors by site, such as pelvic versus nonpelvic. The primary site should be evaluated by MRI, if this had not been done prior to biopsy, and this evaluation should include specific measurements of the tumor and tumor involvement of the marrow so that this information can be used to guide local control therapy.

A complete metastatic evaluation must be undertaken. Computed tomography of the chest with contrast should be done to search for pulmonary or mediastinal disease. A technetium bone scan should be done to search for sites of bone metastases. Recently, total body MRI has been reported to yield information on bone metastases not seen on standard technetium scans; however, the clinical impact of such a costly and intensive evaluation is not known at this time [102]. The bone marrow aspirate and biopsy must be examined: most studies require a single site of aspirate, but there are data demonstrating that sampling of multiple sites increases yield [103]. If the patient presented with neurologic symptoms referable to the spinal cord, metrizimide MRI of the spine or myelogram should be performed urgently. If there is metastatic disease in the lungs, or clinical suspicion of CNS disease, a computed tomogram of the brain should be considered. Ewing tumors accumulates both gallium and thallium; thallium in particular has been recommended to assess chemotherapy response [98]. Several reports suggest that MRI scanning is useful for monitoring response to chemotherapy [104–106]. In a small number of patients, positron emission tomography has been shown to correlate with histological response to chemotherapy and may become a useful modality of evaluation of chemotherapy response [107].

Other elements of the initial evaluation are directed toward gathering information that will allow the clinician to start treatment with minimal delay. Physiologic assessment of the patient prior to chemotherapy must include evaluation of liver function, renal function (serum creatinine and, if abnormal, creatinine clearance), and cardiac function (electrocardiogram and echocardiogram or radionuclide cardiac scan). The radiation therapist, surgeons, and rehabilitation specialists should meet with the patient and family as early as possible in the course of treatment to plan therapy for local control. A multidisciplinary evaluation of the patient's and family's emotional and social needs are essential to planning appropriate care. It is also essential to understand that the impact of intensive combined modality therapy upon family functioning is enormous; without family cooperation, compliance with the treatment regimen is more likely to be compromised, perhaps compromising the outlook for the patient.

13. Treatment principles

The obvious goal of treatment is to cure the patient; the unstated aim is to do so while minimizing the negative late effects and maximally preserving function. In order to amplify possibilities for the patient, it is critical that each patient's care is directed by a team of pediatric or medical oncologists working with surgeons and radiation oncologists who are familiar with the disease and its treatment. This therapeutic term must work in concert with support staff, including experienced nurses, social workers and psychologists, and physical rehabilitation staff, so that the patient is offered a full range of medical, psychosocial, and rehabilitation services. State-of-the-art therapy should be offered: given the rarity of ESFT, participation in the most current clinical research trial available is ideal.

In order to effect cure of a Ewing family tumor, attention must be given to both systemic and local control. Initiation of chemotherapy after diagnosis begins the local control by reducing tumor size and initiates the eradication of overt or micrometastatic disease. After induction chemotherapy, local control is planned and performed; thereafter, chemotherapy continues. Discussion of chemotherapy regimens employed for ES and PNET of bone is followed by a discussion of local control regimens.

14. Chemotherapy of Ewing's sarcoma and peripheral primitive neuroectodermal tumors

The survival of patients with ES of bone was dismal when treatment consisted only of local measures: less than 10% survived [108]. Single-agent studies performed in the 1960s demonstrated that cyclophosphamide, vincristine, and actinomycin-D were effective agents against ES (table 3). A 1967 report of 54 patients treated with radiation to the entire bone cited a 24% five-year survival; however, it was noted that 4 of the 13 survivors also received chemotherapy with either nitrogen mustard and/or actinomycin-D [109]. Other

Chemotherapy [Refs]	# patients	% CR + PR	Comments
Cyclophosphamide [113–119]	36	47%	
Doxorubicin [197–203]	60	42%	
5-fluorouracil [131,204]	10	40%	
Vincristine [119,124–126]	10	40%	
BCNU [119,205]	18	33%	
Ifosfamide [120–123]	60	32%	
Etoposide [127,128]	10	30%	
Actinomycin-D [117,129,130]	16	19%	
Cisplatin [206,207]	27	7%	
Ifosfamide/etoposide [161,162]	92	42%	ES and PNET/VACD pretreated patients
Ifosfamide/etoposide [208]	26	96%	Upfront window in chemotherapy naive patients
Ifosfamide/etoposide/cisplatin [209]	2	100%	Pretreated VACD, VACD +/−IE

Abbreviations: CR, complete response; PR, partial response; ES, Ewing's sarcoma; PNET, primitive neuroectodermal tumor; VACD, vincristine, actinomycin-D, cyclophosphamide, doxorubicin; IE, ifosfamide, etoposide.

reports of chemotherapy activity against ES ushered in an era of prospective trials of combined modality therapy; survivals of more than two years were demonstrated [110–112]. Some of the successes of the relatively early trials ultimately proved to be enduring; for example, the National Cancer Institute (NCI) trial initiated in 1968 resulted in a 33% 15-year survival rate [93]. These early trials engendered several prospective clinical trials designed to develop regimens that would increase long-term survivorship.

Table 3 lists agents with activity against Ewing's sarcoma. The agents shown to be most active include the classical alkylating agents, cyclophosphamide and ifosfamide [113–119,120–123]. High-dose melphalan was also shown to be highly active, but primarily in doses better suited to marrow ablation programs [210,212]. Vincristine [119,124–126] and etoposide [127,128] each show good single-agent activity. Actinomycin-D showed relatively lower response rates [117,129,130] but was one the earliest agents associated with survivorship and was thus integrated into all the early multiple agent trials. BCNU yielded good response rates [119,205] but is associated with relatively prolonged myelosuppression, making its integration into multiple agent trials of newly diagnosed patients difficult; it has been successfully employed in programs for relapsed or very-high-risk patients, in combination with marrow rescue. Cisplatin showed little activity compared to the other agents, but it should be noted that the earlier phase II trials most likely included patients less intensively treated prior to the investigation of the new agent. Although 5-fluorouracil yielded a response rate of 40%, when added to a regimen for metastatic patients there was no evidence of increased efficacy [132], so it has not been incorporated into current regimens.

15. Multiagent multimodality trials for localized Ewing's sarcoma

Table 4 summarizes the major multimodality, multiagent chemotherapy trials for the treatment of Ewing's sarcoma. These trials, unless otherwise noted, were open only to ES of bone. However, it should be noted that evidence of neural differentiation was not uniformly sought on most trials; thus, unless PNET was specifically excluded, it is likely that the trials included some PNET of bone patients as well. The NCI trial initiated in 1968 demonstrated a 33% long-term survival [133], but it must be noted that the chemotherapy doses employed were modest by today's standards. In 1973, the first Intergroup Ewing's Sarcoma Study (IESS) opened. Patients eligible for study had localized bone primaries; patients with amputation prior to study entry were excluded from randomization. The trial opened with the concept that one third of the patients would be randomized not to receive initial adjuvant chemotherapy, but after two of the first three patients so enrolled relapsed, the trial was refigured so that all patients received one of three regimens: vincristine, actinomycin-D, and cyclophosphamide (VAC), or VAC + bilateral prophylactic pulmonary radiation, or VAC + doxorubicin (VACD) [76]. The five-year relapse-free survival (RFS) rates reported in 1990 were 24%, 44%, and 60%, respectively; thus, the regimen of VAC with doxorubicin was found to be significantly better than either of the other regimens [76] (figure 7). Patients with pelvic primaries treated on this study fared worse than those with nonpelvic primaries — so much so that the difference among the three regimens could not be demonstrated in this subset. Looking at all three regimens together, 44% of patients developed metastases (51% of these were bone and pulmonary), and 15% are reported to have suffered local recurrence (10% were combined with metastatic disease). Interestingly, the patients who underwent pulmonary radiation did not have an incidence of pulmonary metastases significantly different from patients on the alternate regimens. Other information gleaned from this study was confirmation of the poorer prognosis in pelvic patients and that patients younger than age 10 fared best [76].

The second IESS study opened in 1978 and compared high-dose intermittent chemotherapy to moderate-dose chemotherapy given 'continuously' for patients with localized nonpelvic primaries. Patients were stratified for proximal versus distal site, biopsy only versus resection, and gender, based on preliminary data from the IESS-I. Both arms consisted of VACD. The high-dose intermittent arm prescribed vincristine and doxorubicin alternating with vincristine and cyclophosphamide every three weeks for six cycles and then vincristine and actinomycin-D alternating with vincristine and cyclophospha-

Table 4. Multimodality multiagent chemotherapy trials for Ewing's sarcoma

Institution [refs] (years trial open)	Patient population	# of patients	Chemotherapy	Outcome
NCI [133] (1968–80)	Localized/ES bone	80	VC or VC + A or D	33% 15-yr DFS
	Metastatic/ES bone	27	VC or VC + A or D	7% >5-yr DFS
NCI [145] (1983–86)	Localized/ES bone	18	All received	58% 30-mo DFS
	Metastatic/ES bone	13	VAC +/− TBI and ABMT	10% 4-yr DFS
IESS-I [76] (1973–78)	Localized/ES bone	331	Randomized to:	
			VAC or	24% 5-yr RFS
			VAC + pulmonary XRT or	44% 5-yr RFS
			VAC + D	60% 5-yr RFS
	By site:			
	Pelvic	68	randomized as above	34% 5-yr DFS
	Nonpelvic	263		57% 5-yr DFS
IESS-II [134] (1978–82)	Localized, nonpelvic/ES bone	214	VAC + D:	68% 5-yr DFS
			high-dose intermittent	48% 5-yr DFS
			low-dose continuous	
IESS-II [81] (1978–82)	Pelvic/ES bone	59	VAC + D: high-dose intermittent	55% 5-yr DFS
St. Jude [83] (1978–86)	Localized/ES bone	52	CD (low-intensity induction) followed by	
	<8cm	15	VA/CD +/BCNU	82% 3-yr DFS
	≥8cm	52		64% 3-yr DFS
MSKCC [144] (1970–79)	Localized/ES bone	67	3 protocols:	79% 2-yr DFS
	Pelvic sites only		VAC + D or	
	All other sites		VAC + D + Bleo + MTX +/BCNU	

Study	Population	N	Regimen	Outcome
CESS 81 [86,136] (1981–85)	Localized/ES bone (PNET excluded)	93	VACD	55% 69-mo DFS
CESS 86 [86,136,137] (1986–91)	Localized/ES or PNET of bone <100 cm³/extremity >100 cm³ or central	177	VACD VAID (intense) VAC or VACD	69% 5-yr OS
SFOP [141,142] (1978–84)	Localized/ES bone	95	VACD	51% 5-yr DFS
SFOP [142] (1984–87)	Localized/ES bone (PNET excluded)	65	VDI	52% 5-yr DFS
Rizzoli [138] (1972–82)	Localized/ES bone	All 85 59	All (1972–82) VDC (1972–78) VADC (1979–82)	41% 9-yr DFS 32% 9-yr DFS 54% 9-yr DFS
CCG/POG [7,8] (1988–92)	Localized ES or PNET bone	95	VACD VACD alternating with IE	50% 3-yr EFS 69% 3-yr EFS
NCI [143] (1986–92)	ES-PNET bone Localized/ES-PNET bone Metastatic/ES-PNET bone	53 31 23	VDC/IE	42% 5-yr EFS 64% 5-yr EFS 13% 5-yr EFS
IESS-MD [132] (1975–77)	Metastatic and/or regional extension/ES bone	39	VACD	30% 5-yr S
IESS-MD [132] (1980–83)	Metastatic and/or regional extension/ES bone	48	VACD + 5 FU	28% 5-yr S

Abbreviations: S, survival; EFS, event-free survival; DFS, disease-free survival; NCI, National Cancer Institute; MSKCC, Memorial Sloan Kettering Cancer Institute; IESS, Intergroup Ewing's Sarcoma Study; CCG/POG, Pediatric Oncology Group/Children's Cancer Study Group; V, vincristine; D, doxorubicin; C, cyclophosphamide; I, ifosfamide; E, etoposide; A, actinomycin-D; 5-FU, 5-fluorouracil; Bleo, bleomycin; XRT, radiation.

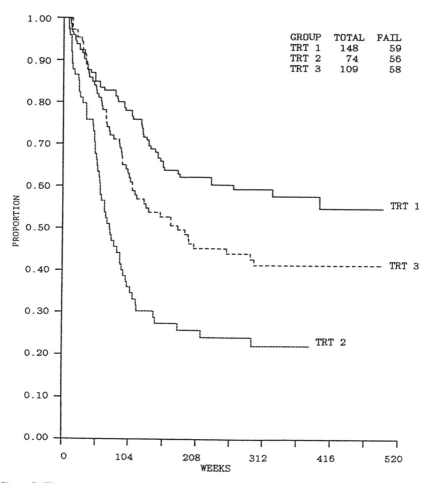

Figure 7. Time to relapse (local recurrence, first metastases or death) by treatment on IESS-I. TRT 1, VAC + doxorubicin; TRT 2, VAC; TRT 3, VAC + bilateral pulmonary radiotherapy.

mide. The 'continuous arm' prescribed lower-dose cyclophosphamide and vincristine weekly; actinomycin-D was introduced at week 6, and doxorubicin was introduced at week 15. At five years, the DFS was 68% in the high-dose intermittent arm, compared to 48% for the continuous arm [134]. Analysis of this study demonstrated that the dose intensity of doxorubicin in the high-dose arm was the most important factor relating to the better outcome [135]. Although on the surface the 68% five-year DFS seems a major improvement over the first IESS trial, it must be remembered that the IESS-I included pelvic patients. On the IESS-I, the overall five-year RFS for nonpelvic patients was 57%; the five-year RFS in the VAC and doxorubicin arm approached 70% [76]. In IESS-II, the site (which in this group excluded pelvic patients), the patient's gender, and the extent of surgery were not shown to be significant variables.

278

All patients with localized pelvic Ewing's sarcoma treated on the IESS-II program received the high-dose intermittent arm of VACD. The five-year RFS in this set of 59 patients was 55% [81], with a 12% local relapse rate (8% were local plus distant metastases, and 3% were only local relapse). The low local relapse rate may have been attributed to a higher complete resection rate than earlier programs; however, it is also likely that the local recurrence rate was underestimated, since imaging methods at that time were less sensitive than current methods and since the primary site was not biopsied when pulmonary or distant bone metastases were identified.

Almost cotemporal with the IESS-II, the St. Jude investigators were evaluating a relatively nontoxic program employing oral cyclophosphamide for seven days followed by intravenous doxorubicin on day 8 as induction therapy. The early results on this program were very promising [83]. Among 24 metastatic and nonmetastatic patients, 19 had no gross residual tumor after induction chemotherapy. In a follow-up study of 53 localized patients who received the same induction, 50 proceeded on to local therapy with surgery and radiation, with radiation doses based on the initial chemotherapy response.

A single-arm trial of VACD initiated by the German Cooperative Ewing's Sarcoma Study (CESS), CESS-81, yielded a 55% DFS for 93 patients at 69 months [86,136]. In this program, local control was surgery, surgery with 36 Gy to incompletely resected tumors, or 50–60 Gy radiation to central tumors and 46 versus 60 Gy for unresected extremity tumors; patients in this study had relatively high local relapse rates, attributed to problems in radiation quality control [86,136,137]. Factors significantly associated with poor prognosis in this study were initial tumor volume greater than 100 mL and more than 10% viable tumor at the time of resection (in the subset undergoing surgery for local control).

Bacci and colleagues published a series of 144 patients treated on two sequential programs; the first 85 patients received vincristine, doxorubicin, and cyclophosphamide, and the second 59 received this regimen and actinomycin-D. In a comparison of the two groups, it appeared that the patients who received all four drugs had an improved survival [138]. However, this trial was not randomized, and the four-drug regimen employed higher doxorubicin and cyclophosphamide doses than the three-drug regimen.

Most investigators agree, based on the preceding data, that doxorubicin is a critical agent in the treatment of ESFT. However, two reports challenge the conventional wisdom, at least in regard to extraosseous ES. The Intergroup Rhabdomyosarcoma Study (IRS) I, II, and III (1972–1991) included some extraosseous ES patients. A report describing the outcome of paraspinal tumors registered on IRS I and II states that extraosseous ES paraspinal tumors composed 32% of the patients and that as a group these patients achieved five-year disease-free survival of about 60% [139], despite the fact that many of them received VAC only, and others were randomized between VA, VAC +/− doxorubicin. Among the 2792 patients registered on IRS I–III, there were 130 (5%) patients with extraosseous ES [140]. Of these, 12% had metastases at diagnosis. At 10 years, 62%, 61%, and 77% of the patients of IRS I, II, and III, respectively, were alive. There were 63 patients who were irradiated for local control because of gross residual disease at the time of diagnosis, and 39 were treated with VAC and 24 VAC + doxorubicin. An advantage among the patients who received doxorubicin could not be discerned [140]. From this small group of patients, it is impossible to conclude decisively that doxorubicin is not valuable in extraosseous ES, as it appears to be in osseous ES.

The role of ifosfamide and ifosfamide in combination with etoposide was first investigated, with promising results, in the setting of relapsed patients (see table 3). Two single-arm, historically controlled trials investigated the role of ifosfamide in multimodality trials. The CESS-86 study [86,137] prescribed a 36-week program of vincristine, actinomycin-D, cyclophosphamide, and doxorubicin (VACD) alternating with vincristine, actinomycin-D, ifosfamide, and doxorubicin (VAIA) for induction. Local control was decided clinically: either surgery, resection + 46 Gy radiation, or 60 Gy radiation. After local control, treatment with VACD/VAID resumed. In contrast to the CESS 81, there was no difference in survival based on the local control method, and a somewhat better survival overall was noted in the VAID regimen, compared to the regimen without ifosfamide [86,136,137]. In contrast, the French found no benefit in substituting ifosfamide for cyclophosphamide when compared to a historical control group [141,142]. In this study there was also an unexpected high rate of cardiac toxicity: three patients developed acute cardiac failure after having received 420–480 mg/m^2 doxorubicin [141,142]. A report from the National Cancer Institute detailed the treatment of 54 patients with ESFT of bone or soft tissue treated with a 51-week program of vincristine, doxorubicin, and cyclophosphamide alternating with ifosfamide and etoposide. Local control with radiation and/or surgery was performed after week 12 of therapy [143]. Forty-three of the patients on this program had metastatic disease at diagnosis; 54% were bone tumors. The five-year disease-free survival was 42% overall, 64% for localized tumors, and 13% for metastatic tumors. Congestive heart failure occurred in 7% at a cumulative dose of doxorubicin of 480 mg/m^2; two patients died, one underwent cardiac transplant, and one resolved. One patient developed myelodysplastic syndrome [143].

The CCG–POG intergroup study (1988–1992) of ES and PNET of bone was a prospective randomized trial comparing a high-dose intermittent regimen of vincristine, doxorubicin, or actinomycin-D (VACD) and a regimen of the same agents and doses alternating with ifosfamide and etoposide. The treatment regimen lasted 51 weeks. Local control measures were radiation, surgery, or surgery followed by radiation for inadequate margins. In this program [7,8], the three-year survival for nonmetastatic patients was 80% for patients who received the arm including ifosfamide and etoposide and 56% for patients who received VACD. The most remarkable difference was seen in patients with pelvic primaries. There was no demonstrable improvement, however, in the outcome of metastatic patients, and a difference between the regimens when examining only extremity patients was not significant. This study also demonstrated a significant effect of age on outcome, with patients 9 years of age or younger having a improved outlook. In summary, single-arm or historically controlled studies give mixed results regarding the role of ifosfamide and/or etoposide in newly diagnosed patients [136,137,141,142]. The POG–CCG randomized trial supports the addition of ifosfamide and etoposide, particularly for the nonmetastatic pelvic patients.

The duration of treatment and the total doses of drugs required to effectively treat patients with ESFT is not entirely clear. The IESS I–II [76,134] employed no less than one year of therapy. The most recent reported SFOP program was approximately one year of therapy [141,142]. In contrast, the CESS trials prescribed about 36 weeks of therapy [136,137], and others have reported trials of six months of intensive therapy [145,146]. Significant differences in outlook between these trials are difficult to discern. Therefore, there is presumptive evidence that sufficiently intensive shortened-duration programs are likely to be as effective as programs of longer duration. The ongoing CCG–POG intergroup trial is comparing a five-drug regimen (vincristine, cyclophosphamide, and doxorubicin alternating with ifosfamide and etoposide) of 51 weeks duration to a dose-intensified 30-week regimen; the regimens prescribe equal total drug doses, and both regimens employ cytokine support. This program is open to patients with all Ewing family tumors, and patients with bone and soft tissue tumors are eligible.

16. Primitive neuroectodermal tumors

Few reports attempt to isolate the experience with extracranial PNET tumors; the majority of studies for ES undoubtedly include some PNET patients. A report from Memorial Sloan-Kettering in New York reviews the clinical data of patients with PNET seen over a 20-year period [147]. Over half the patients reported in this series presented with thoracopulmonary primary tumors. The progress-free survival (PFS) in this set of patients was only 25% at 24 months; the authors conclude that PFS was correlated with extirpative surgery within three months of diagnosis, dose-intensive use of alkylating agents, and radiation therapy to treat residual microscopic disease [147]. However, early surgery may simply equate with accessible and perhaps smaller tumors, and high alkylator dose is likely to correlate with more aggressive trends in the more recently treated patients. Investigators from St. Jude reported a survival rate of 35% for 26 patients with PNET treated from 1962 to 1987 [148]. However, a more recent report from the same institution demonstrates three-year RFS of 67% in 22 patients treated on programs recommended for ESFT that included chemotherapy with VACD and ifosfamide/etoposide and excision and/or radiation [149]. Other centers report survivals similar to that seen with ES tumors when patients are treated on regimens including VACD and/or ifosfamide, as employed for ES [150,151]. Current recommendations are to treat PNET patients as one would treat ES patients.

17. Soft tissue ESFT

There are few data that isolate results for soft tissue ESFT. Most ESFT have been treated on a variety of soft tissue sarcoma programs. Most investigators assume that the soft tissue ESFT will respond to the same treatment as the bone ESFT. As previously discussed, one controversial issue is the role of doxorubicin in the treatment of soft tissue extraosseous ES. More than half (30 of 56) of the paraspinal soft tissue sarcoma patients treated on the IRS studies I and II (1978–1984) were extraosseous ES; the 10-year survival for these patients was greater than 60%, despite the fact that a significant number of them did not receive doxorubicin [139]. A review of IRS I–III (1972–1991) identified 130 patients with extraosseous ES of various sites treated on the IRS programs. In the group of 63 patients with localized tumors with gross residual disease at the start of induction chemotherapy, there was no evidence that patients who received doxorubicin had an improved prognosis compared to those who did not (65% alive at 10 years versus 62%) [140]. It is also interesting to note that among 114 extraosseous ES patients treated on the IRS with localized disease, 21 had a complete resection at diagnosis and a 10-year survival rate of 86%. Patients with microscopic residual received 41.4 Gy radiation, and those with gross residual were treated with 40–55 Gy (dose based on age and tumor size); the respective 10-year survival rates were 78% and 60%, respectively [140]. The five-year survival rate for patients with metastatic extraosseous ES treated on IRS I–II was 25% [140]. These survival rates are not very different than that seen on treatment programs for ES of bone. The data concerning the outlook of patients with soft tissue ESFT as compared to bone tumors should be forthcoming from the currently open CCG–POG intergroup trial enrolling all ESFT patients. The role of doxorubicin will not be defined in this program, since all patients will receive doxorubicin.

18. Treatment of metastatic disease

It is generally acknowledged that patients with metastases fare poorly on current standard regimens. A comparison of two sequential Intergroup studies of Ewing's sarcoma of bone [132] demonstrated a very poor outlook for patients with metastatic disease. The five-year survival was 30% in the first study and 28% in the second. Patients older than age 10 had the poorest outlook, with a less than 20% survival in the IESS-II. In a study of 18 patients treated at St. Jude with a regimen of oral cyclophosphamide for seven days followed by doxorubicin, surgery and radiation, and maintenance therapy consisting of BCNU and VA and VC, 10 patients remained disease free for 16–82 months [152]. This success has been difficult to duplicate. In both the

IESS and St. Jude trials, some of the long-term survivors were patients with rib primaries and pleura as the metastatic site; most current trials consider these patients to have regional rather than metastatic disease. The recently closed POG–CCG intergroup trial (1988–1992) of VACD compared to VACD alternating with IE showed a survival of less than 20% for metastatic patients [7,8]. A group of patients treated at the NCI with an intensive VAC plus IE program has yielded similar poor results for metastatic with a 13% EFS at five years [143].

Efforts to combat metastatic disease have included the addition of radiation to all sites of disease, the use of sequential hemibody radiation (for high-risk and/or metastatic patients [153–155]) or total body radiation [145], and even more intensive chemotherapy regimens. Treatment plans employing TBI and intensive chemotherapy are discussed below in section 20 (Megatherapy). Standard treatment programs usually mandate the use of radiation to sites of metastatic disease. With the exception of the St. Jude protocol [152], most regimens reported for patients with pulmonary metastases included radiation to the lung. Radiation doses to the lung of 15–18 Gy in 150 cGy fractions are generally recommended [132]. Some investigators have recommended boost doses to 40–50 Gy to gross pulmonary lesions, provided that the field is small. The CESS reported that survival in patients with lung metastases appeared to be better in patients who received higher doses of pulmonary radiation: 1 of 6 who received no radiation survived, as did 4 of 10 who received 12–16 Gy and 5 of 6 who received 18–21 Gy [156]. Radiation to bone metastases with a dose of 40–50 Gy has been recommended; some investigators limit radiation of bone metastases to four sites or less in order to limit the dose to marrow-bearing bone.

There is a paucity of data regarding the role of surgery for metastatic disease existing at the time of diagnosis. There are no reports specifically relating to resection of bony metastases. Retrospective reviews of pulmonary metastatectomy in ES are difficult to interpret, since these studies include patients with pulmonary metastases at diagnosis and relapse, as well as patients treated on a variety of chemotherapy and salvage regimens. In a review of 19 NCI patients with ES who underwent thoracotomy, 53% were rendered surgically disease free; for these patients, the five-year disease-free survival rate was 15%, with a median survival of 28 months [157]. A retrospective review of pulmonary metastatectomy from the Netherlands included 12 patients with ES; the median survival after resection was 18 months, but all the patients eventually succumbed [158]. An updated review from the NCI included 28 patients with ES who had a 1.7-year median survival after metastatectomy; patients who had three or more nodules or an incomplete resection had a shorter survival [159]. It is impossible to say, from the data available, whether metastatectomy contributes to survival in newly diagnosed ESFT patients beyond that which one would expect from the more standard approach of pulmonary radiation.

19. Treatment of recurrent disease

Local recurrence is suggested by a recurrent mass, pain, or both. In patients whose local treatment consisted of radiation, new cortical destruction or lytic lesions on plain film or increased uptake on bone scan is suspicious of recurrence [160]. MRI and CT scans may be difficult to interpret in irradiated patients because of persistent edema and fibrosis. In patients who have had surgery, CT or MRI is often not possible or difficult to interpret because of metal prostheses or other hardware. Although biopsy, particularly of irradiated bone or at a surgical site, is not without complication, confirmation of local recurrence should be sought if at all possible. If local recurrence is suspected, the patients should also be evaluated for metastatic disease with a CT scan of the chest and a complete bone scan. If local and/or metastatic disease is confirmed, bone marrow aspiration and biopsy should also be performed.

Treatment of recurrent local disease is directed by the prior therapy. Patients who were initially treated with radiation generally require surgery for control of local recurrence. Limb sparing is generally unsatisfactory after radiation; thus, in patients with recurrent extremity tumors, amputation must be considered. Patients who underwent surgery for local control may benefit from radiation, but for extremity lesions, amputation should also be considered. Inasmuch as repeated local control therapy without additional systemic therapy would be highly unlikely to be curative, a chemotherapy trial to assess response should be considered prior to surgery. The role of aggressive surgery for second local control should be evaluated based on the expectation of cure. A patient who did not receive initial intensive therapy or all active drugs, or one who relapses locally a considerable time after chemotherapy was completed, is most likely to benefit [152]. One must consider reserving radical surgery for patients in whom an aggressive chemotherapy and/or radiation salvage regimen is possible.

Resection of pulmonary metastases has been reported to prolong life in selected patients with one to three resectable lesions [157–159]; however, cure with resection alone would be exceedingly unlikely. CT scans generally underestimate the extent of pulmonary disease, and thus the chance of a complete resection may be less than one would expect based on imaging studies. The primary role of the surgeon for patients with pulmonary metastases is for biopsy and, in rare cases, resection. Whole lung radiation should be considered; doses of 15–18 Gy are standard. Higher doses of pulmonary RT (18–21 Gy) may be considered [156].

Chemotherapy for recurrent disease should be based on an assessment of previous treatment. Patients who relapse after a significant time off therapy may respond to the same agents [152], but dose intensification should be considered. Patients initially treated with VACD only are likely to benefit from ifosfamide and etoposide [120–123,127,128,161,162]. Patients who have received VACD and ifosfamide and etoposide who relapse on therapy or shortly after completing therapy may benefit from entry in ongoing phase II trials of investigational agents. Patients whose tumors are responsive to chemotherapy may be considered for intensive 'megatherapy' retrieval programs, ideally in organized investigational programs.

20. Megatherapy

Poor results for patients with metastases at diagnosis, high-risk tumors such as bulky pelvic lesions, and relapsed patients have led to trials of intensive chemotherapy, as well as trials of intensive chemotherapy and total body irradiation (TBI), most with autologous marrow or peripheral stem cell support. The efficacy of these programs are somewhat difficult to interpret, since most published reports include a mixture of newly diagnosed and relapsed patients. Table 5 summarizes some notable trials, and reviews of trials, of intensive chemotherapy and/or radiotherapy. Burdach and colleagues in Germany reported a 45% six-year DFS after transplantation for 17 patients with chemotherapy-responsive metastatic or relapsed ES [163]. An optimistic report from the SFOP reported a three-year DFS of 41% for a group of 44 metastatic patients enrolled in a program of standard induction chemotherapy, after which the 34 good responders went on to receive high-dose busulfan and melphalan supported by autologous stem-cell reconstitution [164]. A review of megatherapy for metastatic or relapsed ES patients over 11 years at a single institution (Vienna) demonstrated only a 23% survival [165]; the investigators now advocate aggressive radiation of all lesions, as defined by pretherapy total bone MRI and marrow PCR analysis, in order to improve results [102]. A summary of the European experience from the European Bone Marrow Transplant Registry (see table 5) reports an event-free survival (EFS) of 21% at five years in patients metastatic at diagnosis; relapsed patients entering BMT in a second complete response had a 32% EFS at five years [166]. Based on these data, it is not possible to conclude that these programs salvage significant numbers of relapsed and/or metastatic patients: the published reports include few patients, and the abstracts generally have short follow-up. The long-term survivals reported for metastatic patients do not appear to be better than those reported with more standard chemotherapy regimens. Chemotherapy-sensitive patients in second complete remission or partial remission may benefit from megatherapy; however, patients who relapse on the current aggressive regimens are less likely to enter a second remission compared to patients treated in the past. Therefore, it is difficult to assume that these data will apply to patients being treated on current regimens. An alternative to megatherapy with PSC or autologous marrow support is intensive therapy with cytokine support, as is currently being investigated by the POG. For the data on the role of megatherapy to be meaningful, it is imperative that patients are enrolled on investigational programs so that the data can be appropriately interpreted and analyzed.

Table 5. Representative trials of intensive therapy for high-risk ESFT

Institution [ref] (years)	Description of patients	#	Treatment/ conditioning regimen	Local and metastatic site control methods	Outcome
London [210] (1978–81)	Relapsed ES	5	Melphalan + ABMT	Variable	4 of 5: CR; of 4CR, 3 relapse
NCI [211] (1977–80)	High-risk ES (20) Relapsed ES (4)	24	Intensive VAC Low-dose TBI Intensive VACD, ABMT followed by VACD maintenance	RT 50Gy to primary	83% CR 30% 2-yr DFS
Gainesville/Cleveland [212]	Relapsed ES	8	Melphalan + ABMT (1 patient Ara-c)	3 of 8 received RT	6 PR 2NR
Helsinki [213]	Recurrent ES/PNET	3	HD thioptepa + ABMT	None	1 PR
Hopkins [214] (1985–88)	Recurrent ES/PNET	7	Busulfan/cytoxan + 4HC purged autologous BM	Pre-ABMT: 3 RT, 2 S	Survival: 3–23 mo (med 14 mo)
Vienna [163] (1987–92)	ES: Multifocal primary or early or multiple relapse	7 10	Melphalan + VP (+ 4 CP) + 12 Gy TBI ABMT or PBSC: 13 Allogenic BM: 4	May have had surgery or RT prior to megatherapy All in CR or PR at time of ABMT	45% 6-yr RFS 8 of 17 alive in CR

Study	Diagnosis	N	Treatment	Local therapy	Outcome
NCI [215,216] (1981–86)	Newly diagnosed high-risk/metastatic ESFT bone/soft tissue		3 sequential protocols: all VACD; those with CR after local control went on to TBI + autologous BM	50–60 Gy Local RT	25% 6-yr EFS (excluding 20% of patients who did not achieve CR after induction)
SFOP [164] (1991–93)	Metastatic	44	Standard induction busulfan/melphalan followed by BPSC	RT or surgery before MC: only responders to induction therapy go on to HDC	41% 3-yr EFS
Memorial [217] (1992–94)	Metastatic or replapsed ES/PNET	9	Melphalan + TBI 4HC purged BM or PBSC	RT to all sites	2 patients NED: 6, 18 mo
EBMT [166] (1982–92)	High-risk ES in CR Recurrent ES in CR	63	20 different regimens: 93% with melphalan; 30% TBI ABMT 45 (16 + 4HC purge) PBSC 10 BM + PBSC 6 alloBM 2	Multiple regimens	21% 5-yr EFS: CR1 32% 5-yr EFS: CR2

Abbreviations: NCI, National Cancer Institute; SFOP, French Pediatric Oncology Society; EBMT, European Bone Marrow Transplant Registry; ABMT, autologous bone marrow transplant; VAC, vincristine, actinomycin-D, cyclophosphamide; VACD, vincristine, actinomycin-D, cyclophosphamide, doxorubicin; 4HC, 4-hydroxyperoxycyclophosphamide; VP, etoposide; CP, carboplatin; Ara-c, cytosine arabinoside; AlloBM, allogeneic bone marrow; PBSC, peripheral blood stem cells; HDC, high-dose chemotherapy.

21. Local control

Options for local control of the primary tumor in the ESFT are radiation therapy, surgery, or both modalities used sequentially. There has never been a prospective randomized trial directly comparing local control modalities with reference to local failure rates, survival, and functional outcome. Thus, it is not surprising that there is continuing controversy over which, if any, method is preferred [167,168]. Surgery partisans cite trends towards improved survival in patients who have been treated with surgery; however, it must be noted that all such data are derived from retrospective reviews, which are marred by the fact that patients who undergo surgery are more likely to be those patients with smaller and more accessible tumors. Beyond claims of superior local control and survival, presumed advantages of surgery are a lessened risk of secondary sarcoma due to radiation and a likelihood of less interference with growth potential in young patients. Possible advantages of radiation as sole local control are the lack of limitation imposed by inaccessible site or bulk thought to be too great for surgical control. Some believe that combining radiation and surgery may improve local control and ultimately survival. Surgeons and radiation therapists both claim results with functional superiority, yet there is no comparative prospective study analyzing functional results. Some investigators advocate a planned approach employing both surgery and radiation, particularly in high-risk patients; however, this approach is problematic, since the patient is then subject to the disadvantages of both radiation and surgery. The combination of surgery followed by radiation is generally employed for patients with positive or close margins after surgery or who demonstrate a poor histologic response to chemotherapy. Radiation may be employed to treat an unresectable lesion, which if responsive to radiation may then be resected at a later date; the utility of this approach with reference to decreased local failure rates and improved survival has not been proven. Some investigators advocate marginal resection followed by radiation and consider lower doses of radiation for microscopic residual, but significantly lower does for microscopic residual is not uniformly accepted as adequate for local control. The following section will review some of the data that exist regarding local control modalities and outcomes in ESFT of bone.

Table 6 summarizes the local failure rates for radiation therapy as reported in major clinical trials for ESFT of bone. It should be noted that local control rates as reported may be underestimated, since it is possible that some patients reported as suffering from metastatic relapse as first events may also have persistent or progressive disease at the local site that was not noted. Excluding the CESS 81, which reported problems with radiation compliance, local control rates with radiation appear acceptable for nonpelvic tumors. For bulky pelvic tumors, radiation control rates are less satisfactory. It is not surprising that local tumor control with radiation is less in pelvic lesions, since local control has been shown to decrease with increasing tumor size, e.g., tumors larger than 8 cm [83,169]. It is important to note that it was shown that failure of local control with radiation generally occurred within the bone, not at the margins, indicating that the failures were not due to inadequate fields [169]. Most programs have reported less than 10% isolated local failures (see table 6) in nonpelvic tumors. Thus, if freedom from relapse were the only yardstick used to judge radiation as therapy for local control of ESFT of bone, radiation would be acceptable, at least for nonpelvic or less than bulky lesions [170,171].

An important question is this: Even if local control rates reported for patients treated with radiation as the sole local control were acceptable, does survival increase if surgery or surgery plus radiation is employed? The answer to this question is not known. Survival and disease-free survival among patients who have had surgery appears better in several trials, but selection bias remains a significant problem. A report from the Mayo Clinic [75] that reviewed the records of 140 patients treated between 1969 and 1982 found that the survival rate in this group was 74% at five years for patients who underwent surgery and 34% for those who did not. It must be noted that all patients received radiation therapy as well, so these data cannot be used to state that surgery alone is a preferred modality. Investigators from Bologna [172] report that among 182 patients treated between 1979 and 1982, disease-free survival was 30.3% in those who were treated with radiation only, 47.9% in those who received radiation and surgery, and 59.1% for those who were treated only with surgery. The authors themselves state that these numbers are significantly biased by the selection of more favorable patients for surgical procedures. A review by Sailor and colleagues reported a 91% five-year survival rate for patients undergoing surgery with or without radiation, but only 54% for those who were treated with radiation only [173]. The CESS-81 [86,136] reported a distinct advantage for patients who underwent surgery, but admittedly the radiation therapy compliance problems in this study were unacceptably high. The CESS-86 [86,137] achieved better local control rates, yet despite an improved local control rate, surgery was not shown to significantly impact overall survival. A review of the impact of surgery and surgical margins that included ES patients from the CESS-81, -86 and -91P demonstrated that surgery improved the 10-year local control rate: the local or combined (local plus metastatic) relapse rate was 31% after irradiation alone and 7% after surgery with or without radiation [174]. However, it should be noted that this review included patients from the CESS-81 series, with whom there may have been problems with irradiation [86]. The local or combined relapse rate after surgery with radical or wide margins was 5%, compared to 12% for patients with marginal or intralesional resections [174]. Despite these data, there was no statistically demonstrable difference in survival based on the extent of excision, because there was an increased incidence of metastases in the patients who underwent surgery. The authors have hypothesized that patients who undergo surgery and have viable tumor in place are at higher risk of disseminating tumor at the time of surgery; they propose radiation followed by later surgery in high-risk patients [174].

289

Table 6. Local failure rates in Ewing's sarcoma in patients treated with radiation and chemotherapy

Institution [refs] (years trial open)	Patient categories	# of patients	RT dose (Gy)	Local failure (%)[a] Comments
NCI [133] (1968–80)	Localized/ES bone	80	50	20% / 33% (pelvic site)
NCI [145] (1983–86)	Central/proximal ES bone / Distal/ES bone	8 / 10	55–60 (rib 45) [+ TBI 4/day × 2 days for HR patients]	25% (pelvic) / 30% (pelvic)
IESS-I [76] (1973–78)	Localized/ES bone / Pelvic site only	331 / 68	45–65 (dose by age)	15% (pelvic) / 33% (pelvic)
IESS-II [134] (1978–82)	Localized, nonpelvic/ES bone	214	45–55	9% (17% of patients had CR or amputation)
IESS-II [81] (1978–82)	Pelvic/ES bone	58	55	11% (pelvic) (19% CR; 14% IncR)
St. Jude [83] (1978–86)	Localized/Es bone	39	30–35 if no soft tissue residual after induction / 50–55 if gross residual	34% (all > 8 cm.) / 42% RT only / 0% RT + S
CESS 81 [86,136] (1981–85)	Localized/ES bone (PNET excluded)	29 RT + S / 32 RT only	36 RT + S / 46–60 RT only	50% RT only / 17% RT + S
CESS 81 [86,137] (1986–91)	Localized/ES or PNET of bone	63 RT + S / 31 RT	46–60 randomized q day v. bid	5% / 14%

Study	Patient type	Treatment	Dose (cGy)	Local failure[a]
MSKCC [144] (1970–79)	Localized/ES bone	34 RT	45–70 gross residual	21%
		20 RT + S	30 after resection	No local failure
SFOP [142] (1984–87)	Localized/ES bone	26 RT	45–60	31%
		24 RT + S	40–60	13%
Rizzoli [138] (1972–82)	Localized/ES bone	86 RT	40–60	36%
		48 RT + S	35–45	8%
	(subset: pelvic only)	(20 RT)	(40–60)	(50%)
		(10 RT + S)	(35–45)	(40%)
Bologna [172] (1979–86)	Localized/ES bone	43 RT	45–64	31%
		27 RT + S	45–64	7%
POG [181,182] (1983–87)	Localized/ES–PNET bone	97	55–56	24% (Tailored port)
NCI [143] (1986–92)	ES–PNET bone/soft tissue (localized/metastatic)	54 (53 eval.) (31/23)	27–63	19% (includes metastatic patients)
Gainesville [180] (1971–82)	Localized/extremity/ES bone	31	47–61 (150 cGy q day) 50.4–60 (120 cGy BID) (+/– TBI to 8 or 12)	23% 19%
Gainesville [183] (1982–87)	Localized/metastatic/ES bone	33 RT	55.2–60 (120 cGy BID) (+/– 800 cGy TBI)	12%

[a] Local failure and/or simultaneous metastasis.

Abbreviations: NCI, National Cancer Institute; IESS, Intergroup Ewing's Sarcoma Study; CESS, Cooperative Ewing's Sarcoma Study; MSKCC, Memorial Sloan-Kettering Cancer Center; SFOP, French Society of Pediatric Oncology; RT, radiation therapy; S, surgery; CR, complete resection; IncR, incomplete resection; eval, evaluable.

Several authors have tried to mitigate the effect of selection bias by reviewing local control results at selected anatomic sites. Although helpful, these studies also yield conflicting results. Further, these reviews are flawed because the patients are heterogeneous with regard to chemotherapy programs and differ with reference to the techniques available for both radiation and surgery over the time periods surveyed. In an attempt to exclude patients with obviously expendable bones, or very bulky pelvic lesions, Terek and colleagues reviewed 32 patients with Ewing's sarcoma of the femur treated between 1970 and 1985. Local recurrence occurred in 5 of 10 treated with radiation, 0 of 9 treated with surgery, and 1 of 13 treated with surgery and radiation [175]. Although an advantage for surgery with regard to local control seems apparent, the local therapy choice had no statistically significant impact on overall survival: the five-year survival was 31% [175].

Resection of pelvic lesions has generated interest. Since most pelvic lesions are bulky and are less easily controlled with radiation alone, it seems intuitive that a reduction in tumor bulk would decrease local relapse rates and improve survival. A study from Memorial [176] reported that twice as many pelvic patients who underwent resection survived compared to patients treated with radiation. Frassica and colleagues also reported an apparent difference in outcome correlated with resection: 75% five-year survival in resected patients (with radiation) and 18% in patients receiving radiation alone [177]. In contrast, an improved outlook in pelvic patients undergoing surgery was not demonstrated in the IESS studies [81], nor in a series from Italy [178]. A recent retrospective review of 39 patients with ES of the pelvis showed no significant diffference in disease-free and overall survival between those undergoing surgery and those treated with radiation [179].

In summary, there is no definitive general answer to the question of which form of local control is best. The first imperative is that the local control choice should be designed to eradicate the primary tumor. Functional considerations should be given weight in decision-making, but it is paramount that the ultimate survival of the patient is the most important goal: systemic therapy should not be compromised in order to improve orthopedic function. The choice of local control method must be based on a careful assessment of the individual patient. Factors to be weighed include the skeletal maturity of the patient, the bulk of the tumor, and the site of the tumor. Each patient should be evaluated by a team consisting of oncologists, surgeons, and radiotherapists able to recommend a local control regimen tailored to the patient's needs.

22. Radiation therapy

Issues regarding the implementation of radiation therapy include the timing of radiation, fractionation of doses, and the extent of the radiation field. Early programs such as the IESS-I initiated radiation at the start of treatment, since chemotherapy had not yet been definitively proven to be useful [76]. Subsequent programs have prescribed the start of radiation therapy after induction chemotherapy. The duration of induction therapy prior to radiation may be as short as six weeks as in the IESS-II [134], nine weeks as in many published trials [7,86,136,137], or as long as 12 weeks in the recently reported NCI program [143]. There is no evidence to indicate that local control is compromised by a delay of up to 12 weeks. Completion of induction therapy initiates systemic control and provides a way to assess the response to chemotherapy. Exceptions to planned delay of radiation until after induction chemotherapy are rare, but should be noted: patients who present with spine or paraspinal lesions with neurological symptoms at diagnosis may require emergency radiation as soon as the diagnosis is confirmed, and very rarely patients with chest disease causing respiratory distress will require emergency radiation after diagnosis is confirmed.

In the past, it had been thought that whole bone radiation was required because ES always involves the marrow cavity. Whole bone radiation, however, is not without significant morbidity, particularly in patients with significant growth ahead of them. The IESS-II prescribed 5-cm margins [134]. Investigators at St. Jude [169] demonstrated excellent local control rates for lesions less than 8 cm when they employed radiation to the initial bone tumor, the soft tissue residual after induction chemotherapy, and a 3-cm margin [83,169]. Investigators from Gainesville [180] treated the initial tumor plus a 4-cm margin, sparing at least one epiphysis in standard-risk patients. In 1983, the POG started a randomized trial of standard whole bone radiation compared to radiation to the initial tumor plus a 2-cm margin. As the study was ongoing, interim analysis showed that tailored port radiation was successful, and the study was modified so that all patients received tailored port radiation. Final data from this report are not available, but interim analysis supports the use of tailored port radiation [181,182]. The current POG–CCG trial employs less than whole bone radiation, based on these preliminary results. There is no published series to date that confirms the adequacy of less than whole bone radiation for lesions greater than 8 cm.

Treatment dose also varies somewhat among reported regimens. In the IESS-I [170,171], dose was modified according to patient age, with patients less than 5 years old receiving 45 Gy to whole bone and 10 Gy boost to the tumor, while those older than 15 received 55 Gy whole bone and 10 Gy boost to the tumor site. There was no correlation between treatment dose and local control. In CESS-81, 45–60 Gy was given for primary radiation and 30–36 Gy for postoperative radiation [86,136]. In CESS-86, 60 Gy was given unless critical organs were in the field [86,137]. Patients with lesions larger than 8 cm were treated with 35 Gy at St. Jude, and 90% local control was achieved, but in these patients with lesions larger than 8 cm there was a 48% local recurrence after 35 Gy. The conclusion was that the overall control rate for 35 Gy is inadequate [169].

The schedule of radiation in most programs is 1.8–2 Gy per fraction five days a week. The CESS-86 randomized patients between hyperfractionated

(1.6 Gy BID) and standard radiation, and no difference in survival or local relapses was noted [86,137]. Investigators from Gainesville have employed hyperfractionated radiation (1.2 Gy BID to 50.4–60 Gy, depending on response to induction chemotherapy) in a series of three protocols [180,183]. The local control rates reported were good, and functional outcomes were deemed superior to historical controls. Although hyperfractionation appears to be at least as effective as daily fractionation, at this time there are not enough data to warrant the use of twice-a-day radiation outside the context of controlled trials.

Prophylactic lung radiation was employed in the IESS-I study. Pulmonary radiation (15–18 Gy) in combination with VAC chemotherapy was superior to VAC alone but was less effective than the addition of doxorubicin to VAC in this study [76]. No current protocols routinely employ prophylactic pulmonary radiation. Pulmonary radiation for pulmonary metastases is appropriate at a dose of 12–21 Gy in standard fractions (see discussion of treatment of metastases above). Total body radiation has been employed in trials of megatherapy, as discussed above. Hemibody radiation used as part of systemic therapy has also been employed [153–155], but there are no data demonstrating results superior to chemotherapy trials, in which radiation is restricted to local disease.

23. Surgical approaches

The initial surgical approach should be biopsy, done in a manner consistent with obtaining adequate tissue and assuring that the biopsy site is consistent with the potential for later excision and/or radiation. In certain circumstances, fine-needle aspiration may be sufficient for diagnosis [101]. In the case of extremity lesions, the biopsy should be placed so that the possibility of limb sparing remains open. Ideally, the biopsy should be done in the institution that will treat the patient so that the material can be processed for all the required immunochemistry and molecular studies. If a lesion involves a weight-bearing bone, biopsy of soft tissue may be preferable to bone biopsy in order to lessen the risk of pathological fracture. One study demonstrated an increased risk of complications in patients whose biopsy was performed at the referring rather than the treating institution [184].

There is no evidence that prechemotherapy excision confers an advantage over surgical resection after chemotherapy induction for ESFT. In fact, an attempt at prechemotherapy excision is likely to result in increased morbidity and a higher risk of positive margins, which will mandate either a second surgery or radiation. The concept of surgery after neoadjuvant chemotherapy is generally accepted by orthopedic surgeons who are accustomed to the role of neoadjuvant chemotherapy before limb sparing. For chest wall and rib lesions, there is a tendency among surgeons to recommend resection prior to chemotherapy; however, recent reports question this model and urge preoperative chemotherapy, which is highly likely to reduce the morbidity and extent of surgery and perhaps to spare the patient radiation therapy without compromising the patient's outlook [99,100]. Specific data regarding the appropriate timing of surgery for soft tissue lesions are not as clear, but it should be noted that patients with extraosseous ES treated on the IRS programs with group III (unresected) tumors had survival rates similar to those of patients with bone ESFT [140], indicating that immediate surgical excision is not required in soft tissue ESFT. Delay of surgery until after induction chemotherapy provides the treatment team with valuable information regarding response to chemotherapy. Induction chemotherapy is generally complete from 9 to 12 weeks after diagnosis. If surgery is the choice of local control, surgery should be done after recovery from induction chemotherapy.

The goal of resection should be a compete excision with clean margins, for both soft tissue and bone tumors. Radical or wide resection is ideal, but in order to minimize functional deficit and growth deficits, margins considered acceptable are 5 cm for bone, 5 mm for fat planes, and 2 mm for fascial planes. These recommendations are similar to those used for limb sparing in osteosarcoma. Patients with closer margins will require radiation therapy after recovery from surgery. Some investigators have recommended irradiation after surgery for patients with poor histologic response as well [137,174]. Some consider radiation first for bulky lesions, to be followed by surgery [174].

Recommendations for surgery by site are generally detailed in open protocols. For extremity and pelvic lesions, standard orthopedic limb-sparing approaches are recommended. Custom prosthesis, allograft, and vascularized autograft are reconstruction options to be considered. It should be noted, however, that if margins are likely to be close or positive, postoperative radiation will be required and may have a negative impact on wound healing and bone graft survival. Rib primaries may have discontinuous lesions, and therefore it is generally recommended that the entire involved rib be removed. In the past, it has been recommended that a rib below and above also be resected, but current thinking holds this to be unnecessary; it should be borne in mind that induction chemotherapy improves the ability to resect rib and chest wall lesions significantly [99,100].

Some unusual presentations require modification of the standard surgical biopsy approach. For example, patients who present with cord compression syndrome may have a diagnosis made by needle biopsy, and emergency radiation therapy and prompt initiation of chemotherapy may obviate the need for laminectomy. If a diagnosis cannot be made by needle biopsy and laminectomy is required, decompression as needed is indicated, but complete excision will not spare the patient radiation under most circumstances. Spine lesions are often associated with paravertebral and/or epidural extension, and therefore it is recommended that patients with spine lesions always receive radiation therapy in lieu of or in addition to surgery.

After surgical resection with negative margins, radiation is not generally recommended in most trials. However, in the CESS studies, patients who had less than 90% histologic response received radiation even if a wide or radical resection had been accomplished [86,136,137]. If there is gross or microscopic residual after resection, it is standard to add radiation therapy.

24. Late effects

The late effects of chemotherapy for patients with ES are primarily those related to treatment with alkylating agents and anthracyclines. A risk of cardiac dysfunction and infertility are among the most well-documented and serious consequences of chemotherapy. Secondary malignancies are a devastating consequence of therapy, and will be discussed below. Survivors of ESFT should be monitored for late effects by oncologists familiar with the late complications of chemotherapy.

Orthopedic and functional late effects vary depending upon the method of local control and the age of the patient at the time of treatment. Radiation, particularly in doses greater than 60 Gy, may be associated with significant problems such as pathologic fracture, growth problems, fibrosis, and poor function. The IESS-I reported pathologic fracture or shortening of 2 cm or more in 25% of survivors followed [185]. A review of 29 patients with ES of lower extremities who received 50 Gy radiation and chemotherapy found that 18 of 22 had mild to moderate functional deficits; one patient had dysfunction severe enough to require amputation [186]. Hyperfractionated radiation therapy has been reported to result in improved functional outcome compared to standard radiation dose fractionation [180,183]. The functional outcomes of patients who have had limb-sparing surgery for extremity lesions, or resection at other sites, vary by site and procedure. There are few data available specifically examining the functional outcomes in ESFT patients treated with surgery, but there is no reason to believe that the outcome in patients who have not had radiation will differ from patients who have undergone limb sparing for other bone tumors such as osteosarcoma. All ESFT patients who have undergone irradiation or limb-sparing procedures should be followed for late effects and offered appropriate physical therapy programs.

Nicholson and colleagues studied overall functional outcome for 29 adult survivors of childhood ES who were five years or more past diagnosis and at least 21 years of age [187]. In this study, siblings were interviewed as controls [187]. The ES survivors perceived their health as only fair or poor, despite no actual increase in the incidence of specific medical conditions. Physical disability and a slightly lower rate of marriage were reported in comparison to matched siblings; however, employment status despite disability and income was not notably different than controls [187]. The most disturbing information uncovered was that 4 of the 29 (7.2%) survivors developed a second malignancy, namely, three osteosarcoma in the radiation field and one cervical cancer.

Several studies have estimated the risk of secondary malignancy in ES survivors. Sarcoma, most often osteosarcoma, in the irradiated field is a known risk of ES; other malignancies, including secondary leukemia, have been reported. An early report estimated the risk of a secondary cancer, primarily bone sarcoma in irradiated fields, to be as high as 35% ($\pm$ 15%) [188]. The risk of secondary bone sarcoma associated with increasing radiation and alkylator dose was described by the Late Effects Study Group, which estimated a 22% risk of developing bone cancer at 20 years after diagnosis of ES [25]. In a study of over 10,000 three-year survivors of childhood cancer, only 1.9% of ES survivors developed a secondary cancer [189]. Using a United Kingdom population-based registry, it has been shown that as many as 5.4% of three-year survivors of ES will develop a second bone cancer, and higher risk was associated with increasing radiation and alkylating agent dose [190]. An analysis based on data reported to United States tumor registries should a 100-fold risk of developing bone cancer in ES survivors [191]. In a report from Stanford, among 25 survivors free of disease for at least three years, one ANLL and one osteosarcoma developed; the actuarial risk of developing bone cancer at five years was estimated to be 4% and the risk of all secondary cancer 8% [192]. In a recent report based on a database of 266 ES survivors, the incidence of secondary sarcoma at 20 years after diagnosis was 6.5% and for all malignancies (including leukemia) was estimated to be 9.2% [193]. The highest risk of bone sarcoma was seen with radiation doses in excess of 60 Gy, which are now relatively uncommon [193]. Although the exact risk of secondary cancer is uncertain, it is clear that survivors of ES must be monitored for secondary malignancy. Radiation doses currently employed are somewhat lower than in the past; however, higher cumulative doses of alkylating agents, anthracyclines, and the addition of etoposide are known risk factors for secondary malignancy [194,195]. It is critical that success in treating ESFT is not impaired by an unacceptable incidence of secondary cancer.

25. Conclusions and considerations for the future

Optimal treatment for patients with ESFT requires both local control of the primary tumor and systemic treatment. Decisions regarding local control must be made by a team of experts in surgery, radiation, and oncology familiar with these tumors. Chemotherapy is essential to cure. Advances in radiation therapy and surgical techniques have improved the functional outlook for ESFT survivors. To amplify our knowledge base and provide state-of-the-art therapy, patients with ESFT tumors should be treated specifically in clinical trials designed for these relatively rare tumors. The treating institutions should be able to provide services in all the disciplines involved: pathology, imaging, oncology, surgery, rehabilitation services, and psychosocial support. Current treatment programs employ increasingly intensive chemotherapy, and it is critical that the treatment be delivered by staff appropriately trained in the delivery of intensive chemotherapy and in management of potential complications.

Investigation into the molecular biology of these tumors has provided us with tools to specify diagnosis. We now enjoy an understanding of the histologic lineage of this family of neuroectodermal tumors. Ongoing investigations into the presence of subclinical disease, as detected by RT-PCR for the molecular transcripts associated with the ESFT, will likely yield prognostic information and may eventually guide us in determining the optimal duration of therapy. Detection of micrometastatic disease by RT-PCR may help us to better define risk groups so that treatment duration or intensity may be better tailored. New treatments based on our current knowledge of the molecular biology of the ESFT are quite speculative; however, antisense gene therapy may be employed to purge marrow, to treat directly, or to target tumors with radioisotope therapy. The ESFTs are among the cancers for which the developments in molecular biology have yielded extraordinary information that has improved our understanding of these tumors. Hopefully, this new knowledge will lead to new methods of therapy. Current programs tend to rely on increasing intensification of standard chemotherapeutic agents. This intensification will undoubtedly remain the mainstay of therapy for the near future, but as we approach a point of diminishing returns for increasing doses of chemotherapy, it is encouraging to know that we may be provided with a new set of tools for the future.

Acknowledgement

The authors would like to thank Dr. Deborah Schofield from the Department of Pathology, Children's Hospital of Boston, for her invaluable assistance.

Dr. Granowetter would like to thank the Dorothy Rodbell Cohen Foundation for Sarcoma Research for their support.

References

1. Ewing J. 1921. Diffuse endothelioma of bone. Proc NY Pathol Soc 21:17–24.
2. Crist WM, Kun LE. 1991. Common solid tumors of childhood. N Engl J Med 324:461–471.
3. Tefft M, Vawter GF, Mitus A. 1969. Paravertebral 'round-cell' tumors in children. Radiology 1501–1509.
4. Askin FB, Rosai J, Sibley RK, Dehner LP, McAlistar WH. 1979. Malignant small cell tumor of the thoracopulmonary region in childhood. Cancer 43:2438–2451.
5. Gurney JG, Davis S, Severson RK, Fang J-Y, Ross JA, Robison LL. 1996. Trends in cancer incidence among children in the U.S. Cancer 78:532–541.
6. Horowitz ME, Delaney TF, Malawer MM, Triche TJ. 1993. Ewing's sarcoma family of tumors: Ewing's sarcoma of bone and soft tissue and the peripheral primitive neuroectodermal tumors. In Pizzo PA, Poplack DG (eds.), Principles and Practice of Pediatric Oncology. Philadelphia: J B Lippincott, pp. 795–822.
7. Grier H, Krailo M, Link M, et al. 1994. Improved outcome in non-metastatic Ewing's sarcoma and PNET of bone with the addition of ifosfamide and etoposide to vincristine,

adriamycin, cyclophosphamide, and actinomycin: a Children's Cancer Group and Pediatric Oncology Group report (abstract). Proc Am Soc Clin Oncol 13:421.

8. Grier HE, personal communication.
9. Siegel RD, Ryan LM, Antman KH. 1988. Adults with Ewing's sarcoma. An analysis of 16 patients at the Dana Farber Cancer Institute. J Clin Oncol 11:614–617.
10. Mooday AM, Norman AR, Tait D. 1996. Paediatric tumors in the adult population: the experience of the Royal Marsden Hospital 1974–90. Med Pediatr Oncol 26:153–159.
11. Klaassen R, Sautre-Garau X, Aurias A, et al. 1992. Ewing's sarcoma of bone in adults: an anatomic-clinical study of 30 cases. Bull Cancer Paris 79:161–167.
12. Polednak AP. 1985. Primary bone cancer incidence in black and white residents of New York State. Cancer 55:2883–2888.
13. Jensen RD, Drake RM. 1970. Rarity of Ewing's sarcoma in negroes. Lancet 1:777.
14. Fraumeni JF, Glass AG. 1970. Rarity of Ewing's sarcoma among U.S. Negro children. Lancet 1:366–367.
15. Li FP, Tu JT, Liu FS, Shiang EL. 1980. Rarity of Ewing's sarcoma in China. Lancet 1:1255.
16. Finkelstein MM. 1994. Radium in drinking water and the risk of death from bone cancer among Ontario youths. Can Med Assoc 151:565–571.
17. Hartley AL, Birch JM, McKinney PA, et al. 1988. The Inter-Regional Epidemiological Study of Childhood Cancer (IRESCC): a case control study of children with bone and soft tissue sarcoma. Br J Cancer 58:838–842.
18. Novakovic B, Goldstein AM, Wexler LE, Tucker MA. 1994. Increased risk of neuroectodermal tumors and stomach cancer in relatives of patients with Ewing's sarcoma family of tumors. J Natl Cancer Inst 86:1702–1706.
19. Hartley AL, Birch JM, Blair V, Teare MD, Marsden HB, Harris M. 1991. Cancer incidence in the families of children with Ewing's tumor. J Natl Cancer Inst 83:955–956.
20. Hartley AL, Birch JM, Marsden HB, et al. 1988. Malignant disease in the mothers of children with Ewing's sarcoma. Med Pediatr Oncol 16:95–97.
21. Zamora P, Garcia de Paredes MI, Baron M, et al. 1986. Ewing's sarcoma in brothers. An unusual observation. Am J Clin Oncol 9:358–360.
22. Hutter RVP, Francis KC, Foote FW. 1964. Ewing's sarcoma in siblings. Am J Surg 107:598–603.
23. Li FP, Fraumeni JF Jr. 1982. Prospective study of a family cancer syndrome. JAMA 247:2692–2694.
24. Newton WA, Meadows AT, Shimada H, Bunin GR, Vawter GF. 1991. Bone sarcomas as second malignant neoplasms following childhood cancer. Cancer 67:193–201.
25. Tucker MA, D'Angio GJ, Boice JD, et al. 1987. Bone sarcomas linked to radiotherapy and chemotherapy in children. N Engl J Med 317:588–593.
26. Fisher R, Kaste SC, Parham DM, Shapiro DN, Pappo AS. 1995. Ewing's sarcoma as a second malignant tumor in a child previously treated for Wilms' tumor. J Pediatr Heamatol Oncol 17:76–80.
27. Jimenez M, Leon P, Castro L, Azcona C, Sierrrasesumage L. 1995. Second tumors in pediatric oncologic patients. Report of 5 cases. Rev Med Univ Navarra 40:72–77.
28. Triche TJ. 1993. Pathology of pediatric malignacies. In Pizzo PA, Poplack DG (eds.), Principles and Practice of Pediatric Oncology. Philadelphia: J B Lippincott, pp. 115–152.
29. Dehner LP. 1993. Primitive neuroectodermal tumor and Ewing's sarcoma. Am J Surg Pathol 17:1–13.
30. Schofield DS, personal communication.
31. Perlman EJ, Dickman PS, Askin FB, Grier HE, Miser JS, Link MP. 1994. Ewing's sarcoma–routine diagnostic utilization of MIC2 analysis: a Pediatric Oncology Group/Children's Cancer Group intergroup study. Hum Pathol 25:304–307.
32. Triche T, Cavazzana A. 1988. Round cell tumors of bone. In Unni KK (ed.), Bone Tumors. New York: Churchill Livingstone, pp. 199–224.
33. Weidner N, Tjoe J. 1994. Immunohistochemical profile of monoclonal antibody O13: anti-

body that recognizes glycoprotein p30/32^{MIC2} and is useful in diagnosing Ewing's sarcoma and peripheral neuroepithelioma. Am J Surg Pathol 18:486–494.

34. Fellinger EJ, Garin-Chesa P, Triche TJ, Huvos AG, Rettig WJ. 1991. Immunohistochemical analysis of Ewing's sarcoma cell surface antigen p30/32^{MIC2}. Am J Pathol 139:317–325.

35. Thiele CJ. 1990. Pediatric peripheral neuroectodermal tumors, oncogenes and differentiation. Cancer Invest 8:629–639.

36. Pagani A, Fischer-Colbrie R, Eder U, Pellin A, Llombart-Bosch A, Bussolath G. 1995. Neural and mesenchymal differentiation in Ewing's sarcoma cell lines. Morphological, immunophenotypic, molecular biological and cytogenetic evidence. Int J Cancer 63:738–743.

37. Ladanyi M, Heinemann FS, Huvos AG, Rao PH, Chen Q, Jhanwar SC. 1990. Neural differentiation in small round cell tumors of bone and soft tissue with the translocation t(11;22)(q24;q12). Hum Pathol 21:1245–1251.

38. Cavazzana AO, Miser JS, Jefferson J, Triche TJ. 1987. Experimental evidence for a neural origin of Ewing's sarcoma of bone. Am J Pathol 127:507–518.

39. Turc-Carel C, Philip T, Berger M-P, et al. 1984. Chromosome study of Ewing's sarcoma (ES) cell lines. Consistency of a reciprocal translocation t(11;22)(q24;q12). Cancer Genet Cytogenet 12:1.

40. Whang-Peng J, Triche TJ, Knutsen T, Miser J, Douglass EC, Israel MA. 1984. Chromosomal translocation in peripheral neuroepithelioma. N Engl J Med 311:584–585.

41. Whang-Peng J, Triche TJ, Knusten T, et al. 1986. Cytogenetic characterization of selected small round cell tumors of childhood. Cancer Genet Cytogenet 21:185–208.

42. Douglass EC, Valentine M, Green AA, Hayes FA, Thompson EI. 1986. t(11;22) and other chromosomal rearrangements in Ewing's sarcoma. J Natl Cancer Inst 77:1211–1213.

43. Aurias A, Rimbaut C, Buffe C, Dubousset J, Mazabraud A. 1983. Chromosomal translocations in Ewing's sarcoma of bone. N Engl J Med 309:496–497.

44. Fletcher JA, Kozakewich HP, Hoffer FA, et al. 1991. Diagnostic relevance of clonal cytogenetic aberration in malignant soft-tissue tumors. N Engl J Med 324:436–442.

45. Delattre O, Zucman J, Melot T, et al. 1994. The Ewing family of tumors — a subgroup of small-round-cell tumors defined by specific chimeric transcripts. N Engl J Med 331:294–299.

46. Zucman J, Delattre O, Desmaze C, et al. 1992. Cloning and characterization of the Ewing's sarcoma and peripheral neuroepithelioma t(11;22) translocation breakpoints. Genes chromosomes Cancer 5:271–277.

47. Delattre O, Zucman J, Plougastel B, et al. 1992. Gene fusion with an ETS DNA-binding domain caused by chroomsome translocation in human tumors. Nature 359:162–165.

48. Zucman J, Melot T, Desmaze C, et al. 1993. Combinatorial generation of variable fusion proteins in the Ewing family of tumors. EMBO J 12:4481–4487.

49. Plougastel B, Zucman J, Peter M, Thomas G, Delattre O. 1993. Genomic structure of the EWS gene and its relationship to EWSR1, a site of tumor-associated chromosomal translocation. Genomics 18:609–615.

50. Zoubek A, Dockhorn-Dworniczak B, Delattre O, et al. 1996. Does expression of different EWS chimeric transcripts define clinically distinct risk groups of Ewing tumor patients? J Clin Oncol 14:1245–1251.

51. Zoubek A, Pfleiderer C, Salzer-Kuntschik M, et al. 1994. Variability of EWS chimaeric transcripts in Ewing tumours: a comparison of clinical and molecular data. Br J Cancer 70:908–913.

52. Jeon I, Davis JN, Braun BS, et al. 1995. A variant Ewing's sarcoma translocation (7;22) fuses the EWS gene to the ETS gene ETV1. Oncogene 10:1229–1234.

53. Urano F, Akihiro U, Hong W, Kikuchi H, Hata J. 1996. A novel chimera gene between EWS and E1A-F, encoding the adenovirus E1A Enhancer-binding protein, in extraosseous Ewing's sarcoma. Biochem Biophys Res Commun 219:608–612.

54. Douglass EC, Rowe ST, Valentine M, et al. 1990. A second non-random translocation, der16 t(1;16)(q21;q13) in Ewing's sarcoma and peripheral neuroectodermal tumors. Cytogenet Cell Genet 53:87.

55. Gerald WL, Rosai J, Ladanyi M. 1995. Characterization of the genomic breakpoint and

chimeric transcripts in the *EWS–WT1* gene fusion of the desmoplastic small round cell tumor. Proc Natl Acad Sci USA 92:1028–1032.

56. Ladanyi M, Gerald W. 1994. Fusion of the EWS and WT1 genes in the desmoplastic small round cell tumor. Cancer Res 54:2837–2840.

57. Immanuel D, Zinszner H, Ron D. 1995. Association of SARFH (Sarcoma-associated RNA-binding Fly Homolog) with regions of chromatin transcribed by RNA polymerase II. Mol Cell Biol 15:4562–4571.

58. Ben-David Y, Giddens EB, Letwin K, Bernstein A. 1991. Erythroleukemia induction by Friend murine leukemia virus: insertional activation of a new member of the *ets* gene family, *Fli-1*, closely linked to *c-ets-1*. Genes Dev 5:908–918.

59. Wasylyk B, Hohn SL, Giovane A. 1993. The Ets family of transcription factors. Eur J Biochem 211:7–18.

60. Gill S, McManus AP, Crew AJ, et al. 1995. Fusion of *EWS* gene to a DNA segment from 9q22–31 in a human myxoid chondrosarcoma. Genes Chromosom Cancer 12:307–310.

61. Paganopoulos I, Hoglund M, Mertens F, et al. 1996. Fusion of the *EWS* and *CHOP* genes in myxoid liposarcoma. Oncogene 12:489–494.

62. Rao VN, Ohno T, Prasad DDK, Bhattacharya G, Reddy ESP. 1993. Analysis of the DNA-binding and transcriptional activation functions of human FLI-1 protein. Oncogene 8:2167–2173.

63. Siddique H, Rao VN, Lee L, Reddy ESP. 1993. Characterization of the DNA binding and transcriptional activation domains of the erg protein. Oncogene 8:1751–1755.

64. Bailly RA, Bosselut R, Zucman J, et al. 1994. DNA-binding and transcriptional activation properties of the EWS-FLI-1 fusion protein resulting from the t(11;22) translocation in Ewing sarcoma. Mol Cell Biol 14:3230–3241.

65. May WA, Lessnick SL, Braun BS, et al. 1993. The Ewing's sarcoma EWS/FLI-1 funsion gene encodes a more potent transcriptional activator and is a more powerful transforming gene than FLI-1. Mol Cell Biol 13:7393–7398.

66. May WA, Gishizsky ML, Lessnick SL, et al. 1993. Ewing sarcoma 11;22 translocation produces a chimeric transcription factor that require the DNA-binding domain encoded by *FLI1* for transformation. Proc Natl Acad Sci USA 90:5852–5856.

67. Mao X, Miesfeldt S, Yang H, Leiden JM, Thompson CB. 1994. The FLI-1 and chimeric EWS-FLI-1 oncoprotein display similar DNA binding specificities. J Biol Chem 269:18216–18222.

68. Ohno T, Rao VN, Reddy ESP. 1993. EWS/Fli-1 chimeric protein is a transcriptional activator. Cancer Res 53:5859–5863.

69. Magnaghi-Jaulin L, Masutani H, Robin P, Lipinski M, Harel-Bellan A. 1996. SRE elements are binding sites for the fusion protein EWS-FLI-1. Nucleic Acids Res 24:1052–1058.

70. Denny CT. 1996. Gene rearrangements in Ewing's sarcoma. Cancer Invest 14:83–88.

71. Braun BS, Frieden R, Lessnick SL, May WA, Denny CT. 1995. Identification of target genes for the Ewing's sarcoma *EWS/FLI* fusion protein by representational difference analysis. Mol Cell Biol 15:4623–4630.

72. West D, Grier H, Swallow M, Demetri G, Granowetter L, Sklar J. 1997. Detection of circulating tumor cells in patients with Ewing's sarcoma and peripheral primitive neuroectodermal tumor. J Clin Oncol 15:583–588.

73. Peter M, Magdelenat H, Michon J, et al. 1995. Sensitive detection of occult Ewing's cells by the reverse transcriptase-polymerase chain reaction. Br J Cancer 72:96–100.

74. Ouchida M, Ohno T, Fujimura Y, Rao VN, Reddy ESP. 1995. Loss of tumorigenicity of Ewing's sarcoma cells expressing antisense RNA to EWS-fusion transcripts. Oncogene 11:1049–1054.

75. Wilkins RM, Pritchard DJ, Burgert EO, Unni KK. 1986. Ewing's sarcoma of bone. Experience with 140 patients. Cancer 58:2551–2555.

76. Nesbit ME, Gehan EA, Burgert O, et al. 1990. Multimodal therapy for the management of primary nonmetastatic Ewing's sarcoma of bone: a long-term follow-up of the First Intergroup Study. J Clin Oncol 8:1664–1674.

77. Grubb MR, Currier BL, Pritchard DJ, et al. 1994. Primary Ewing's sarcoma of the spine. Spine 19:309–313.
78. Ozaki T, Lindner N, Hoffman, et al. 1995. Ewing's sarcoma of ribs. A report from the Cooperative Ewing's Sarcoma Study. Eur J Cancer 31A:2284–2288.
79. Sirvent N, Kanolds J, Levy C, et al. 1996. Non-metastatic Ewing's sarcoma family of tumors of the ribs: experience of the French Society of Pediatric Oncology (SFOP) in 55 patients (abstract). Med Pediatr Oncol 27:261.
80. Trigg ME, Makuch R, Glaubiger D. 1985. Actuarial risk of isolated CNS involvement in Ewing's sarcoma following prophylactic cranial irradiation and intrathecal methotrexate. Int J Radiat Oncol Biol Phys 11:699–702.
81. Evans RG, Nesbit ME, Gehan EA, et al. 1991. Multimodal therapy for the management of localized Ewing's sarcoma of pelvic and sacral bones: a report from the second Intergroup Study. J Clin Oncol 7:1173–1180.
82. Evans R, Nesbit M, Askin F, et al. 1985. Local recurrence, rate and sites of metastases and time to relapse as a function of treatment regimens, size of the primary and surgical history in 62 patients presenting with non-metastatic Ewing's sarcoma of the pelvic bones. Int J Radiat Oncol Biol Phys 11:129–136.
83. Hayes FA, Thompson EI, Meyer WH, et al. 1989. Therapy for localized Ewing's sarcoma of bone. J Clin Oncol 7:208–213.
84. Glaubiger DL, Makuch RW, Schwarz J. 1980. Determination of prognostic factors and their influence on therapeutic results in patients with Ewing's sarcoma. Cancer 45:2213–2219.
85. Bacci G, Avella M, McDonald D, Toni A, Orlandi M, Campanacci M. 1988. Serum lactate dehydrogenase (LDH) as a tumor marker in Ewing's sarcoma. Tumori 74:649–655.
86. Dunst J, Sauer R, Burgers JMV, et al. 1991. Radiation therapy as local treatment in Ewing's sarcoma: results of the cooperative Ewing's sarcoma studies CESS 81 and 86. Cancer 67:2818–2825.
87. Mendenhall CM, Marcus RB Jr, Enneking WF, Springfield DS, Thar TL, Million RR. 1983. The prognostic significance of soft tissue extension in Ewing's sarcoma. Cancer 51:913–917.
88. Schmidt D, Hermann C, Jurgens H, Hanns D. 1991. Malignant peripheral neuroectodermal tumor and its necessary distinction from Ewing's sarcoma: a report from the Kiel pediatric tumor registry. Cancer 68:2251–2259.
89. Hartman KR, Triche TJ, Kinsella TJ, Miser JS. 1991. Prognostic value of histopathology in Ewing sarcoma — long term follow-up of distal extremity primary tumors. Cancer 67:163–171.
90. Terrier PH, Henry-Amar M, Triche T, et al. 1995. Is neuroectodermal differentiation of Ewing's sarcoma of bone associated with an unfavorable prognosis? Eur J Cancer 31A:307–414.
91. Oberlin O, Patte C, Demeococq F, et al. 1985. The response to initial chemotherapy as a prognostic factor in localized Ewing's sarcoma. Eur J Cancer 21:463–467.
92. Picci P, Rougaff BT, Bacci JR, et al. 1993. Prognostic significance of histopathologic response to chemotherapy in nonmetastatic Ewing's sarcoma of the extremities. J Clin Oncol 11:1763–1769.
93. Kinsella TJ, Miser JS, Waller B, et al. 1991. Long-term follow-up of Ewing's sarcoma of bone treated with combined modality therapy. Int J Radiat Oncol Biol Phys 20:389–395.
94. Primary malignant bone tumors. In Greenfield GB, Arrington JA (eds.), Imaging of Bone Tumors: A Multidisciplinary Approach. Philadelphia: JB Lippincott.
95. Williams MP, Husband JE, Mc Elwain TJ. 1989. Role of computed tomography scanning in the management of Ewing's sarcoma. Med Pediatr Oncol 17:414–417.
96. Boyko OB, Cory DA, Cohen MD, Proviser A, Mirkin D, DeRosa GP. 1987. MRI imaging of osteogenic and Ewing's sarcoma. Am J Radiol 148:317–322.
97. Estes DN, Magill LH, Thompson EI, Hayes FA. 1990. Primary Ewing sarcoma: follow-up with Ga-67 scintigraphy. Radiology 177:449–553.
98. Ramanna L, Waxman A, Binney G, Waxman S, Mirra J, Rosen G. 1990. Thallium-210

scintigraphy in bone sarcoma: comparison with gallium-67 and technetium-MDP in the evaluation of chemotherapeutic response. Radiology 175:791–796.

99. Shamberger RC, Tarbell NJ, Perez-Atayde A, Grier HE. 1994. Malignant small round cell tumor (Ewing's–PNET) of the chest wall in children. J Pediatr Surg 29:179–196.

100. Rao BN, Hayes FA, Thompason EI, et al. 1995. Chest wall resection for Ewing's sarcoma of the rib: an unnecessary procedure. 1988. Updated in 1995. Ann Thorac Surg 60:1454–1455.

101. Hoffer FA, Gianturco LE, Fletcher JA, Grier HE. 1994. Percutaneous biopsy of peripheral primitive neuroectodermal tumors and Ewing's sarcomas for cytogenetic analysis. AJR 162:1141–1142.

102. Kronberger M, Mostbeck G, Zoubek A, et al. 1996. Extended pretherapeutic staging by total-bone MRI and PCR analysis of bone marrow in patients with Ewing tumors (abstract). Med Pediatr Oncol 27:237.

103. Oberlin O, Bayle C, Hartmann O, Terrier-Lacombe MJ, Lemerle J. 1995 Incidence of bone marrow involvement in Ewing's sarcoma: value of extensive investigation of the bone marrow. Med Pediatr Oncol. 24:343–6.

104. Holscher HC, Bloem JL, Nooy MA, et al. 1990. The value of MR imaging in monitoring the effect of chemotherapy on bone sarcomas. AJR 154:763–769.

105. Erlemann R, Sciuk J, Bosse A, et al. 1990. Response of osteosarcoma and Ewing sarcoma to preoperative chemotherapy: assessment with dynamic and static MRF imaging and skeletal scintography. J Nucl Med 31:567–572.

106. Golfieri R, Baddeley H, Pringle JS, Leung AWL, Greco A, Siouihami R. 1991. MRI in primary bone tumors: therapeutic implications. J Radiol 12:201–207.

107. Ravindranath Y, Dicarli M, Abella E, et al. 1996. Positron emission tomography (PET) scanning with [18]fluorodeoxyglucose (FDG), correlates with histological response in children with osteosarcoma (OS) and Ewing's sarcoma (ES) (abstract). Med Pediatr Oncol 22:244.

108. Wang CC, Schultz MD. 1953. Ewing's sarcoma. N Engl J Med 248:571–576.

109. Philips RE, Higinbotham NL. 1967. The curability of Ewing's endothelioma of bone in children. J Pediatr 70:391–397.

110. Hustu HO, Holton C, James D Jr, Pinkel D. 1968. Treatment of Ewing's sarcoma with concurrent radiotherapy and chemotherapy. J Pediatr 73:249–251.

111. Johnson RE, Pomeroy TC. 1972. Integrated therapy for Ewing's sarcoma. Radiology 114:532–535.

112. Rosen G, Wollner N, Tan C, et al. 1974. Disease-free survival in children with Ewing's sarcoma treated with radiation therapy and adjuvant four-drug sequential chemotherapy. Cancer 33:384–393.

113. Samuels MI, Howe CD. 1967. Cyclophosphamide in the management of Ewing's sarcoma. Cancer 20:961–966.

114. Haggard ME. 1967. Cyclophosphamide (NSC-2627) in the treatment of children with malignant neoplasms. Cancer Chemother Rep 51:403–405.

115. Sutow WW, Sullivan MP. 1962. Cyclophosphamide in children with Ewing's sarcoma. Cancer. Chemother Rep 23:55–60.

116. Finkelstein JZ, Hittle RE, Hammond D. 1969. Evaluation of a high dose cyclophosphamide regimen in childhood tumors. Cancer 23:1239–1242.

117. Goepert H, Rochlin DB, Smart CR. 1967. Palliative treatment of Ewing's sarcoma. Am J Surg 113:246–250.

118. Pinkel D. 1962. Cyclophosphamide in children with cancer. Cancer 15:42–49.

119. Stutow WW, Vietti TJ, Fernbach DJ, Lane DM, Donaldson MH, Lonsdale D. 1971. Evaluation of chemotherapy in children with metastatic Ewing's sarcoma and osteogenic sarcoma. Cancer Chemother Rep 55:67–78.

120. Scheulen ME, Niederle N, Bremer K, et al. 1983. Efficacy of ifosfamide in refractory malignant disease and uroprotection by mesna: results of a clinical phase II study with 151 patients. Cancer Treat Rev 10 (Suppl A):93–101.

121. Antman KH, Montella D, Rosenbaum C, Schwen M. 1985. Phase II trial of ifosfamide with mesna in previously treated metastatic sarcoma. Cancer Treat Rep 69:499–504.

122. Magrath IT, Sandlund JT, Raynor A, Rosenberg S, Arasi V, Miser J. 1986. A phase II study of ifosfamide in the treatment of recurrent sarcomas in young people. Cancer Chemother Pharmacol 18 (Suppl):S25–S28.

123. Pratt CB, Douglass EC, Etcubanas EL, et al. 1989. Ifosfamide in pediatric malignant solid tumors. Cancer Chemother Pharmacol 24 (Suppl):S24–S27.

124. Sutow WW. 1968. Vincristine (NSC-67574) therapy for malignant solid tumors in children (except Wilms' tumor). Cancer Chemother Rep 52:485–487.

125. James DH, George P. 1964. Vincristine in children with malignant solid tumors. J Pediatr 64:534–541.

126. Selawry OS, Holland JF, Wolman IJ. 1968. Effect of vincristine (NSC-67574) on malignant solid tumors in children. Cancer Chemother Rep 52:497–500.

127. Chard RL, Krivit W, Bleyer WA, Hammond D. 1979. Phase II study of VP-16-213 in childhood malignant disease: a Children's Cancer Study Group Report. Cancer Treat Rep 63:1755–1759.

128. O'Dwyer PJ, Leyland-Jones C, Alonso MT, Marsoni S, Wittes RE. 1985. Etoposide (VP-16-213). Current status of an active anticancer drug. N Engl J Med 312:692–700.

129. Humphrey EW, Hymes AC, Ausman RK, Ferguson DJ. 1961. An evaluation of actinomycin D and mitomycin C in patients with advanced cancer. Surgery 50:881–885.

130. Senyszyn JJ, Johnson RE, Curran RE. 1970. Treatment of metastatic Ewing's sarcoma with actinomycin D (NSC-3053). Cancer Chemother Rep 54:103–107.

131. Krivit W, Bentley HP. 1960. Use of 5-fluorouracil in the management of advanced malignancies in childhood. Am J Dis Child 100:217–227.

132. Cangir A, Vietti TJ, Gehan EA, Burgert OE, Thomas P, et al. 1990. Ewing's sarcoma metastatic at diagnosis: results and comparisons of two intergroup Ewing's sarcoma studies. Cancer 66:887–893.

133. Kinsella TJ, Miser JS, Waller B, et al. 1991. Long-term follow-up of Ewing's sarcoma of bone treated with combined modality therapy. Int J Radiat Oncol Biol Phys 20:389–395.

134. Burgert O, Nesbitt ME, Garnsey LA, et al. 1990. Multimodal therapy for the management of nonpelvic, localized Ewing's sarcoma of bone: Intergroup study IESS-II. J Clin Oncol 8:1514–1524.

135. Smith MA. 1991. The impact of doxorubicin dose intensity on survival of patients with Ewing's sarcoma. J Clin Oncol 9:889–891.

136. Jurgens H, Exner U, Gadner H, et al. 1988. Multidisciplinary treatment of primary Ewing sarcoma of bone: a 6-year experience of a European Cooperative Trial. Cancer 61:23–32.

137. Dunst J, Jurgens H, Sauer R, Pape H, Paulussen M, Winkelmann W, Rube C. 1995. Radiation therapy in Ewing's sarcoma: an update of the CESS 86 Trial. Int J Radiat Oncol Biol Phys 32:919–930.

138. Bacci G, Toni A, Avella M, et al. 1989. Long term results in 144 localized Ewing's sarcoma patients treated with combined therapy. Cancer 63:1477–1486.

139. Ortega JA, Wharam M, Gehan EA, et al. 1991. Clinical features and results of therapy for children with paraspinal soft tissue sarcoma: a report of the Intergroup Rhabdomyosarcoma Study. J Clin Oncol 9:796–801.

140. Raney BR, Asmar L, Newton WA, et al. 1997. Ewing's sarcoma of soft tissues in childhood; a report from the Intergroup Rhabdomyosarcoma Study 1972–1991. J Clin Oncol 15:574–582.

141. Oberlin O, Patte C, Demeococq F, et al. 1985. The response to initial chemotherapy as a prognostic factor in localized Ewing's sarcoma. Eur J Cancer Clin Oncol 21:463–467.

142. Oberlin O, Habrand J-L, Zucker JM, et al. 1992–••. No benefit of Ifosfamide in Ewing's sarcoma: a nonrandomized study of the French Society of Pediatric Oncology. J Clin Oncol 10:1407–1412.

143. Wexler LH, DeLaney TF, Tsokos M, Avila N, Steinberg SM, Weaver-McClure L, Jacobson J, Jaronski P, Hijazi YM, Balis FM, Horowitz ME. 1996. Ifosfamide and etoposide plus

vincristine, doxorubicin, and cyclophosphamide for newly diagnosed Ewing's sarcoma family of tumors. Cancer 78:901–911.

144. Rosen G, Capparros B, Nirenberg A, Marcove RC, Huvos AG, Kosloff C, Lane J, Murphy ML. 1981. Ewing's sarcoma: ten-year experience with adjuvant chemotherapy. Cancer 47:2204–2213.

145. Miser JS, Kinsella TJ, Triche TJ, et al. 1988. Preliminary results of treatment of Ewing's sarcoma of bone in children and young adults: six months of intensive combined modality therapy without maintenance. J Clin Oncol 6:484–490.

146. Kushner BH, Meyers PA, Gerald WL, et al. Very-high dose short-term chemotherapy for poor-risk peripheral primitive neuroectodermal tumors, including Ewing's sarcoma, in children and young adults. J Clin Oncol 13:2796–2804.

147. Kushner BH, Hajdu SI, Gulati S, et al. 1991. Extracranial primitive neuroectodermal tumors. The Memorial Sloan-Kettering Cancer experience. Cancer 67:1825–1829.

148. Marina NM, Etcubanas E, Parham DM, Bowman LC, Green A. 1989. Peripheral primitive neuroectodermal tumor (peripheral neuroepithelioma) in children. A review of the St. Jude experience and controversies in diagnosis and management. Cancer 64:1952–1960.

149. Gururangan S, Marina N, Luo X, et al. 1994. Improved outcome for patients with peripheral neuroepithelioma (PN) (abstract). Proc Am Soc Clin Oncol 13:418.

150. Miser JS, Kinsella TJ, Triche TJ, et al. 1987. Treatment of peripheral neuroepithelioma in children and young adults. J Clin Oncol 5:1752–1758.

151. Jurgens H, Bier V, Harma D, et al. 1988. Malignant peripheral neuroectodermal tumors: a retrospective analysis of 42 patients. Cancer 61:349–357.

152. Hayes FA, Thompson EI, Parvey L, et al. 1987. Metastatic Ewing's sarcoma: remission induction and survival. J Clin Oncol 5:1199–1204.

153. Jenkin RD, Rider WD, Sonley MJ. 1970. Ewing's sarcoma: a trial of total body irradiation. Radiology 96:151–155.

154. Lombardi F, Lattuada A, Gasparini M, Gianni C, Marchesini R. 1982. Sequential half-body irradiation as systemic treatment of progressive Ewing sarcoma. Int J Radiat Oncol Biol Phys 8:1679–1682.

155. Berry MP, Jenkin RD, Harwood AR, et al. 1986. Ewing's sarcoma: a trial of adjuvant chemotherapy and sequential half-body irradiation. Int J Radiat Oncol Biol Phys 12:19–24.

156. Dunst J, Paulussen M, Jurgens H. 1993. Lung irradiation for Ewing's sarcoma with pulmonary metastases at diagnosis: results of the CESS-studies. Strahlenther Onkol 169:621–623.

157. Lanza LA, Miser JA, Pass HI, Roth JA. 1987. The role of resection in the treatment of pulmonary metastases from Ewing's sarcoma. J Thorac Cardiovasc Surg 94:181–187.

158. Heji HA, Vos A, de Kraker J, Voute PA. 1994. Prognostic factors in surgery for pulmonary metastases in children. Surgery 115:687–693.

159. Temeck BK, Wexler LA, Steinberg SM, McClure LL, Horowitz M, Pass HI. 1995. Metastatectomy for sarcomatous histologies: results and prognostic factors. Ann Thorac Surg 59:1385–1390.

160. Hugenholz EAL, Piers Da, Kamps WA, et al. 1994. Bone scintigraphy in nonsurgically treated Ewing's sarcoma at diagnosis and follow-up: prognostic information of the primary tumor site. Med Pediatr Oncol 22:236–239.

161. Miser JS, Kinsella TJ, Triche TJ, et al. 1987. Ifosfamide with mesna uroprotection and etoposide: an effctive regimen in the treatment of recurrent sarcomas and other tumors of children and young adults. J Clin Oncol 5:1191–1198.

162. Kung FH, Pratt CB, Vega RA, et al. 1993. Ifosfamide/etoposide combination in the treatment of recurrent malignant solid tumors of childhood. A Pediatric Oncology Group Phase II Study. Cancer 71:1898–1902.

163. Burdach S, Jurgens H, Peters C, Nurnberger W, Mauz-Korholz C, Korholz D, Paulussen M, Pape H, Dillo D, Koscielniak E, Gadner H, Gobel U. 1993. Myeloablative radiochemotherapy and hematopoietic stem-cell rescue in poor-prognosis Ewing's sarcoma. J Clin Oncol 11:1482–1488.

164. Valteau-Couanet D, Michon J, Plouvier M, et al. 1996. Treatment of metastatic Ewing's sarcomas (ES) with busulfan and melphalan consolidation chemotherapy (HDCT). A study of the French Society of Pediatric Oncology (SFOP) (abstract). Med Pediatr Oncol 27:238.

165. Ladenstein R, Peters C, Zoubek A, et al. 1996. The role of megatherapy (MGT) followed by stem cell rescue (SCR) in high risk Ewing tumors (ET). 11 Years single center experience (abstract). Med Pediatr Oncol 27:237.

166. Ladenstein R, Lasset C, Pinkerton R, et al. 1995. Impact of megatherapy in children with high-risk Ewing's tumours in complete remission: a report from the EBMT solid tumour registry. Bone Marrow Transplant 15:697–705.

167. Horowitz ME, Neff JR, Kun LE. 1991. Ewing's sarcoma. Radiotherapy versus surgery for local control. Pediatr Clin North Am 38:365–380.

168. Marcus RB. 1996. Current controversies in pediatric radiation oncology. Orthoped Clin North Am 27:551–557.

169. Arai Y, Kun L, Brooks T, et al. 1991. Ewing's sarcoma: local tumor control and patterns of failure following limited-volume radiation therapy. Int J Radiat Oncol Biol Phys 21:1501–1508.

170. Razek A, Perez C, Tefft M, et al. 1980. Intergroup Ewing's sarcoma study. Local control related to radiation dose, volume, and site of primary lesion in Ewing's sarcoma. Cancer 46:516–521.

171. Tefft M, Razek A, Perez C, et al. 1978. Local control and survival related to radiation dose and volume and to chemotherapy in non-metastatic Ewing's sarcoma of pelvic bones. Int J Radiat Oncol Biol Phys 4:367–372.

172. Barbieri E, Emiliani E, Zini G, et al. 1990. Combined therapy of localized Ewing's sarcoma of bone: analysis of results in 100 patients. Int J Radiat Oncol Biol Phys 119:1165–1170.

173. Sailer SL, Harmon DC, Mankin HJ, et al. 1988. Ewing's sarcoma: surgical resection as a prognostic factor. Int J Radiat Oncol Biol Phys 15:43–52.

174. Ozaki T, Hillman A, Hoffman C, et al. 1996. Significance of surgical margin on the prognosis of patients with Ewing's sarcoma. A report from the Cooperative Ewing's sarcoma study. Cancer 78:892–900.

175. Terek RM, Brien EW, Marcove RC, Meyers PA, Lane JM, Healey JH. 1996. Treatment of femoral Ewing's sarcoma. Cancer 78:70–78.

176. Li WK, Lane JM, Rosen G, et al. 1983. Pelvic Ewing's sarcoma. Advances in treatment. J Bone Joint Surg 65A:738–747.

177. Frassica FJ, Frassica DA, Pritchard DJ, et al. 1993. Ewing sarcoma of the pelvis. J Bone Joint Surg 75A:1457–1465.

178. Bacci G, Picci P, Gitelis S, et al. 1982. The treatment of localized Ewing's sarcoma. Cancer 49:1561–1570.

179. Scully SP, Temple HT, Keefe RJ, et al. 1995. The role of surgical resection in pelvic Ewing's sarcoma. J Clin Oncol 13:2336–2341.

180. Marcus RB Jr, Cantor A, Heare TC, et al. 1991. Local control and function after twice-a-day radiotherapy for Ewing's sarcoma of bone. Int J Radiat Oncol Biol Phys 21:1509–1515.

181. Donaldson S, Shuster J, Andreozzi C, et al. 1989. The Pediatric Group (POG) experience in Ewing's sarcoma of bone (abstract). Med Pediatr Oncol 17:283.

182. Donaldson S, personal communication.

183. Bolek TW, Marcus RB Jr, Mendenhall NP, Scarborough MT, Graham-Ple J. 1996. Local control and functional results after twice daily radiotherapy for Ewing's sarcoma of the extremities. Int J Radiat Oncol Biol Phys 35:687–692.

184. Mankin HF, Lange TA, Spanier SS. 1982. The hazards of biopsy in patients with malignant primary bone and soft tissue tumors. J Bone Joint Surg 68:1121–1127.

185. Thomas PRM, Perez CA, Neff JR. 1984. The management of Ewing's sarcoma: role of radiotherapy in local tumor control. Cancer Treat Rep 68:703–710.

186. Jentzsh K, Binder H, Cramer H, et al. 1981. Leg function after radiotherapy for Ewing's sarcoma. Cancer 47:1267–1278.

187. Nicholson SH, Mulvihill JJ, Byrne J. 1992. Late effects of therapy in adult survivors of osteosarcoma and Ewing's sarcoma. Med Pediatr Oncol 20:6–12.

188. Strong LC, Herson J, Osborne BM, Sutow WW. 1979. Risk of radiation-related subsequent neoplasms in survivors of Ewing's sarcoma. J Natl Cancer Inst 62:1401–1406.

189. Hawkins MM, Draper GJ, Kingston JE. 1987. Incidence of second primary tumors among childhood cancer survivors. Br J Cancer 56:339–347.

190. Hawkins MM, Kinnier Wilson LM, Burton HS, et al. 1996. Radiotherapy, alkylating agents, and risk of bone cancer after childhood cancer. J Natl Cancer Inst 88:270–278.

191. Travis LB, Curtis RE, Hankey BF, Fraumeni JF. 1994. Letter to the Editor: second cancers in patients with Ewing's sarcoma. Med Pediatr Oncol 22:296–297.

192. Smith LM, Cox RS, Donalson SS. 1992. Second cancers in long-term survivors of Ewing's sarcoma. Clin Orthoped 275–281.

193. Kuttesh JF Jr, Wexler LE, Marcus RB, et al. 1996. Second malignancies after Ewing's sarcoma: radiation dose-dependency of secondary sarcomas. J Clin Oncol 14:2818–2825.

194. Winick NJ, McKenna RW, Shuster JJ, et al. 1993. Secondary acute myeloid leukemia in children with acute lymphoblastic leukemia treated with etoposide. J Clin Oncol 111:209–217.

195. Pui C, Behm FG, Raimondi SC, et al. 1989. Secondary leukemia in children treated for acute lymphoid leukemia. N Engl J Med 321:136–142.

196. Zucman J, Delattre O, Demaze C, et al. 1993. *EWS* and *ATF-1* gene fusion induced by t(12;22) translocation in malignant melanoma of soft parts. Nature Geneti 4:341–345.

197. Oldham RK, Pomeroy TC. 1972. Treatment of Ewing's sarcoma with Adriamycin (NSC-123127). Cancer Chemother Rep 56:635–639.

198. Evan AE, Baehner RL, Chard RL, et al. 1974. Comparison of daunorubicin (NSC 83142) with Adriamycin (NSC-123127) in the treatment of late stage childhood solid tumors. Cancer Chemother Rep 58:671–676.

199. Pratt CB, Shanks EC. 1974. Doxorubicin in treatment of malignant solid tumors in children. Am J Dis Child 127:534–536.

200. Bonnadonna G, Beretta G, Tancici G, et al. 1975. Adriamycin (NSC-123127) studies at the Instituto Nazionale Tumori, Milan. Cancer Chemother Rep 6:231–245.

201. Ragab AH, Sutow WW, Komp DM, Starling KA, Lyon GM Jr, George S. 1975. Adriamycin in the treatment of childhood solid tumors. Cancer 36:1567–1571.

202. Tan CTC, Rosen G, Ghavimi F, et al. 1975. Adriamycin (NSC-123127) in pediatric malignancies. Cancer Chemother Rep 6:259–266.

203. Wang J, Holland JF, Sinks LF. 1975. Phase II study of Adriamycin (NSC 123127) in childhood solid tumors. Cancer Chemother Rep 6:267–270.

204. Haggard ME, Cangir A, Ragab AH, et al. 1977. 5-Fluoruracil in childhood tumors. Cancer Treat Rep 61:69–71.

205. Palma J, Gakan S, Freeman A, Sinks L, Holland JF. 1972. Treatment of metastatic Ewing's sarcoma with BCNU. Cancer 30:909–913.

206. Kamalaker P, Freeman AI, Higby DJ, Wallace HJ Jr, Sinks L. 1977. Clinical response and toxicity with cisdichlorodiammineplatinum (III) in children. Cancer Treat Rep 61:835–839.

207. Baum ES, Gaynon P, Greenberg L, Krivit W, Hammond D. 1981. Phase II trial of cisplatin in refractory childhood cancer: Children's Cancer Study Group Report. Cancer Treat Rep 65:815–822.

208. Meyer WH, Kun L, Marina N, et al. 1992. Ifosfamide and etoposide in newly diagnosed Ewing's sarcoma of bone. J Clin Oncol 10:1737–1742.

209. Van Hoff J, Grier HE, Douglass EC, Green DM. 1995. Etoposide, ifosfamide, and cisplatin therapy for refractory childhood solid tumors. Cancer 75:2966–2970.

210. Cornbleet MA, Corringham RET, Prentice HG, Boesen EM, McElwain TJ. 1981. Treatment of Ewing's sarcoma with high-dose melphalan and autologous bone marrow transplantation. Cancer Treat Rep 65:241–244.

211. Kinsella TJ, Glaubiger D, Diesseroth A, et al. 1983. Intensive combined modality therapy

307

including low-dose TBI in high-risk Ewing's sarcoma patients. Radiat Oncol Biol Phys 9:1955–1960.

212. Graham-Pole J, Coccia P, Lazarus HM, Weiner R, Herzig RH, Strandjord S, Gross S. 1984. High-dose melphalan therapy for the treatment of children with refractory neuroblastoma and Ewing's sarcoma. Am J Pediatr Hematol Oncol 6:17–26.

213. Saarinen UM, Hovi L, Makipernaa, Riikonen P. 1991. High-dose thioptepa with autologous bone marrow rescue in pediatric solid tumors. Bone Marrow Transplant 8:369–376.

214. Graham ML, Yeager AM, Leventhal BG, et al. 1992. Treatment of recurrent and refractory pediatric solid tumors with high-dose busulfan and cyclophosphamide followed by autologous bone marrow rescue. J Clin Oncol 10:1857–1864.

215. Bader JL, Horowitz ME, Dewan R, et al. 1989. Intensive combined modality therapy of small round cell and undifferentiated sarcomas in children and young adults: local control and patterns of failure. Radiother Oncol 16:189–201.

216. Horowitz ME, Kinsella TJ, Wexler LH, et al. 1993. Total-body irradiation and autologous bone marrow transplant in the treatment of high-risk Ewing's sarcoma and rhabdomyosarcoma. J Clin Oncol 11:1911–1918.

217. Meyers PA, Gardner S, Lindsley K, Leibel S, Kushner B. 1995. High-risk Ewing's sarcoma (ES)/primitive neuroectodermal tumor (PNET) of bone: consolidation with total body irradiation (TBI), melphalan, and autologous stem cell reconstitution (abstract). Proc Am Soc Clin Oncol 14:451.

308

10. Rhabdomyosarcoma: biology and therapy

Alberto S. Pappo and David N. Shapiro

1. Introduction

Rhabdomyosarcoma, a malignant tumor of skeletal muscle, is the most common soft tissue sarcoma in people younger than 21 years, accounting for 5% to 8% of all cases of childhood cancer [1,2]. The traditional histologic classification scheme for rhabdomyosarcoma is primarily based on the degree of resemblance to normal fetal skeletal muscle prior to innervation [3]. These tumors are classified into two broad histiotypes, namely, embryonal and alveolar, that each have characteristic pathologic, cytogenetic, and clinical features [4]. Embryonal rhabdomyosarcomas occur in young children and account for approximately 60% of the cases; the primary tumor is usually located in specific anatomic sites, including the head and neck region, genitourinary tract, and orbit. The tumor is characterized by histologically variable numbers of malignant spindle and primitive round cells that may contain the cross-striations typical of skeletal muscle. By contrast, alveolar rhabdomyosarcomas often occur during adolescence as primary tumors of the extremities or trunk. This histologic variant is characterized by the presence of fibrovascular septa that form alveolar-like spaces filled with primitive, poorly cohesive, monomorphous, malignant cells. Patients with tumors of alveolar histology are generally considered to have a poorer clinical prognosis than do those with embryonal rhabdomyosarcomas [5].

2. Biology and genetics

Recent studies characterizing the complex genetic program controlling normal skeletal muscle development and efforts toward the molecular characterization of tumor-specific cytogenetic alterations have substantially improved our understanding of rhabdomyosarcoma tumorigenesis. Although rhabdomyoblasts share many structural features with their normal skeletal muscle counterparts, the presence of specific genetic lesions leads to the altered growth and behavioral characteristics of these tumors. The results of these investigations, discussed below, will yield important diagnostic tools for improving the classi-

D.O. Walterhouse and S.L. Cohn (eds), DIAGNOSTIC AND THERAPEUTIC ADVANCES IN PEDIATRIC ONCOLOGY. Copyright © 1997. Kluwer Academic Publishers, Boston. All rights reserved.

fication scheme for this tumor, facilitate the sensitive and specific detection of residual disease, and offer the possibility of novel therapeutic interventions designed to target tumor-specific gene products.

2.1. Biology

Consistent with their origin from skeletal muscle precursors, rhabdomyosarcomas share patterns of expression of muscle-specific genes with their normal cognate tissue, fetal skeletal muscle. For example, rhabdomyosarcomas express transcripts for the MyoD family of muscle-specific regulatory factors [6–8]. Members of the MyoD family (MyoD [*MYF3*], myogenin [*MYF4*], *MYF5*, and herculin) have a conserved basic helix–loop–helix (HLH) motif that mediates DNA binding, protein dimerization, and transcriptional activity [9]. These muscle-specific transcription factors are sufficient to orchestrate skeletal myogenesis and directly regulate expression of essential skeletal muscle-specific structural genes [10]. Further, expression of MyoD family members is considered to be consistent with commitment to the myogenic lineage and therefore is a useful marker of skeletal muscle precursors. Expression of MyoD transcripts has been demonstrated repeated in all rhabdomyosarcomas examined; occasionally, myogenin, *MYF5*, and herculin are also expressed [11–14]. Interestingly, recent data have suggested that endogenous MyoD protein is only a weak transcriptional activator in rhabdomyosarcoma, perhaps due to a deficiency of a cooperating factor in the tumor cells [15]. Although no correlation between tumor histology and the expression pattern of these transcription factors has been reported, their restricted expression to cells of myogenic lineage has proven to be a useful adjunct in the pathologic diagnosis of rhabdomyosarcoma and in the differentiation of these tumors from other primitive pediatric neoplasms [16].

2.2. Genetics

Cytogenetic analysis has become increasingly important for the characterization of childhood tumors and has provided a reliable means of grouping dissimilar forms of the same disease. The results of more than 60 detailed cytogenetic studies of rhabdomyosarcomas have been reported; approximately two thirds of the cases were alveolar in histology. Chromosomal abnormalities were demonstrated in both embryonal and alveolar tumors [17–24]. Importantly, several chromosomal regions appear to show nonrandom involvement in specific structural rearrangements, allowing the positional cloning of important genes adjacent to these breakpoints.

In 1982, the characteristic chromosomal translocation t(2;13)(q35;q14) was first described in alveolar rhabdomyosarcoma [25]. Subsequent studies have confirmed the presence of this translocation in more than 70% of the successfully karyotyped alveolar rhabdomyosarcomas, and it is now considered spe-

310

cific for tumors of this histology [20]. A less frequent variant abnormality, t(1;13)(p36;q14), has also been described and occurs in 10% to 15% of alveolar tumors [20,23,24]. This translocation involves a cytogenetically indistinguishable region on chromosome 13q14. The pathologic and clinical features of patients with the t(1;13) may differ from those of children with the more common t(2;13), since these patients with the t(1;13) tend to be younger and their tumors more often involve extremity sites [26].

As determined by flow cytometry, approximately two thirds of alveolar tumors have near-tetraploid DNA content. The remaining cases are usually diploid [20,23,24,27–32]. This result is not unexpected because karyotypic evidence supports the development of tetraploidy by endoreduplication of a primary diploid tumor line [17]. Interestingly, near-tetraploidy is almost never observed in embryonal rhabdomyosarcomas; it is apparently pathognomonic for tumors of alveolar histology [28].

Various chromosomal abnormalities have been reported for embryonal rhabdomyosarcoma, including deletion of chromosome 1p with hyperdiploidy, trisomy 2; and ring chromosome 13 [19,20,33–38]. The complexity and variety of these cytogenetic abnormalities argue against the nonrandom, karyotypically apparent structural rearrangements seen in alveolar tumors. However, characteristic ploidy patterns have been noted with embryonal tumors. These studies have shown that about two thirds of embryonal rhabdomyosarcomas have hyperidiploid DNA content; the remainder are usually diploid [28–32]. Of potential importance, these investigations have also shown that diploid embryonal rhabdomyosarcomas frequently respond poorly to standard chemotherapeutic regimens.

Identification of the genes disrupted by the t(2;13) breakpoint relied upon somatic cell hybrid mapping studies, which place the candidate *PAX3* gene within the same region of chromosome 2q as the breakpoint [39,40]. *PAX3* is a member of a large superfamily of developmental control genes that encode transcription factors containing a characteristic DNA-binding domain, termed the *paired box* [41]. The paired box was first found in three *Drosophila* segmentation genes and subsequently was detected in mouse, human, nematode, zebrafish, and chick genomes [42–45]. Cloning and analysis of the murine homologue, *Pax-3*, revealed both a 128-amino-acid paired box and a 78-amino-acid paired-type homeodomain in the 5' half of the gene. Together, these regions are associated with coordinate, sequence-specific DNA binding activity [46]. *PAX3* structural rearrangements in alveolar rhabdomyosarcoma were then confirmed to be direct consequences of the tumor-specific translocation, which disrupts the gene downstream of the paired box and homeodomain. Fine-mapping showed that all rearrangements occur within the 20-kb intron between the last two *PAX3* exons. In all cases, these rearrangements result in translocation of the 5' region of *PAX3* to the tumor-derived der(13) chromosome and of the 3' region of *PAX3* to the tumor-derived der(2) chromosome. Interestingly, mutations (rather than translocations) of the *PAX3* paired box are found in patients with Waardenburg syndrome, a developmental disorder characterized by sensorineural deafness and pigmentary disturbances [47–52].

Isolation and characterization of cDNA clones has shown that the *PAX3* rearrangement leads to a novel chimeric gene comprising the 5′ *PAX3* sequences juxtaposed to 3′ sequences derived from a member of the forkhead family of transcription factors that is located on chromosome 13q14 (designated *ALV* or *FKHR*). This rearrangement creates an 836-amino-acid fusion protein (predicted molecular mass of 97 kDa) composed of the paired box and homeodomains from *PAX3* with the conserved forkhead DNA binding domain and the unique *FKHR* carboxyl-terminal region [53,54]. More than 40 forkhead genes have been identified among species ranging from yeast to human; all forkhead family members share a highly conserved 100-amino-acid motif, termed the *forkhead domain*, which has sequence-specific DNA binding activity [55–59]. Structural analysis of this domain has identified two potential helix-forming regions in the amino-terminal region and a basic region near the carboxyl terminal — features that are similar among members of the helix–loop–helix family of transcription factors [60,61]. Other regions of the protein confer potent transcription regulatory activity in several of the forkhead family members [62–64]. In addition, genetic and functional studies of forkhead genes have demonstrated their contributions to control of embryonic development and adult tissue-specific gene expression [65–68].

Based upon amino acid sequence homology within the DNA binding domain, *FKHR* is closely related to a group of forkhead-like genes including the *Drosophila fkh*, *slp-1*, and *slp-2* genes and the rat and human *BF1* genes [69–71]. Interestingly, *FKHR* shows the highest degree of identity with *AFX1*; this forkhead family member was recently identified fused in frame to *MLL* as the result of the t(X;11) in acute lymphoblastic leukemia [72]. Encoding a 655-amino-acid protein with a predicted molecular mass of 72 kDa, the 6.6-kb *FKHR* transcript is expressed in nearly all fetal and adult tissues.

Reverse transcriptase polymerase chain reactions (RT-PCR) and Northern analyses were performed on several independently derived alveolar rhabdomyosarcoma cell lines; all lines demonstrated the t(2;13). Chimeric transcripts arising from the der(13) chromosome were detected in all lines tested [53,54]. The uniform size of these transcripts suggests that the translocation breakpoints occur within equivalent introns of *PAX3* and *FKHR*. Sequence analysis has confirmed that the *PAX3* fragment (which is truncated after ASP[391]) is fused in frame to 3′ *FKHR* sequences.

The der(13) allele, which expresses the PAX3–FKHR fusion transcript, is most likely central to the etiology of alveolar rhabdomyosarcoma for several reasons. First, the reciprocal der(2) gene product lacks both the *PAX3* paired box and homeodomains. The paired box and homeodomains together seem to affect DNA binding specificity differently than does either domain alone [73–75]. Second, although both types of chimeric transcripts have been identified in many alveolar rhabdomyosarcoma cell lines, sensitive RT-PCR analysis failed to detect the der(2) transcript in other lines. These observations are consistent with Northern analyses of tumor cell RNA showing that the der(13) transcript is significantly more abundant in tumors expressing both chimeric transcripts. Finally, only the der(13)-derived 97-kDa fusion protein has been identified by immunoprecipitation [53]. Together, these data suggest that the der(13) encodes the protein product involved in tumorigenesis of alveolar rhabdomyosarcomas.

The PAX3–FKHR protein has several important structural features that may be important to its function. The avian retroviral oncogene *qin* and its human homologue recently were identified as forkhead family members, suggesting that under certain conditions, the mammalian forkhead genes may possess transforming activity [76,77]. In light of functional and structural studies demonstrating that the amino terminus of the forkhead domain is essential for DNA binding, the t(2;13) fusion protein (which contains only the carboxyl portion of the domain) is unlikely to contribute to sequence-specific DNA interactions [60,64]. However, the extreme carboxyl terminus of *FKHR* contains an acidic domain that may be important for protein function because this domain is similar to the transcriptional regulatory domains of other transcription factors such as AP-1 and JUN [78]. By contrast, retention of the intact *PAX3* paired box and homeodomain suggests that they contribute to the DNA binding specificity of the fusion protein. Further, the reported in vitro transforming potential of the PAX genes depends on the structural integrity of the paired domain and retention of its DNA-binding capacity [79]. Therefore, the fusion protein may bind normally to *PAX3* genomic targets but aberrantly activate or repress transcription by its action through novel *FKHR* 3′ regulatory sequences. This hypothesis has been confirmed in vitro and in vivo: t(2;13) fusion proteins can bind to and transcriptionally activate model *PAX3* binding sites in the absence of demonstrable contribution from the bisected *FKHR* domain [80,81]. Consistent with this observation, a potent transactivation domain located within the 60 carboxyl-terminal amino acids of the FKHR protein has been identified [80].

Alternatively, the t(2;13) may lead to activation of the oncogenic potential of *PAX3* and/or *FKHR* simply through increased protein levels. Perhaps translocation causes juxtaposition of FKHR sequences with positive regulatory elements (e.g., enhancers or RNA stabilization sequences). This hypothesis is consistent with expression of chimeric *PAX3–FKHR* transcripts in cells that lack normal *PAX3* transcripts, which could be generated from the unrearranged allele on chromosome 2. Conversely, expression of the chimeric protein could also be increased by elimination of *PAX3* 3′ negative regulatory elements. Data supporting either of these models of augmented chimeric protein expression are unavailable as yet.

Although the (2;13)(q35;q14) translocation has been found in most alveolar rhabdomyosarcomas, several cases that contain a variant (1;13)(p36;q14) translocation have been reported [20,23,24]. Similar to the consequences of the t(2;13), the t(1;13) fuses the *PAX7* gene on chromosome 1 to *FKHR* sequences on chromosome 13 [82]. This fusion results in a chimeric transcript encoding the *PAX7* paired box and homeodomain with the carboxyl terminal *FKHR* transactivation domain. The predicted amino acid sequences of the *PAX7* paired box are 94% homologous to the *PAX3* paired box, and the homeodomain of *PAX7* is 97% identical to that of *PAX3* [83]. This high degree of similarity suggests that the *PAX3* and *PAX7* DNA binding domains recognize very similar targets, perhaps regulating a common set of target genes important for rhabdomyosarcoma tumorigenesis.

The involvement of *PAX3* and *PAX7* in the t(2;13) and t(1;13) of alveolar rhabdomyosarcoma is similar to recent data concerning the t(11;22) and t(21;22) of Ewing's sarcoma and peripheral neuroepithelioma [84,85]. In these tumors, the amino-terminal portion of *EWS* is fused to carboxyl-terminal regions of *FLI1* or *ETS*, two members of the ETS family of transcription factors. However, by contrast with Ewing's sarcoma (in which both chimeric transcripts are expressed from the *EWS* promoter), the chimeric transcripts in alveolar rhabdomyosarcoma are expressed from either the *PAX3* or the *PAX7* promoter. In situ hybridization studies of mouse embryogenesis demonstrate that expression of *Pax-3* and *Pax-7* follows distinct but overlapping developmental patterns [46,86]. In addition to their expression in specific regions of the developing nervous system, both genes are expressed in somites around the time of dermomyotome formation. *Pax-3* expression occurs prior to myoblast migration and formation of the skeletal muscle precursors, but *Pax-7* expression begins a few days later and persists during differentiation of the trunk and limb musculature. Expression of *Pax-3* and *Pax-7* in skeletal muscle precursors is consistent with their activity in the development of alveolar rhabdomyosarcoma.

Although the genes involved in both of the most common alveolar rhabdomyosarcoma transloacations have been identified, further understanding of their specific mechanisms of transformation depends on finding their individual or shared targets. In this regard, the specific targets of both *PAX3* and *PAX7* are unknown, and optimal DNA recognition sequences mremain to be identified for most paired box and forkhead genes. Clearly, defining altered patterns of gene expression will be central to elucidating the pathways responsible for tumorigenesis in alveolar rhabdomyosarcoma. Recent data suggest that enforced expression of the PAX3–FKHR fusion protein not only interferes with normal myogenic differentiation program but also can activate genes important for tumor growth and invasiveness [87,88].

Unlike alveolar rhabdomyosarcomas, embryonal rhabdomyosarcomas seem to lack consistent translocations and other characteristic karyotypic abnormalities that could be important mechanisms contributing to tumorigenesis [33,37]. However, other genetic mechanisms, including mitotic nondisjunction and loss (with or without reduplication of the remaining homologue), localized gene conversion, point mutation, small deletion, and mitotic recombination, are all factors that can affect tumor development. The existence of mitotic recombination in initiated progenitor cells giving rise to a specific tumor has suggested the chromosomal location for numerous tumor suppressor loci (even in the absence of known cytogenetic aberrations) by delineating the smallest overlapping region of somatic homozygosity shared among tumors of a similar phenotype.

In this regard, restriction fragment length polymorphism analysis of embryonal rhabdomyosarcomas has shown consistent loss of heterozygosity (LOH) through mitotic recombination for loci on chromosome 11p; this loss has not been observed for alveolar rhabdomyosarcomas [11,89]. The smallest region affected in these cases encompasses 11p15.5-pter and includes the loci for the hemoglobin-β gene cluster, tyrosine hydroxylase, *H19*, insulin, insulin-like growth factor 2, and the *HRAS* oncogene [90,91]. Importantly, this region has also been implicated in the development of other embryonal tumors, including Wilms' tumor, adrenal carcinoma, and hepatoblastoma, as well as tumors of the lung, bladder, ovary, and breast [92,93]. Further, the gene for Beckwith–Wiedemann syndrome, an autosomal-dominant syndrome characterized by generalized somatic hyperplasia and a predisposition for the development of embryonal tumors (including Wilms' tumor and rhabdomyosarcoma), has been mapped to the same chromosomal region as that lost through LOH in embryonal rhabdomyosarcoma [94].

Functional evidence of a rhabdomyosarcoma tumor suppressor gene at 11p15.5 has been obtained through experiments using microcell hybridization to transfer an intact chromosome 11 into an embryonal rhabdomyosarcoma with LOH in this region [95]. In the microcell hybrids, selective retention of either the short or long arms of chromosome 11 resulted in dramatic loss of proliferative capacity without loss of tumorigenicity. Thus, in addition to the suppressor locus at 11p15.5, these results suggest the existence of a tumor suppressor on 11q that had not been recognized in previous molecular analyses [96].

Recent microcell fusion experiments incorporating smaller segments of chromosome 11p have further localized the 11p15.5 suppressor [97]. The suppressor locus lies within an approximately 4500-kb region between the anonymous genomic markers D11S719 and D11724. The gene appears to reside between and is excluded from the centrometric region near the calcitonin gene and the more telomeric region near *IFG2*, two chromosomal segments once thought to contain the suppressor. Interestingly, the 4500-kb region lies directly between a cluster of germline trnaslocation breakpoints associated with Beckwith–Wiedemann syndrome and the region of unparental disomy found in some patients with this disorder [98,99].

The evidence for a tumor suppressor locus at 11p15.5 appears incontrovertible, but the mechanism by which this gene is inactivated has yet to be established. Studies investigating the parental origin of alleles in this genomic region in familial and sporadic cases of embryonal rhabdomyosarcoma have shown that isodisomic chromosome 11p alleles are consistently paternal in origin [100]. Thus, genomic imprinting of the paternal allele in embryonal rhabdomyosarcoma may be an alternative first step to inactivation by muta-

315

tion for achieving nullizygosity at the 11p15.5 suppressor locus. Similar presumed epigenetic modifications from preferentially inherited parental alleles have been reported for several other tumors, including retinoblastoma, Wilms' tumor, and osteosarcoma [101–103].

Molecular analyses have clearly demonstrated that rhabdomyosarcoma, which has traditionally been classified by histologic criteria, can also be defined according to specific and characteristic genetic lesions. Alveolar tumors harbor tumor-specific translocations, which result in the formation of chimeric transcription factors. By contrast, embryonal tumors have loss of heterozygosity in a region of chromosome 11p15.5, implying inactivation of a tumor suppressor gene. Although other molecular defects (e.g., mutations of the *P53* tumor suppressor gene, activating point mutations in the *NRAS* and *KRAS* cellular oncogenes, imprinting of *IGF2*, and occasional *NMYC* gene amplification) have been described in rhabdomyosarcomas, none of these is specific for these tumors, and therefore these defects presumably lack etiologic importance for initial rhabdomyosarcoma tumor development [104–107]. Future understanding of the role of these molecular defects in rhabdomyosarcoma tumorigenesis will undoubtedly result in improved targeted treatment strategies for this malignancy.

3. Therapeutic considerations

Prior to the introduction of combined modality therapy (comprising chemotherapy, radiotherapy, and surgery), fewer than one third of children with rhabdomyosarcoma survived [108–111]. By contrast, nearly 70% of children with this disease are cured with current therapies [112]. The improved outcomes for these children can largely be attributed to refinements in risk stratification, supportive care, and the use of multimodal therapy. As described previously, the recent identification of nonrandom chromosomal translocations within distinct histologic subtypes of rhabdomyosarcoma and the cloning of the genes associated with these translocations offer the opportunity to better understand the mechanisms involved in the pathogenesis of this disease [11,54,113,114]. These findings will improve diagnosis, staging, and monitoring of these patients and will facilitate development of novel specific therapies for children who are at increased risk for relapse.

3.1. Prognostic factors and clinical staging

Accurate identification of prognostic factors in children with rhabdomyosarcoma can help distinguish groups of patients who are at risk for treatment failure. The presence of specific clinical and laboratory features at initial diagnosis can help refine staging systems and develop specific risk-based therapies for these children. The system used most widely to stage patients with rhabdomyosarcoma is the surgicopathologic system developed by the Intergroup Rhabdomyosarcoma Study (IRS; table 1). In this system, patients are stratified according to the amount of residual tumor after initial surgery. Another clinical staging scheme, the Tumor–Node–Metastasis (TNM) system, stratifies patients according to the extent of tumor present at diagnosis and is not dependent upon the efficacy of the initial surgical intervention (table 2). The TNM system has been widely applied to the staging of adult patients with a variety of solid tumors.

Extent of disease (clinical group or stage) and primary site have consistently been shown to predict survival in children with rhabdomyosarcoma (Figure 1). In a study of 1688 patients registered on two consecutive IRS trials, patients whose localized tumors could be surgically extirpated had an excellent outcome (five-year overall survival, 82%), but those with metastatic disease fared poorly (five-year overall survival, 24%) [5]. In addition, multivariate analysis of patients enrolled in the first two IRS trials showed that certain clinical features within specific clinical groups also can help predict clinical outcome [5]. For example, patients with group I disease whose tumors had embryonal or botryoidal histology had a superior outcome. For patients in clinical group III, primary tumors of the orbit were associated with a favorable prognosis. For group IV patients, the presence of a primary tumor in the genitourinary tract conferred a relatively good prognosis. These findings prompted development of risk-based therapies in which extent of disease, anatomic location, and histologic subtype influence the intensity and duration of treatment.

The prognostic significance of the pretreatment TNM staging system has been examined by IRS investigators. Among the 505 patients with rhabdomyosarcoma who were enrolled in IRS studies from 1978 to 1982, certain subgroups of patients had significantly improved survival. These groups included patients whose tumors were confined to the organ or tissue of origin (T_1), those with small nonmetastatic lesions (<5 cm in diameter), and those whose primary tumors were in nonparameningeal head and neck regions, the genitourinary tract, or the orbit [115]. In a subsequent international collaborative study of 951 children with nonmetastatic rhabdomyosarcoma, TNM status and primary site both were prognostically significant [116]. These

Table 1. IRS clinical grouping classification

Group I:	Localized disease, completely resected
Group II:	Gross total resection with evidence of regional spread
(a)	Gross resection of tumor with microscopic residual disease
(b)	Complete resection of primary tumor, regional nodes involved
(c)	Regional disease with involved nodes — microscopic residual disease and/or histologic involvement of the dissected regional node most distal to the primary tumor site
Group III:	Incomplete resection with gross residual disease
Group IV:	Distant metastatic disease present at onset (lung, liver, bones, bone marrow, brain, and distant muscle and nodes)

317

Table 2. A. TNM pretreatment staging classification

Stage	Sites	T	Size	N
1	Orbit	T_1 or T_2	a or b	N_o or N_1
	Head and neck (excluding parameningeal)			
	GU–nonbladder/nonprostate			
2	Bladder/prostate	T_1 or T_2	a	N_o or N_x
	Extremity			
	Cranial Parameningeal			
	Other (includes trunk, retroperitoneum, etc.)			
3	Bladder/prostate	T_1 or T_2	a	N_1
	Extremity		b	N_o or N_1
	Cranial parameningeal			
	Other (includes trunk, retroperitoneum, etc.)			
4	ALL	T_1 or T_2	a or b	N_o or N_1

B. Definitions

Tumor
T_1 Confined to anatomic site of origin
  (a)   <5 cm in diameter
  (b)   ≥5 cm in diameter
T_2 Extension and/or fixation to surrounding tissue
  (a)   <5 cm in diameter
  (b)   ≥5 cm in diameter

Regional Nodes
N_o Regional nodes not clinically involved
N_1 Regional nodes clinically involved by neoplasm
N_x Clinical status of regional nodes unknown (especially for sites that preclude lymph node evaluation)

Metastasis
M_o No distant metastasis
M_1 Metastasis present

findings were confirmed recently in 189 patients with extremity lesions who were treated in IRS-III [117]. Patients with stage 2 disease (unfavorable site, tumors <5 cm, no nodal metastases) fared significantly better than those with stage 3 disease (≥5 cm, nodal disease; table 2).

3.2. Treatment of pediatric rhabdomyosarcoma

The outcome for children with rhabdomyosarcoma has improved dramatically over the past 30 years. In the late 1950s and early 1960s, after local therapies such as surgery and irradiation, fewer than one third of children with rhabdomyosarcoma survived [2,108,110,111]. Exceptions included patients with tumors in selected primary sites (orbit and bladder) who were treated with radical surgery (orbital exenteration or cystectomy); survival rates as high as 70% were reported for these patients [118,119]. Because most rhabdomy-

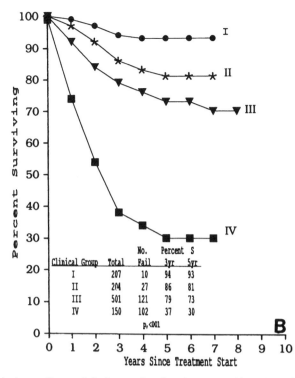

Clinical Group	Total	No. Fail	Percent S 3yr	5yr
I	207	10	94	93
II	204	27	86	81
III	501	121	79	73
IV	150	102	37	30

p, <001

B

Figure 1. Survival according to clinical group for all patients treated in IRS-III. (Reproduced with permission from Crist WM et al., J Clin Oncol 13:610–630, 1995.)

osarcoma treatment failures were systemic, testing of chemotherapeutic agents for control of macroscopic and microscopic distant disease was initiated. Vincristine, dactinomycin, and cyclophosphamide (VAC; singly or in combination) yielded promising results during the 1960s [4,108,120,121]. Soon thereafter, the value of adjuvant chemotherapy was tested in a prospective study by the Children's Cancer Study Group A. In this trial, patients whose tumors were completely resected received postoperative radiotherapy; they then were randomized to receive either adjuvant dactinomycin and vincristine for one year or observation only. Approximately 82% of patients treated with adjuvant chemotherapy remained in remission after two years, compared to 47% of the control group [11]. Other pioneering work documented that the use of combined modality therapy increased response rates and improved survival among children with rhabdomyosarcoma [122–124]. These early encouraging results in limited numbers of patients, combined with the heterogeneity and rarity of childhood rhabdomyosarcoma, prompted implementation in 1972 of the first national cooperative trial. Relevant contributions from these national and international cooperative trials are discussed below.

The IRS committee has reported the results of three consecutive trials: IRS-I (1972–1978, $n = 686$), IRS-II (1978–1984, $n = 999$), and IRS-III (1984–1991, $n = 1062$) [112,125,126]. For each of these three studies, two thirds of eligible patients were younger than 10 years, and there was a slight male predominance. The primary sites and extent of disease at diagnosis are shown in figure 2. Nearly 50% of children presented with unresectable disease (clinical group III). The most common anatomic location was the head and neck region (including the orbit and parameninges). The estimated five-year overall survival rate has steadily and significantly increased in each of the three successive IRS trials — 55% in IRS-I, 63% in IRS-II, and 71% in IRS-III. In IRS-I, treatment assignment was based on the postsurgical extent of disease, with no stratification for specific risk subgroups, However, several subsequent studies have documented differences in clinical outcome according to primary site, histology, and clinical group [127–134].

The second IRS study recognized the prognostic significance of certain well-characterized risk factors (clinical group, site, and histology) and stratified patients accordingly (table 3). Patients with group I and II alveolar tumors of the extremities and those with primary tumors in 'special pelvic' sites (bladder, prostate, vagina, uterus) received VAC chemotherapy. IRS-III further expanded upon these observations and stratified patients into nine distinct risk subgroups according to extent of disease, primary tumor site, and histology (table 3). Therapy assignment in IRS-IV varies with clinical group and pretreatment TNM characteristics (table 2). Findings from the first three IRS studies and the treatment protocols of IRS-IV are summarized below and in table 1.

3.3.1. Clinical group I. This group comprises children whose tumors were completely resected and who were expected to have an excellent prognosis

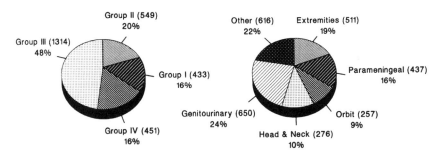

Figure 2. Distribution of patients who were enrolled in IRS-I, IRS-II, and IRS-III according to clinical group and primary site. (Reproduced with permission from Pappo A et al., J Clin Oncol 13:2123–2139, 1995.)

320

Table 3. Findings of the Intergroup Rhabdomyosarcoma Study trials

Patient Strata	IRS-I[a] Treatment (regimen)	Survival (%)	IRS-II Treatment (regimen)	Survival (%)	IRS-III Treatment (regimen)	Survival (%)
Clinical group I (favorable histology)	VAC × 2 yr (A)	93	VAC × 2 yr (21)	85	Cyclic-sequential VA for 1 yr (31)	93
	VAC + RT × 2 yr (B)	81	VA × 1 yr (22)	84		
	Amputees, VAC × 2 yr (G)	83				
Clinical group II (favorable histology)	VA + RT × 1 yr (C)	73	VA + RT × 1 yr (23)	88	VA + RT × 1 yr (32)	54
	VAC + RT × 2 yr (D)	70	Pulsed VAC + RT × 1 yr (24)	79	VA + ADR + RT × 1 yr (33)	89
Clinical group III (excluding special pelvic, orbit, and selected head sites[b])	VAC + RT × 2 yr (E)[c]	53	Pulsed VAC + RT × 2 yr (25)[c]	—	Pulsed VAC + RT × 2 yr (34)[d,c]	70
	VAC + ADR + RT × 2 yr (F)[c]	51	Pulsed VADRC-VAC + RT × 2 yr (26)	—	Pulsed VADRC-VAC + CDDP + RT × 2 yr (35)	63
	E + F	52	25 + 26	59[g]	Pulsed VADRC-VAC + CDDP + VP-16 + RT × 2 yr (36)	64
					34 + 35 + 36	65[h]
Clinical group IV	VAC + RT × 2 yr (E)[c]	14	Pulsed VAC + RT × 2 yr (25)[c]	—	Pulsed VAC + RT × 2 yr (34)[d,c]	27
	VAC + ADR + RT × 2 yr (F)[c]	26	Pulsed VADRC-VAC + RT × 2 yr (26)	—	Pulsed VADRC-VAC + CDDP + RT × 2 yr (35)	31
	E + F	20	25 + 26	27	Pulsed VADRC-VAC + CDDP + VP-16 + RT × 2 yr (36)	29
					34 + 35 + 36	30
Clinical group III (special pelvic sites[b])	—	71	Pulsed VAC ± RT ± surgery × 2 yr (27)	72[g]	Pulsed VADRC-VAC + CDDP ± AMD + VP16 ± RT ± surgery × 2 yr[d] (37 A & B)	83[h]
Clinical group I & II (unfavorable histology-alveolar)	—	57[j]	Pulsed VAC ± RT × 1 yr (25)	71	Pulsed VADRC-VAC + CDDP + RT × 1 yr (38)	80
Orbit and selected head sites[f] (favorable histology)					VA + RT × 1 yr (32)	

Table 3 (continued)

Patient Strata	IRS-I[a]		IRS-II		IRS-III	
	Treatment (regimen)	Survival (%)	Treatment (regimen)	Survival (%)	Treatment (regimen)	Survival (%)
Group II	—		VA + RT or VAC + RT × 1 yr (23–24)		VA + RT × 1 yr (32)	
Group III	—		VAC or VADRC + RT × 1 yr (25–26)		VA + RT × 1 yr (32)	
			Regimens 23–26 (overall results combined).	91[g]	Overall results regimen 32	91[h]
Paratesticular (group II, favorable, histology)	—		VA + RT or VAC + RT × 1 yr (23–24)	81	VA + RT × 1 yr (32)	81
Overall results		55		63		71

Note: Detailed descriptions of treatment may be found in Maurer et al. [10,11] and Crist et al. [6].

Abbreviations: VAC, vincristine–dactinomycin–cyclophosphamide; yr, year(s); RT, radiation therapy; VA, vincristine–dactinomycin; ADR, doxorubicin; VADRC, vincristine, doxorubicin, and cyclophosphamide; CDDP, cisplatin.

[a] All patients were randomized by clinical group only; prognostically important subgroups were not recognized until IRS-II.

[b] Bladder, prostate, vagina, and uterus.

[c] For all sites.

[d] Second-look surgery recommended of week 20 for all patients in partial or complete remission. Patients in partial remission were to receive ADR plus DTIC (regimen 34) or AMD plus VP-16 (regimens 35 and 37 A and B), or AMD plus DTIC (regimen 26).

[e] Differences in outcome between regimens 25 v 26 in IRS-II, and 34 v 35 v 36 in IRS-III were not statistically significant.

[f] Oral cavity, cheek, oropharynx, larynx, scalp, and parotid.

[g] Overall 5-year survival for all group III patients treated in IRS-II is 66%.

[h] Overall 5-year survival for all group III patients treated in IRS-III is 74%.

[i] Three-year estimate.

Reproduced with permission from Pappo A, et al J Clin Oncol 13:2123–2139, 1995.

[112,125,126]. Following surgical resection, patients or the first IRS trial were randomized to receive VAC chemotherapy alone with radiotherapy to the tumor bed. The five-year overall and disease-free survival estimates did not differ significantly between these two groups. Therefore, it was concluded that radiotherapy could be omitted without significantly jeopardizing outcome of children with clinical group I tumors.

IRS-II addressed whether cyclophosphamide could be deleted from the vincristine–dactinomycin–cyclophosphamide combination in patients with group I nonextremity nonalveolar tumors (these patients fared well in IRS-I). This trial showed that VA chemotherapy was equivalent to VAC chemotherapy in this subset of patients. In the third IRS study, intensified VA therapy was administered for 12 months to patients with favorable histology tumors (regardless of primary site). This treatment combination was as effective as prolonged treatment with the more intensive VAC regimen used in IRS-II. Thus, patients with completely resected favorable histology tumors can be safely and effectively treated with two drugs (VA) without the need for alkylators or radiation therapy.

In IRS-IV, patients with orbital and paratesticular primary lesions receive VA chemotherapy. Patients with tumors with unfavorable features (as defined by site, size, and/or nodal disease) are randomized to receive one of three different chemotherapeutic regimens (VAC; vincristine, ifosfamide, and etoposide [VIE]; or vincristine, dactinomycin, and ifosfamide [VAI]). Radiotherapy is reserved for patients with stage 3 disease (large tumors or nodal disease).

3.3.2. Clinical group II. Children in this category usually received postoperative radiotherapy at various points during treatment, resulting in a local control rate of 90% [112,125,126]. In IRS-I, the addition of cyclophosphamide to the VA regimen failed to improve outcome for these patients. In IRS-II, intensifying therapy with a VAC regimen also failed to improve outcome among patients with nonectremity nonalveolar tumors. In IRS-III, children with clinical group II favorable histology tumors (excluding orbit, head, and paratesticular primaries) were randomized to receive VA or VA and doxorubicin. The five-year progression-free and overall survival rates were, respectively, $77 \pm 6\%$ and $89 \pm 5\%$ for the VA and doxorubicin arm compared to $56 \pm 10\%$ and $54 \pm 13\%$ for the VA arm ($p = 0.08$ and 0.03, respectively). However, the beneficial effect of adding doxorubicin became less dramatic ($p = 0.18$) when the results of the two VA-containing regimens in IRS-II and IRS-III were combined. The value of doxorubicin in these children therefore requires further clarification. Based on these findings. VA with radiotherapy remains the therapeutic standard for children with clinical group II disease who present with a favorable histology tumor in a favorable site. In IRS-IV, patients with primary lesions of the orbit receive VA chemotherapy; all others are randomized to receive either VAC, VAI, or VIE.

3.3.3. Clinical group III.

Children with inoperable rhabdomyosarcoma represent the largest group of patient enrolled in the IRS trials [112,125,126]. Among all clinical groups, these patients have shown the most dramatic improvements in five-year overall (IRS-I, 52 ± 3%; IRS-III, 74 ± 2%) and progression-free (IRS-I, 48.3%; IRS-III, 66.2%) survival rates. In IRS-I, all group III patients were randomized to receive either VAC chemotherapy and radiation of VAC with doxorubicin (VADRC-VAC) and radiation. Addition of doxorubicin to the VAC regimen failed to significantly improve complete response rates (67% vs. 72%), five-year overall survival (53% vs. 51%), or five-year disease-free survival (39% vs. 43%).

In IRS-II, all patients (excluding those with tumors in special pelvic sites) were randomized to receive intensified VAC or VADRC-VAC therapy. Prognosis did not differ significantly for these two regimens. However, compared to their less intensive counterparts in IRS-I, the intensified VAC and VADRC-VAC regimens were superior in inducing complete responses and prolonged survival.

Excluding those with tumors in special pelvic sites, the orbit, and selected head sites (scalp, parotid, oral cavity, larynx, oropharynx, cheek), patients in IRS-III were randomized to receive either pulsed VAC chemotherapy or VADRC–VAC–cisplatin or VADRC–VAC–cisplatin–VP16. At five years, the progression-free and overall survival rates for the three regimens were similar (table 3). Several patients among these study arms received alternate induction chemotherapy with one of three drug pairs (doxorubicin-DTIC, dactinomycin-VP16, or dactinomycin-DTIC) and second-look surgery. Although the precise impact of each of these treatments on clinical outcome could not be assessed, outcome for these children was improved compared to that of patients who were treated in IRS-II (five-year overall survival, 65 ± 3% vs. 59 ± 3%; five-year progression-free survival, 61 ± 3% vs. 52 ± 3%).

Preliminary data from the IRS-IV pilot showed that significant toxicity was evident with the administration of escalating cyclophosphamide doses when growth factor support was omitted from this regimen. The overall incidence of toxic deaths was 7.6%, comprising one death at 1.8g/m^2 dose level and eight among patients who received 2.2g/m^2. In addition, hepatic veno-occlusive disease has been recently recognized as a complication of high-dose VAC therapy in these patients [135].

3.3.4. Clinical group IV.

The outcome for patients with metastatic disease continues to be poor, despite intensification of therapy or new drug combinations. The combined-agent regimens used in the first three IRS studies have consistently led to five-year overall and progression-free survival rates below 30%. Because of the dismal prognosis for these group IV patients, IRS-IV and IRS-V are investigating novel drugs, including melphalan, ifosfamide, and topotecan, that have shown promising activity in preclinical models. To facilitate evaluation of their efficacy, either alone or in combination with other active agents, these drugs are given in an 'up-front widow' to newly diagnosed patients with metastatic disease [136–139].

3.3.5. Bladder/prostate tumors. The favorable outcome of children with primary genitourinary tumors was recognized in IRS-I (five-year overall survival, 74%) [125]. However, this outcome was achieved at the expense of numerous bladder extirpations for patients with genitourinary primary tumors; only 23% of the patients had functional bladders three years after therapy [140]. The treatment strategy in IRS-II shifted to a primary chemotherapeutic approach, and four months of VAC chemotherapy was followed by delayed radiation and/or surgery in an attempt to reduce the side effects typically associated with these treatment modalities. This treatment approach failed to improve the bladder salvage rate (three-year bladder function retention rate, 25%) and led to survival rates similar to those of IRS-I [141].

In IRS-III, induction chemotherapy was followed by radiotherapy, which was initiated at week 6. Second-look surgery at week 20 was recommended, and alternate induction therapy with dactinomycin and VP16 was initiated if tumor remained. The three-year bladder preservation rate (60%), five-year progression-free survival estimate (74 ± 5%), and overall survival rate (83 ± 4%) associated with IRS-III were strikingly superior to those of IRS-I and IRS-II [112,125,126,142].

3.3.6. Unfavorable histology clinical groups I and II tumors. The poor outcome for children with clinical group I alveolar tumors was recognized in IRS-I [125]. All these patients therefore received intensive VAC chemotherapy in IRS-II [126]. This treatment modification increased the three-year disease-free survival rate from 43% to 69%. Therapy was further intensified in IRS-III by using a VADRC–VAC–cisplatin–containing regimen. The five-year progression-free (71 ± 6%) and overall survival (80 ± 6%) rates for IRS-III significantly improved over those for comparable patients treated on IRS-II (59 ± 5% and 71 ± 5%, respectively; $p = 0.002$ and 0.01) [125].

3.3.7. Parameningeal tumors. The treatment prescribed in IRS-I for all patients with clinical group III or IV disease included VAC or VADRC–VAC chemotherapy with radiation of the primary tumor to a 2-cm margin beginning at week 6. Of the 57 patients with parameningeal tumors in this study, 20 (35%) had direct meningeal extension either at diagnosis ($n = 10$) or within the first 12 months of therapy ($n = 10$); 18 (90%) of these patients died [134]. Characteristics associated with an increased risk of direct meningeal extension included intracranial extension of the primary tumor, erosion of the base of skull, and cranial nerve palsy. These findings prompted a protocol modification in 1977 to initiate radiation therapy concurrently with induction chemotherapy (encompassing the entire cranial neuraxis and primary tumor) for high-risk patients and intermittent intrathecal chemotherapy [128]. These changes were associated with substantial improvements in overall survival (67% vs. 47%) and reduced the incidence of CNS relapse [126,128].

Compared to patients in IRS-II, those in IRS-III with limited meningeal involvement (cranial nerve palsy or base-of-skull erosion without intracranial extension) received a reduced volume of radiotherapy [112]. The higher five-year progression-free survival rate in IRS-III (69 $\pm$ 4%) compared to IRS-II (61 $\pm$ 4%) suggests that this treatment modification did not compromise outcome [112]. In IRS-IV, intrathecal chemotherapy has been omitted, and patients with limited intracranial extension receive limited-volume radiotherapy.

3.3.8. Favorable histology paratesticular group II tumors. Patients with tumors in the paratesticular area account for 7% of rhabdomyosarcoma cases [131]. Because these children fared well in the first two IRS studies (estimated three-year overall survival rate, 90%), they were not randomized in IRS-III and were treated with reduced therapy that included VA and radiotherapy for one year. The five-year overall survival estimate (81%) was similar to that reported for a randomized VAC or VA study in IRS-II (75%) [112]. These findings suggest that less intensive therapy is appropriate for children with group II paratesticular tumors.

3.3.9. Favorable histology orbit and head tumors (groups II and III). The favorable prognosis for children with orbital (five-year overall survival, >90%) and nonparameningeal head sites (five-year overall survival, 75% to 80%) was recognized in IRS-I and IRS-II [129]. In IRS-III, patients with group II or III tumors were treated with VA and radiotherapy for one year. Outcome for these patients (five-year overall survival, 91%; five-year progression-free survival, 78%) was similar to those observed in IRS-I and IRS-II, which used more intensive therapies [112].

3.4. The SIOP trials (1975–1989)

The International Society of Pediatric Oncology (SIOP) has conducted three consecutive trials (SIOP 75, MMT 84, and MMT 89) of treatments for rhabdomyosarcoma [116,143–148]. Risk stratification was based primarily on patient characteristics (according to the TNM system) prior to treatment. Investigators in these trials used a primary chemotherapeutic approach for controlling local and distant disease while attempting to decrease the late sequelae associated with radical surgery and radiotherapy. These therapies resulted in outcomes similar to those of the IRS studies, but local recurrence was significantly higher.

The first SIOP trial (1975–1983) enrolled 281 patients with nonmetastatic rhabdomyosarcoma and mandated a VADR–VAC-based regimen. Children with completely resected. localized stage I disease received VAC–VADR for 18 months; patients with incomplete excision also received 45 Gy of radiotherapy. For stages II or III disease, primary chemotherapy with VADR–VAC was compared to primary radiotherapy; the four-year survival rate for the entire group was 56%. Overall survival did not differ between the treatment arms, suggesting that primary chemotherapy only can be used in selected patients without compromising survival [116,143,149].

Based upon their pretreatment TNM stage and initial response to therapy, 286 patients with rhabdomyosarcoma received 3 to 10 courses of an ifosfamide-containing regimen (VAI) during the second SIOP trial (MMT 84). If the response to initial chemotherapy was inadequate, patients received second-line therapy with cisplatin and doxorubicin. Local therapy was given to all patients with parameningeal primary tumors but was omitted in all others unless they failed to achieve a complete response. The four-year overall survival estimate for nonmetastatic patients was 69%. This regimen produced high response rates (78%) and avoided radiotherapy in 40% to 75% of selected patients [148]. The SIOP MMT 89 study enrolled 362 nonmetastatic rhabdomyosarcoma and 56 patients with metastatic disease [146,147,150]. The treatment approach included stratification according to site and stage and VAI with or without carboplatin, epirubicin, or etoposide as front-line therapy [151,152]. Patients with completely resected stage I tumors received VA therapy, whereas those with incompletely resected stage I tumors and those with stage II or III disease received VAI therapy. The three-year estimate of overall survival was 78% for patients with no metastases and 25% for those with metastatic disease [147,150].

3.5. The CWS trials (1981–1986)

The German Cooperative Soft Tissue Sarcoma (CWS) trials stratified patients according to the IRS surgicopathologic staging system and implemented a risk-directed therapeutic approach based on initial chemotherapeutic response. The first study (CWS-81) used VAC–VADRC chemotherapy and demonstrated a correlation between the degree of tumor response after the first seven weeks of chemotherapy [153]. For patients who experienced a complete response at week 7, the five-year PFS rates were 82% compared to 50% for patients whose tumor volume decreased by more than two thirds and 32% for those with a volume reduction of less than one third. The results of second-look surgery after two cycles of chemotherapy mandated the amount of radiotherapy. Children with nonmetastatic disease fared well, demonstrating a five-year disease-free survival rate of 68 ± 4%, and patients with metastatic disease had a poor prognosis (five-year disease-free survival estimate, 11 ± 5%).

In the CWS-86 study, cyclophosphamide was replaced by ifosfamide in an attempt to produce a more effective regimen. Radiotherapy prior to second-look surgery dramatically improved local control rates among patients with macroscopic residual tumor. In addition, the VAIADR regimen increased the proportion of patients with responsive disease (71% vs. 55%) [154]. The five-

327

year disease-free survival estimate for patients with nonmetastatic disease was 69%.

3.6. The Italian RMS studies

The first Italian rhabdomyosarcoma trial compared the efficacy of a standard VAC regimen comprising five days of divided dactinomycin doses to that of a VAC-M regimen in which the dactinomycin dose was given as a single, high-dose injection [155]. Toxicity and response were similar for both treatment arms. A subsequent trial demonstrated encouraging early responses in children with group III or IV rhabdomyosarcoma who received VAIADR [156].

3.7. Local therapy: lessons from multi-institutional trials

Although rhabdomyosarcoma is a chemosensitive tumor, drugs alone cannot cure most children who have this disease. Surgical resection alone or in combination with irradiation is necessary for local control of the tumor. Radiotherapy has been used to eradicate residual microscopic or macroscopic tumor cells following surgery or chemotherapy. In response to the results of several trials, radiotherapy doses now vary according to patient age, tumor site, and amount of residual tumor.

As discussed previously, early introduction of radiotherapy has improved survival among patients with parameningeal rhabdomyosarcomas [128]. Intensified chemotherapy and second-look surgery have decreased the use of radiotherapy and extensive primary surgery for patients with vaginal and vulvar rhabdomyosarcomas [157]. In addition, the use of early radiotherapy, aggressive chemotherapy, and second-look surgery has dramatically decreased the use of radical surgery to treat children with genitourinary rhabdomyosarcoma [112,142,157]. Currently, microscopic residual disease is treated with 40 Gy of radiation to the tumor bed and a 2-cm margin. In IRS-IV, radiotherapy of completely resected tumors with unfavorable features (large size, unfavorable site, nodal involvement) is mandated. Gross residual disease requires higher doses — 45 to 55 Gy, depending on the site and size of tumor.

Further, to increase local control and decrease the acute and late adverse effects of radiotherapy, IRS-IV initiated a pilot protocol evaluating hyperfractionated radiotherapy n patients with unresected or metastatic rhabdomyosarcoma [158]. Severe or life-threatening toxicities occurred in 154 of the 204 group III cases (75%) and in 52 of the 80 group IV cases (65%). These frequencies are similar to the 81% incidence of significant toxicity following conventionally fractionated radiotherapy in IRS-III. This study suggests that hyperfractionated radiotherapy is feasible and is associated with tolerable side effects in children with unresected or metastatic rhabdomyosarcoma. A prospective randomized trial to compare the efficacy of conventional versus hyperfractionated radiotherapy is underway.

Surgical approaches to the treatment of rhabdomyosarcoma also have been influenced by information gathered from multi-institutional trails. For example, because nodal involvement has been shown to be particularly common among patients with extremity and genitourinary tumors, nodal sampling should be strongly considered at the time of initial staging [159]. If performed within 35 days of the primary procedure, surgical reexcision may benefit patients with microscopic positive residual tumor in extremity locations [160]. Paratesticular masses should be resected using either an inguinal orchiectomy or hemiscrotectomy (which should be reserved for patients with neoplastic fixation or for those who had a previous transcrotal procedure) [161].

3.8. Late effects of therapy

Because of the improved long-term survival of children treated for rhabdomyosarcoma, several serious and potentially life-threatening therapy-related complications have emerged. In IRS-IV, incorporation of ifosfamide into front-line therapeutic protocols for children with unresectable rhabdomyosarcoma was associated with a 14% incidence of renal toxicity. Factors contributing to renal tubular injury included high doses of ifosfamide ($>72 g/m^2$), age younger than 3 years, and preexisting renal abnormalities (e.g., hydronephrosis) [162].

Among 50 patients treated for orbital rhabdomyosarcoma in IRS-I, 90% developed cataracts, 61% showed growth retardation, 50% had bone hypoplasia and facial asymmetry, and 10% developed learning disabilities [163]. Among the 86 boys with paratesticular rhabdomyosarcoma who were treated in IRS-I and IRS-II, 10% had bowel obstruction and decreased ejaculatory function. Further, lymphedema was seen in 5% of these patients, and 4% had bony hypoplasia in the field of radiotherapy. One third of these boys developed hemorrhagic cystitis, and half of the patients for whom adequate follow-up was available developed elevated FSH levels or azoospermia [162]. Of the 109 patients with bladder and prostate tumors who were treated in IRS-I and II, 29% developed posttherapy hematuria, 29% showed evidence of delayed pubertal development, and 10% had growth retardation [164].

There were 162 patients with nonorbital head and neck rhabdomyosarcomas enrolled in IRS-II and -III. Among these children, 75% had abnormal statural growth and 20% were receiving growth hormone replacement. Of the 162 patients, 10% developed cataracts, 50% had impaired auditory function, and 30% had cosmetic and/or dental abnormalities [165].

The occurrence of second malignant neoplasms is one of the most devastating late sequelae of successful contemporary therapy. Of the 1770 patients enrolled in IRS-I and IRS-II, 22 developed second malignant neoplasms (10-year cumulative incidence rate, 1.7%). The most common second malignancies were bone sarcomas ($n = 11$) and acute nonlymphoblastic leukemia ($n = 5$); the median time to development of these two neoplasms was 7 and 4 years, respectively [166]. Investigators at Memorial Sloan Kettering Cancer Center reported a 10-year cumulative risk (6%) among 130 long-term survivors of rhabdomyosarcoma; high doses of dactinomycin, cyclophosphamide, and radiotherapy were associated with the increased risk of this complication [167].

4. Conclusions

Recent advances in understanding the unique biological and genetic features of this tumor as well as in new drug development and scheduling have substantially improved the outlook for children with rhabdomyosarcoma. However, despite these improvements, numerous challenges remain regarding the treatment of patients with rhabdomyosarcoma. Among these are the refinement of risk-directed therapy based upon the recognition of newly recognized, prognostically important biological and clinical features. Dose intensification with the administration of hematopoietic growth factor therapy offers the possibility of improved therapy for children with metastatic or recurrent disease. Finally, because none of the agents currently used in the treatment of rhabdomyosarcoma is tumor specific, the recent identification of translocation-specific gene products (*PAX3-FKHR* and *PAX7-FKHR*) in alveolar tumors provides an attractive molecular target for future therapies.

Acknowledgments

This work was supported in part by PHS grants CA23099 and CA21765 from the National Cancer Institute and by the American Lebanese Syrian Associated Charities (ALSAC). We thank Amy L.B. Frazier for expert editorial assistance.

References

1. Miller RW, Young JL, Novakovic B. 1994. Childhood cancer. Cancer 75:395–405.
2. Pappo AS, Shapiro DN, Crist WM, Maurer HM. 1995. Biology and therapy of pediatric rhabdomyosarcoma. J Clin Oncol 13:2123–2139.
3. Horn RC, Enterline HT. 1958. Rhabdomyosarcoma: a clinicopathological study identification and classification. Cancer 11:181–199.
4. Raney RB Jr, Hays DM, Tefft M, Triche TJ. 1993. Rhabdomyosarcoma and the undifferentiated sarcomas. In Pizzo PA, Poplack DG (eds.), Principals and Practice of Pediatric Oncology, 2nd ed. Philadelphia: J B Lipincott, pp. 769–794.
5. Crist WM, Garnsey L, Beltangady MS, Gehan E, Ruymann F, Webber B, Hays DM, Wharam M, Maurer HM. 1990. Prognosis in children with rhabdomyosarcoma: a report of the Intergroup Rhabdomyosarcoma Studies I and II. J Clin Oncol 8:443–452.
6. Li L, Olson EN. 1992. Regulation of muscle cell growth and differentiation by the MyoD family of helix–loop–helix proteins. Adv Cancer Res 58:95–119.
7. Olson EN. 1990. MyoD family: a paradigm for development? Genes Dev 4:1454–1461.
8. Olson EN, Klein WH. 1994. bHLH factors in muscle development: dead lines and commitments, what to leave in and what to leave out. Genes Dev 8:1–8.

330

9. Weintraub H, Davis R, Tapscott S, et al. 1991. The myoD gene family: nodal point during specification of the muscle cell lineage. Science 251:761–766.

10. Tapscott SJ, Weintraub H. 1991. MyoD and the regulation of myogenesis by helix–loop–helix proteins. J Clin Invest 87:1133–1138.

11. Scrable H, Witte D, Shimada H, Seemayer T, Sheng WW, Soukup S, Koufos A, Houghton P, Lampkin B, Cavenee W. 1989. Molecular differential pathology of rhabdomyosarcoma. Genes Chromosomes Cancer 1:23–35.

12. Clark J, Rocques PJ, Braun T, et al. 1991. Expression of members of the myf gene family in human rhabdomyosarcomas. Br J Cancer 64:1039–1042.

13. Hosoi H, Sugimoto T, Hayashi Y, Inaba T, Horii Y, Morioka H, Fushiki S, Hamazaki M, Sawada T. 1992. Differential expression of myogenic regulatory genes, MyoD1 and myogenin, in human rhabdomyosarcoma sublines. Int J Cancer 50:977–983.

14. Tonin PN, Scrable H, Shimada H. 1991. Muscle-specific gene expression in rhabdomyosarcoma, and stages of human fetal skeletal muscle development. Cancer Res 51:5100–5106.

15. Tapscott SJ, Thayer MJ, Weintraub H. 1993. Deficiency in rhabdomyosarcomas of a factor required for MyoD activity and myogenesis. Science 259:1450–1453.

16. Dias P, Parham DM, Shapiro DN, Webber BL, Houghton PJ. 1990. Myogenic regulatory protein (MyoD1) expression in childhood solid tumors: diagnostic utility in rhabdomyosarcoma. Am J Pathol 137:1283–1291.

17. Douglass EC, Valentine M, Etcubanas E, Parham D, Webber BL, Houghton PJ, Houghton JA, Green AA. 1987. A specific chromosomal abnormality in rhabdomyosarcoma [published erratum appears in Cytogenet Cell Genet 1988;47(4): following 232]. Cytogenet Cell Genet 45:148–155.

18. Lizard-Nacol S, Mugneret F, Volk C, Turc-Carel C, Favrot M, Philip T. 1987. Translocation (2;13)(q37;q14) in alveolar rhabdomyosarcoma: a new case (letter). Cancer Genet Cytogenet 25:373–374.

19. Whang-Peng J, Triche TJ, Knutsen T, Miser J, Kao-Shan S, Tsai S, Israel MA. 1986. Cytogenetic characterization of selected small round cell tumors of childhood. Cancer Genet Cytogenet 21:185–208.

20. Whang-Peng J, Knutsen T, Theil K, Horowitz ME, Triche T. 1992. Cytogenetic studies in subgroups of rhabdomyosarcoma. Genes Chromosomes Cancer 5:299–310.

21. Turc-Carel C, Lizard-Nacol S, Justrabo E, Favrot M, Philip T, Tabone E. 1986. Consistent chromosomal translocation in alveolar rhabdomyosarcoma. Cancer Genet Cytogenet 19:361–362.

22. Nojima T, Abe S, Yamaguchi H, Matsuno T, Inoue K. 1990. A case of alveolar rhabdomyosarcoma with a chromosomal translocation, t(2;13)(q37;q14). Virchows Arch [A] 417:357–359.

23. Douglass EC, Rowe ST, Valentine M, Parham DM, Berkow R, Bowman WP, Maurer HM. 1991. Variant translocations of chromosome 13 in alveolar rhabdomyosarcoma. Genes Chromosomes Cancer 3:480–482.

24. Biegel JA, Meek RS, Parmiter AH, Conard K, Emanuel BS. 1991. Chromosomal translocation t(1;13)(p36;q14) in a case of rhabdomyosarcoma. Genes Chromosomes Cancer 3:483–484.

25. Seidal T, Mark J, Hagmar B, Angervall L. 1982. Alveolar rhabdomyosarcoma: a cytogenetic and correlated cytological and histological study. Acta Pathol Microbiol Immunol Scand [A] 90:345–354.

26. Kelly KM, Womer RB, Sorensen P, Xiong Q-B, Barr FG. 1996. Common and variant gene fusions predict clinical phenotype in rhabdomyosarcoma (RMS) (meeting abstract). Proc Am Soc Clin Oncol 15:462.

27. Molenaar WM, Dam-Meiring A, Kamps WA, Cornelisse CJ. 1988. DNA-aneuploidy in rhabdomyosarcomas as compared with other sarcomas of childhood and adolescence. Hum Pathol 19:573–579.

28. Pappo AS, Crist WM, Kuttesch J, Rowe S, Ashmun RA, Maurer HM, Newton WA, Asmar

331

L, Luo X, Shapiro DN. 1993. Tumor-cell DNA content predicts outcome in children and adolescents with clinical group III embryonal rhabdomyosarcoma. J Clin Oncol 11:1901–1905.

29. Shapiro DN, Parham DM, Douglass EC, Ashmun R, Webber BL, Newton WA Jr, Hancock ML, Maurer HM, Look AT. 1991. Relationship of tumor-cell ploidy to histologic subtype and treatment outcome in children and adolescents with unresectable rhabdomyosarcoma [published erratum appears in J Clin Oncol 1991 May;9(5):893]. J Clin Oncol 9:159–166.

30. Wijnaendts LC, van der Linden JC, van Diest P, van Unnik AJ, Delemarre JF, Voute PA, Meijer CJ. 1993. Prognostic importance of DNA flow cytometric variables in rhabdomyosarcomas. J Clin Pathol 46:948–952.

31. Mathieu MC, Niggli F, Vielh P, Oberlin O, Stevens M, Boccon-Gibod L, Flamant F. 1994. Prognostic value of flow cytometric DNA ploidy in childhood rhabdomyosarcomas enrolled in SIOP–MMT 89 study. Med Pediatr Oncol 23:223–230.

32. Niggli FK, Powell JE, Parkes SE, Ward K, Raafat F, Mann JR, Stevens MC. 1994. DNA ploidy and proliferative activity (S-phase) in childhood soft-tissue sarcomas: their value as prognostic indicators. Br J Cancer 69:1106–1110.

33. Potluri VR, Gilbert F. 1985. A cytogenetic study of embryonal rhabdomyosarcoma. Cancer Genet Cytogenet 14:169–173.

34. Hayashi Y, Sugimoto T, Horii Y, et al. 1990. Characterization of an embryonal rhabdomyosarcoma cell line showing amplification and over-expression of the N-myc oncogene. Int J Cancer 45:705–711.

35. Kubo K, Naoe T, Utsumi KR, Ishiguro Y, Ueda K, Shiku H, Yamada K. 1991. Cytogenetic and cellular characteristics of a human embryonal rhabdomyosarcoma cell line, RMS-YM, Br J Cancer 63:879–884.

36. Magnani I, Faustinella F, Nanni P, Nicoletti G, Larizza L. 1991. Karyotypic characterization of a new human embryonal rhabdomyosarcoma cell line. Cancer Genet Cytogenet 54:83–89.

37. Olegard C, Mandahl N, Heim S, Willen H, Leifsson B, Mitelman F. 1992. Embryonal rhabdomyosarcoma with 100 chromosomes but no structural aberrations. Cancer Genet Cytogenet 60:198–201.

38. Voullaire LE, Petrovic V, Sheffield LJ, Campbell P. 1991. Two forms of ring 13 in a child with rhabdomyosarcoma. Am J Med Genet 39:285–287.

39. Barr FG, Holick J, Nycum L, Biegel JA, Emanuel BS. 1992. Localization of the t(2;13) breakpoint of alveolar rhabdomyosarcoma on a physical map of chromosome 2. Genomics 13:1150–1156.

40. Barr FG, Galili N, Holick J, Biegel JA, Rovera G, Emanuel BS. 1993. Rearrangement of the PAX3 paired box gene in the paediatric solid tumour alveolar rhabdomyosarcoma. Nature Genet 3:113–117.

41. Gruss P, Walther C. 1992. Pax in development. Cell 69:719–722.

42. Noll M. 1993. Evolution and role of Pax genes. Curr Biol 3:595–605.

43. Burri M, Tromvoukis Y, Bopp D, Frigerio G, Noll M. 1989. Conservation of the paired domain in metazoans and its structure in three isolated human genes. EMBO J 8:1183–1190.

44. Bopp D, Burri M, Baumgartner S, Frigerio G, Noll M. 1986. Conservation of a large protein domain in the segmentation gene paired and in functionally related genes of Drosophila. Cell 47:1033–1040.

45. Bopp D, Jamet E, Baumgartner S, Burri M, Noll M. 1989. Isolation of two tissue-specific Drosophila paired box genes, Pox meso and Pox neuro. EMBO J 8:3447–3457.

46. Goulding MD, Chalepakis G, Deutsch U, Erselius J, Gruss P. 1991. Pax-3, a novel murine DNA binding protein expressed during early neurogenesis. EMBO J 10:1135–1147.

47. Baldwin CT, Hoth CF, Amos JA, da-Silva EO, Milunsky A. 1992. An exonic mutation in the HuP2 paired domain gene causes Waardenburg's syndrome. Nature 355:637–638.

48. Baldwin CT, Hoth CF, Macina RA, Milunsky A. 1995. Mutations in PAX3 that cause Waardenburg syndrome type I: ten new mutations and review of the literature. Am J Med Genet 58:115–122.

49. Hoth CF, Milunsky A, Lipsky N, Sheffer R, Clarren SK, Baldwin CT. 1993. Mutation in the

paired domain of the human PAX3 gene cause Klein–Waardenburg Syndrome (WS-III) as well as Waardenburg Syndrome Type I (WS-I). Am J Hum Genet 52:455–462.

50. Farrer LA, Grundfast KM, Amos J, et al. 1992. Waardenburg syndrome (WS) type I is caused by defects at multiple loci, one of which is near ALPP on chromosome 2: first report of the WS consortium. Am J Hum Genet 50:902–913.

51. Tassabehji M, Read AP, Newton VE, Harris R, Balling R, Gruss P, Strachan T. 1992. Waardenburg's syndrome patients have mutations in the human homologue of the Pax-3 paired box gene [see comments]. Nature 355:635–636.

52. Tassabehji M, Newton VE, Leverton K, Turnbull K, Seemanova E, Kunze J, Sperling K, Strachan T, Read AP. 1994. PAX3 gene structure and mutations: close analogies between Waardenburg syndrome and the Splotch mouse. Hum Mol Genet 3:1069–1074.

53. Galili N, Davis RJ, Fredericks WJ, Mukhopadhyay S, Rauscher FJ, Emanuel BS, Rovera G, Barr FG. 1993. Fusion of a fork head domain gene to PAX3 in the solid tumour alveolar rhabdomyosarcoma. Nature Genet 5:230–235.

54. Shapiro DN, Sublett JE, Li B, Downing JR, Naeve CW. 1993. Fusion of PAX3 to a member of the forkhead family of transcription factors in human alveolar rhabdomyosarcoma. Cancer Res 53:5108–5112.

55. Weigel D, Jackle H. 1990. The fork head domain: a novel DNA binding motif of eukaryotic transcription factors? (Letter.) Cell 63:455–456.

56. Weigel D, Jurgens G, Kuttner F, Seifert E, Jackle H. 1989. The homeotic gene fork head encodes a nuclear protein and is expressed in the terminal regions of the Drosophila embryo. Cell 57:645–658.

57. Pierrou S, Hellqvist M, Samuelsson L, Enerback S, Carlsson P. 1994. Cloning and characterization of seven human forkhead proteins: binding site specificity and DNA bending. EMBO J 13:5002–5012.

58. Lai E, Prezioso VR, Tao W, Chen WS, Darnell JE. 1991. Hepatocyte nuclear factor 3alpha belongs to a gene family in mammals that is homologous to the Drosophila homeotic gene fork head. Genes Dev 5:416–427.

59. Hacker U, Grossniklaus U, Gehring WJ, Jackle H. 1992. Developmentally regulated Drosophila gene family encoding the fork head domain. Proc Nat Acad Sci USA 89:8754–8758.

60. Clark KL, Halay ED, Lai E, Burley SK. 1993. Co-crystal structure of the HNF-3/fork head DNA-recognition motif resembles histone H5. Nature 364:412–420.

61. Brennan RG. 1993. The winged-helix DNA-binding motif: another helix–turn–helix takeoff. Cell 74:773–776.

62. Pani L, Overdier DG, Porcella A, Qian X, Lai E, Costa RH. 1992. Hepatocyte nuclear factor 3 beta contains two transcriptional activation domains, one of which is novel and conserved with the Drosophila fork head protein. Mol Cell Biol 12:3723–3732.

63. Weigel D, Seifert E, Reuter D, Jackle H. 1990. Regulatory elements controlling expression of the Drosophila homeotic gene fork head. EMBO J 9:1199–1207.

64. Clevidence DE, Overdier DG, Tao W, Qian X, Pani L, Lai E, Costa RH. 1993. Identification of the nine tissue-specific transcription factors of the hepatocyte nuclear factor 3/forkhead DNA-binding-domain family. Proc Nat Acad Sci USA 90:3948–3952.

65. Lai E, Prezioso VR, Tao W, Chen WS, Darnell JE. 1991. Hepatocyte nuclear factor 3a belongs to a gene family in mammals that is homologous to the Drosophila homeotic gene fork head. Genes Dev 5:416–427.

66. Hromas R, Moore J, Johnston T, Socha C, Klemsz M. 1993. Drosophila forkhead homologues are expressed in a lineage-restricted manner in human hematopoietic cells. Blood 81:2854–2859.

67. Kaestner KH, Lee KH, Schlöndoff J, Hiemisch H, Monaghan AP, Schütz G. 1993. Six members of the mouse forkhead gene family are developmentally regulated. Proc Nat Acad Sci USA 90:7628–7631.

68. Miller LM, Gallegos ME, Morisseau BA, Kim SK. 1993. lin-31, a Caenorhabditis elegans HNF-3/fork head transcription factor homolog, specifies three alternative cell fates in vulval development. Genes Dev 7:933–947.

69. Grossniklaus U, Pearson RK, Gehring WJ. 1992. The Drosophila sloppy paired locus encodes two proteins involved in segmentation that show homology to mammalian transcription factors. Genes Dev 6:1030–1051.

70. Tao W, Lai E. 1992. Telencephalon-restricted expression of BF-1, a new member of the HNF-3/fork head gene family, in the developing rat brain. Neuron 8:957–966.

71. Murphy DB, Wiese S, Burfeind P, Schmundt D, Mattei MG, Schultz-Schaeffer W, Thies U. 1994. Human brain factor 1, a new member of the fork head gene family. Genomics 21:551–557.

72. Parry P, Wei Y, Evans G. 1994. Cloning and characterization of the t(X;11) breakpoint from a leukemic cell line identify a new member of the forkhead gene family. Genes Chromosomes Cancer 11:79–84.

73. Treisman J, Gonczy P, Vashishtha M, Harris E, Desplan C. 1989. A single amino acid can determine the DNA binding specificity of homeodomain proteins. Cell 59:553–562.

74. Chalepakis G, Fritsch R, Fickenscher H, Deutsch U, Goulding M, Gruss P. 1991. The molecular basis of the undulated/Pax-1 mutation. Cell 66:873–884.

75. Czerny T, Schaffner G, Busslinger M. 1993. DNA sequence recognition by Pax proteins: bipartite structure of the paired domain and its binding site. Genes Dev 7:2048–2061.

76. Kastury K, Li J, Druck T, Su H, Vogt PK, Croce CM, Huebner K. 1994. The human homologue of the retroviral oncogene qin maps to chromosome 14q13. Proc Nat Acad Sci USA 91:3616–3618.

77. Li J, Vogt PK. 1993. The retroviral oncogene qin belongs to the transcription factor family that includes the homeotic gene fork head. Proc Nat Acad Sci USA 90:4490–4494.

78. Mitchell PJ, Tjian R. 1989. Transcriptional regulation in mammalian cells by sequence-specific DNA binding proteins. Science 245:371–378.

79. Maulbecker CC, Gruss P. 1993. The oncogenic potential of Pax genes. EMBO J 12:2361–2367.

80. Sublett JE, Jeon IS, Shapiro DN. 1995. The alveolar rhabdomyosarcoma PAX3/FKHR fusion protein is a transcriptional activator. Oncogene 11:545–552.

81. Fredericks WJ, Galili N, Mukhopadhyay S, Rovera G, Bennicelli J, Barr FG, Rauscher FJ. 1995. The PAX3–FKHR fusion protein created by the t(2;13) translocation in alveolar rhabdomyosarcomas is a more potent transcriptional activator than PAX3. Mol Cell Biol 15:1522–1535.

82. Davis RJ, D'Cruz CM, Lovell MA, Biegel JA, Barr FG. 1994. Fusion of PAX7 to FKHR by the variant t(1;13)(p36;q14) translocation in alveolar rhabdomyosarcoma. Cancer Res 54:2869–2872.

83. Jostes B, Walther C, Gruss P. 1990. The murine paired box gene, Pax7, is expressed specifically during the development of the nervous and muscular system. Mech Dev 33:27–38.

84. Zucman J, Melot T, Desmaze C, et al. 1993. Combinatorial generation of variable fusion proteins in the Ewing family of tumours. EMBO J 12:4481–4487.

85. Sorensen PH, Lessnick SL, Lopez-Terrada D, Liu XF, Triche TJ, Denny CT. 1994. A second Ewing's sarcoma translocation, t(21;22), fuses the EWS gene to another ETS-family transcription factor, ERG. Nature Genet 6:146–151.

86. Strachan T, Read AP. 1994. PAX genes. Curr Opin Genet Dev 4:427–438.

87. Epstein JA, Lam P, Jepel L, Maas RL, Shapiro DN. 1995. Pax3 inhibits myogenic differentiation of cultured myoblast cells. J Biol Chem 270:11719–11722.

88. Epstein JA, Shapiro DN, Cheng J, Lam PYP, Maas RL. 1996. Pax3 modulates expression of the c-Met receptor during limb muscle development. Proc Natl Acad Sci USA 93:4213–4218.

89. Scrable HJ, Witte DP, Lampkin BC, Cavenee WK. 1987. Chromosomal localization of the human rhabdomyosarcoma locus by mitotic recombination mapping. Nature 329:645–647.

90. Scrable HJ, Johnson DK, Rinchik EM, Cavenee WK. 1990. Rhabdomyosarcoma-associated locus and MYOD1 are syntenic but separate loci on the short arm of human chromosome 11. Proc Nat Acad Sci USA 87:2182–2186.

334

91. Newsham I, Claussen U, Ludecke HJ, Mason M, Senger G, Horsthemke B, Cavenee W. 1991. Microdissection of chromosome band 11p15.5: characterization of probes mapping distal to the HBBC locus. Genes Chromosomes Cancer 3:108–116.

92. Koufos A, Hansen MF, Copeland NG, Jenkins NA, Lampkin BC, Cavanee WK. 1985. Loss of heterozygosity in three embryonal tumor suggests a common pathogenetic mechanism. Nature 316:330–334.

93. Koufos A, Hanse MF, Lampkin BC, Workman ML, Copeland NG, Jenkins NA, Cavenee WK. 1984. Loss of alleles at loci on human chromosome 11 during genesis of Wilms' tumour. Nature 309:170–172.

94. Weksberg R, Glaves M, Teshima I, Waziri M, Patil S, Williams BR. 1990. Molecular characterization of Beckwith–Wiedemann syndrome (BWS) patients with partial duplication of chromosome 11p excludes the gene MYOD1 from the BWS region. Genomics 8:693–698.

95. Loh WE Jr, Scrable HJ, Livanos E, Arboleda MJ, Cavenee WK, Oshimura M, Weissman BE. 1992. Human chromosome 11 contains two different growth suppressor genes for embryonal rhabdomyosarcoma. Proc Natl Acad Sci USA 89:1755–1759.

96. Weissman BE, Saxon PJ, Pasquale SR, Jones GR, Geiser AG, Stanbridge EJ. 1987. Introduction of a normal human chromosome 11 into a Wilms' tumor cell line controls its tumorigenic expression. Science 236:175–180.

97. Koi M, Johnson LA, Kalikin LM, Little PF, Nakamura Y, Feinberg AP. 1993. Tumor cell growth arrest caused by subchromosomal transferable DNA fragments from chromosome 11. Science 260:361–364.

98. Henry I, Bonaiti-Pelliè C, Chehensse V, et al. 1991. Uniparental paternal disomy in a genetic cancer-predisposing syndrome [see comments]. Nature 351:665–667.

99. Henry I, Puech A, Austruy E, Jeanpierre C, Brugieres L, Ahnine L, Barichard F, Tournade MF, Junien C. 1992. Towards the gene(s) for Beckwith–Weidemann Syndrome and associated tumors in 11p15 (meeting abstract). Proc Am Soc Clin Oncol 11:A226–A226.

100. Scrable H, Cavenee W, Ghavimi F, Lovell M, Morgan K, Sapienza C. 1989. A model for embryonal rhabdomyosarcoma tumorigenesis that involves genome imprinting. Proc Natl Acad Sci USA 86:7480–7484.

101. Sakai T, Tohuchida J, Ohtani N, Yandell DW, Rapport JM, Dryja TP. 1991. Allele-specific hypermethylation of the retinoblastoma tumor-supressor gene. Am J Hum Genet 48:880–888.

102. Tycko B. 1994. Genomic imprinting: mechanisms and role in human pathology. Am J Pathol 144:431–443.

103. Rainier S, Johnson LA, Dobry CJ, Ping AJ, Grundy PE, Feinberg AP. 1993. Relaxation of imprinted genes in human cancer. Nature 362:747–749.

104. Mulligan LM, Matlashewski GJ, Scrable HJ, Cavenee WK. 1990. Mechanisms of p53 loss in human sarcomas. Proc Natl Acad Sci USA 87:5863–5867.

105. Stratton MR, Fisher C, Gusterson BA, Cooper CS. 1989. Detection of point mutations in N-ras and K-ras genes of human embryonal rhabdomyosarcomas using oligonucleotide probes and the polymerase chain reaction. Cancer Res 49:6324–6327.

106. Shapiro DN, Jones BG, Shapiro LH, Dias P, Houghton PJ. 1994. Antisense-mediated reduction in insulin-like growth factor-I receptor expression suppresses the malignant phenotype of a human alveolar rhabdomyosarcoma. J Clin Invest 94:1235–1242.

107. Dias P, Kumar P, Marsden HB, Gattamaneni HR, Heighway J, Kumar S. 1990. N-myc gene is amplified in alveolar rhabdomyosarcomas (RMS) but not in embryonal RMS. Int J Cancer 45:593–596.

108. Sutow WW, Sullivan MP, Ried HL, Taylor HG, Griffith KM. 1970. Prognosis in childhood rhabdomyosarcoma. Cancer 25:1384–1390.

109. Pinkel D, Pickren J. 1961. Rhabdomyosarcoma in children. JAMA 175:293–298.

110. Lawrence W, Jegge G, Foote F. 1964. Embryonal rhabdomyosarcoma. Cancer 17:361–366.

111. Heyn RM, Holland R, Newton WA Jr, Tefft M, Breslow N, Hartmann JR. 1974. The role of combined chemotherapy in the treatment of rhabdomyosarcoma in children. Cancer 34:2128–2142.

112. Crist W, Gehan EA, Ragab AH, et al. 1995. The Third Intergroup Rhabdomyosarcoma Study. J Clin Oncol 13:610–630.

113. Douglass EC, Shapiro DN, Valentine M, Rowe ST, Carroll AJ, Raney RB, Ragab AH, Abella SM, Parham DM. 1993. Alveolar rhabdomyosarcoma with the t(2;13): cytogenetic findings and clinicopathologic correlations. Med Pediatr Oncol 21:83–87.

114. Rabbitts TH. 1994. Chromosomal translocations in human cancer. Nature 372:143–149.

115. Lawrence W Jr, Gehan EA, Hays DM, Beltangady M, Maurer HM. 1987. Prognostic significance of staging factors of the UICC staging system in childhood rhabdomyosarcoma: a report from the Intergroup Rhabdomyosarcoma Study (IRS II). J Clin Oncol 5:46–54.

116. Rodary C, Gehan EA, Flamant F, Treuner J, Carli M, Auquier A, Maurer H. 1991. Prognostic factors in 951 nonmetastatic rhabdomyosarcoma in children: a report from the International Rhabdomyosarcoma Workshop. Med Pediatr Oncol 19:89–95.

117. Andrassy RJ, Corpron CA, Hays D, Raney RB, Wiener ES, Lawrence W Jr, Lobe TE, Bagwell C, Maurer HM. 1996. Extremity sarcomas: an analysis of prognostic factors from the intergroup rhabdomyosarcoma study. J Pediatr Surg 31:191–196.

118. Shapiro E, Strother D. 1992. Pediatric genitourinary rhabdomyosarcoma. J Urol 148:1761–1768.

119. Donaldson SS. 1985. The value of adjuvant chemotherapy in the management of sarcomas in children. Cancer 55:2184–2197.

120. Haddy TB, Nora AH, Sutow WW, Vietti TJ. 1967. Cyclophosphamide treatment for metastatic soft tissue sarcoma: intermittent large doses in the treatment of children. Am J Dis Child 114:301–308.

121. Tan C, Dargeon H, Burchenal J. 1959. Effect of actinomycin D in childhood cancer. Pediatrics 24:544–561.

122. Ghavimi F, Exelby PR, Liebermna PH, Scott BF, Kosloff C. 1981. Multidisciplinary treatment of embryonal rhabdomyosarcoma in children: a progress report. Natl Cancer Inst Monogr 56:111–120.

123. Wilbur JR. 1974. Combination chemotherapy for embryonal rhabdomyosarcoma. Cancer Chemother Rep 58:281–284.

124. Pratt CB, Hustu HO, Fleming ID, Pinkel D. 1972. Coordinated treatment of childhood rhabdomyosarcoma with surgery, radiotherapy, and combination chemotherapy. Cancer Res 32:606–610.

125. Maurer HM, Beltangady M, Gehan EA, et al. 1988. The Intergroup Rhabdomyosarcoma Study-I. A final report. Cancer 61:209–220.

126. Maurer HM, Gehan EA, Beltangady M, et al. 1993. The Intergroup Rhabdomyosarcoma Study-II. Cancer 71:1904–1922.

127. Hays DM, Shimada H, Raney RB Jr, Tefft M, Newton W, Crist WM, Lawrence W Jr, Ragab A, Maurer HM. 1985. Sarcomas of the vagina and uterus: the Intergroup Rhabdomyosarcoma Study. J Pediatr Surg 20:718–724.

128. Raney RB Jr, Tefft M, Newton WA, Ragab AH, Lawrence W Jr, Gehan EA, Maurer HM. 1987. Improved prognosis with intensive treatment of children with cranial soft tissue sarcomas arising in nonorbital parameningeal sites. A report from the Intergroup Rhabdomyosarcoma Study. Cancer 59:147–155.

129. Wharam MD Jr, Foulkes MA, Lawrence W Jr, Lindberg RD, Maurer HM, Newton WA Jr, Ragab AH, Raney RB Jr, Tefft M. 1984. Soft tissue sarcoma of the head and neck in childhood: nonorbital and nonparameningeal sites. A report of the Intergroup Rhabdomyosarcoma Study (IRS)-I. Cancer 53:1016–1019.

130. Ortega JA, Wharam M, Gehan EA, Ragab AH, Crist W, Webber B, Wiener ES, Haeberlen V, Maurer HM. 1991. Clinical features and results of therapy for children with paraspinal soft tissue sarcoma: a report of the Intergroup Rhabdomyosarcoma Study. J Clin Oncol 9:796–801.

131. Raney RB, Tefft M, Lawrence W, Ragab AH, Soule EH, Beltangady M, Gehan EA. 1987. Paratestiular sarcoma in childhood and adolescence. A report from the Intergroup Rhabdomyosarcoma Studies I and II, 1973–1983. Cancer 60:2337–2343.

132. Crist WM, Raney RB, Tefft M, Heyn R, Hays DM, Newton W, Beltangady M, Maurer HM. 1985. Soft tissue sarcomas arising in the retroperitoneal space in children. A report from the Intergroup Rhabdomyosarcoma Study (IRS) Committee. Cancer 56:2125–2132.

133. Hays DM, Raney B, Lawrence W, Soule EH, Gehan EA, Tefft M. 1982. Bladder and prostatic tumors in the Intergroup Rhabdomyosarcoma Study (IRS-I). Results of therapy. Cancer 50:1472–1482.

134. Tefft M, Fernandez C, Donaldson M, Newton W, Moon TE. 1978. Incidence of meningeal involvement by rhabdomyosarcoma of the head and neck in children: a report of the Intergroup Rhabdomyosarcoma Study (IRS). Cancer 42:253–258.

135. Ortega S, Donaldson S, Percy IS, Pappo A, Maurer H. 1995. Venocclusive disease (VOD) of the liver following vincristine-Actinomycin D-cyclophosphamide (VAC) therapy for rhabdomyosarcoma. A report from the Intergroup Rhabdomyosarcoma Study Group (meeting abstract). Proc Am Soc Clin Oncol 14:440.

136. Pappo AS, Etcubanas E, Santana VM, Rao BN, Kun LE, Fontanesi J, Roberson PK, Bowman LC, Crist WM, Shapiro DN. 1993. A phase II trial of ifosfamide in previously untreated children and adolescents with unresectable rhabdomyosarcoma. Cancer 71:2119–2125.

137. Horowitz ME, Etcubanas E, Christensen ML, Houghton JA, George SL, Green AA, Houghton PJ. 1988. Phase II testing of melphalan in children with newly diagnosed rhabdomyosarcoma: a model for anticancer drug development. J Clin Oncol 6:308–314.

138. Houghton PJ, Shapiro DN, Houghton JA. 1991. Rhabdomyosarcoma. From the laboratory to the clinic. Pediatr Clin North Am 38:349–364.

139. Houghton PJ, Cheshire PJ, Myers L, Stewart CF, Synold TW, Houghton JA. 1992. Evaluation of 9-dimethylaminomethyl-10-hydroxycamptothecin against xenografts derived from adult and childhood solid tumors. Cancer Chemother Pharmacol 31:229–239.

140. Hays DM. 1993. Bladder/prostate rhabdomyosarcoma: results of the multi-institutional trials of the Intergroup Rhabdomyosarcoma Study. Semin Surg Oncol 9:520–523.

141. Raney B, Gehan E, Hays D, Tefft M, Newton WJ, Haeberlen V, Maurer HM. 1990. Primary chemotherapy with or without radiation therapy and/or surgery for children with localized sarcomas of the bladder, prostate, vagina, uterus, and cervix. A comparison of results in Intergroup Rhabdomyosarcoma Studies I and II. Cancer 66:2072–2081.

142. Donaldson SS. 1993. Lessons from our children. Int J Radiat Oncol Biol Phys 26:739–749.

143. Flamant F, Rodary C, Voute PA, Otten J. 1985. Primary chemotherapy in the treatment of rhabdomyosarcoma in children: trial of the International Society of Pediatric Oncology (SIOP) preliminary results. Radiother Oncol 3:227–236.

144. Rousseau P, Flamant F, Quintana E, Voute PA, Gentet JC. 1994. Primary chemotherapy in rhabdomyosarcomas and other malignant mesenchymal tumors of the orbit: results of the International SOciety of Pediatric Oncology MMT 84 Study [see comments]. J Clin Oncol 12:516–521.

145. Otten J, Flamant F, Rodary C, Brunat-Mentigny M, Dutou L, Olive D, Quintana E, Voute PA. 1989. Treatment of rhabdomyosarcoma and other malignant mesenchymal tumours of childhood with ifosfamide + vincristine + dactinomycin (IVA) as front-line therapy (a SIOP study). Cancer Chemother Pharmacol 24 (Suppl 1):S30.

146. Stevens M, Flamant F, Rey A. 1991. SIOP Malignant Mesenchymal Tumors (MMT) 1989 Study (meeting abstract). Med Pediatr Oncol 19:435.

147. Stevens MCG, Oberlin O, Rey A, Praguin M-T. 1994. Experience from the SIOP MMT 89 study (meeting abstract). Med Pediatr Oncol 23:171.

148. Flamant F, Rodary C, Rey A, Otten J, Voute PA, Sommelet D, Quintana E, Brunat-Mentigny M, Habrand JL. 1991. Assessing the benefit of primary chemotherapy in the treatment of rhabdomyosarcoma in children. Report from the International Society of Pediatric Oncology: RMS 84 Study (meeting abstract). Proc Am Soc Clin Oncol 10:309.

149. Rodary C, Rey A, Olive D, Flamant F, Quintana E, Brunat-Mentigny M, Otten J, Voute PA. 1988. Prognostic factors in 281 children with nonmetastatic rhabdomyosarcoma (RMS) at diagnosis. Med Pediatr Oncol 16:71–77.

337

150. Carli M, Pinkerton R, Frascella E, Flamant F, Oberlin O, Koscielniak E, Stevens M. 1993. Intensive chemotherapy for metastatic sarcoma in children: SIOP European Intergroup study MMT89 (meeting abstract). Proc Annu Meet Am Soc Clin Oncol 12:A1404.

151. Phillips MB, Flamant F, Sommelet-Olive D, Pinkerton CR. 1995. Phase II study of rapid-scheduled etoposide in paediatric soft tissue sarcomas. Eur J Cancer [A] 31A:782–784.

152. Pritchard-Jones K, Modak S, Mancini AF, Carli M, Pinkerton CR. 1996. Response of previously untreated metastatic rhabdomyosarcoma to combination chemotherapy with carboplatin, epirubicin and vincristine. Eur J Cancer 32A:821–825.

153. Koscielniak E, Jurgens H, Winkler K, Burger D, Herbst M, Keim M, Bernhard G, Treuner J. 1992. Treatment of soft tissue sarcoma in childhood and adolescence. A report of the German Cooperative Soft Tissue Sarcoma Study. Cancer 70:2557–2567.

154. Treuner J, Koscielniak E, Keim M. 1989. Comparison of the rates of response to ifosfamide and cyclophosphamide in primary unresectable rhabdomyosarcomas. Cancer Chemother Pharmacol 24(Suppl 1):S48–50.

155. Carli M, Pastore G, Perilongo G, Grotto P, De Bernardi B, Ceci A, Di Tullio M, Madon E, Pianca C, Paolucci G. 1988. Tumor response and toxicity after single high-dose versus standard five-day divided-dose dactinomycin in childhood rhabdomyosarcoma. J Clin Oncol 6:654–658.

156. Carli M, Perilongo G, Grotto P, Guglielmi M, Mancini A, Dall'Orso S. 1989. High tumor response rate in childhood rhabdomyosarcoma (RMS) with 'modified IVA.' Preliminary report of the Italian Cooperative Study RMS 88 (meetng abstract). Med Pediatr Oncol 17:310.

157. Andrassy RJ, Hays DM, Raney RB, Wiener ES, Lawrence W, Lobe TE, Corpron CA, Smith M, Maurer HM. 1995. Conservative surgical management of vaginal and vulvar pediatric rhabdomyosarcoma: a report from the Intergroup Rhabdomyosarcoma Study III. J Pediatr Surg 30:1034–1037.

158. Donaldson SS, Asmar L, Breneman J, Fryer C, Glicksman AS, Laurie F, Wharam M, Gehan EA. 1995. Hyperfractionated radiation in children with rhabdomyosarcoma — results of an intergroup rhabdomyosarcoma pilot study. Int J Radiat Oncol Biol Phys 32:903–911.

159. Lawrence W Jr, Hays DM, Heyn R, Tefft M, Crist W, Beltangady M, Newton W Jr, Wharam M. 1987. Lymphatic metastases with childhood rhabdomyosarcoma. A report from the Intergroup Rhabdomyosarcoma Study. Cancer 60:910–915.

160. Hays DM, Lawrence W Jr, Wharam M, Newton W Jr, Ruymann FB, Beltangady M, Maurer HM. 1989. Primary reexcision for patients with 'microscopic residual' tumor following initial excision of sarcomas of trunk and extremity sites. J Pediatr Surg 24:5–10.

161. Lawrence JW. 1991. Surgical principles in the management of sarcomas in children. In Maurer HM, Ruyman FB, Pochedly C (eds.), Rhabdomyosarcoma and Related Tumors in Children and Adolescents. Boca Raton: CRC Press, pp. 171–180.

162. Heyn R, Raney RB, Hays DM, Tefft M, Gehan E, Webber B. 1992. Late effects of therapy in patients with paratesticular rhabdomyosarcoma. J Clin Oncol 10:614–623.

163. Heyn R, Ragab A, Raney RB Jr, Ruymann F, Tefft M, Lawrence W Jr, Soule E, Maurer HM. 1986. Late effects of therapy in orbital rhabdomyosarcoma in children. A report from the Intergroup Rhabdomyosarcoma Study. Cancer 57:1738–1743.

164. Raney B Jr, Heyn R, Hays DM, Tefft M, Newton WA Jr, Wharam M, Vassilopoulou-Sellin R, Maurer HM. 1993. Sequelae of treatment in 109 patients followed for 5 to 15 years after diagnosis of sarcoma of the bladder and prostate. A report from the Intergroup Rhabdomyosarcoma Study Committee. Cancer 71:2387–2394.

165. Raney RB, Asmar L, Vassilopoulou-Selin R, Klein MJ, Donaldson SS, Gehan EA, Maurer HM. 1995. Late sequelae in 162 patients with non-orbital soft tissue sarcoma of the head and neck: report from Intergroup Rhabdomyosarcoma Studies II and III (meeting abstract). Proc Am Soc CLin Oncol 14:454.

166. Heyn R, Haeberlen V, Newton WA, Ragab AH, Raney RB, Tefft M, Wharam M, Ensign LG, Maurer HM. 1993. Second malignant neoplasms in children treated for

rhabdomosarcoma. Intergroup Rhabdomyosarcoma Study Committee [see comments]. J Clin Oncol 11:262–270.

167. Scaradavou A, Heller G, Sklar CA, Ren L, Ghavimi F. 1995. Second malignant neoplasms in long-term survivors of childhood rhabdomyosarcoma. Cancer 76:1860–1867.

IV

Late Effects of Childhood Cancer

11. Late effects of cancer therapy

Elaine R. Morgan and Maureen Haugen

1. Introduction

Concern about late effects of chemotherapy is a novel problem for the oncologist. As late as the 1960s, survival from childhood cancer was less than 20% overall, with many subsets of patients demonstrating even worse outcome [1]. However, in the last three decades, treatment for malignancy in children has become far more effective. By the late 1980s, 60% to 70% of children with cancer (figure 1) were surviving their illness [2]. Although outcomes were less favorable for certain types of malignancy (figure 2), it is estimated that by the year 2000, one in 900 young adults will be a survivor of childhood cancer [3]. This has created a new area of concern for pediatricians, oncologists, and internists. Dealing with the late effects of therapy, an unheard- of luxury in the 1960s, has now become a dilemma for patients, practitioners, and families of patients and must take a prominent position in the practice of pediatric oncology.

Chemotherapy, radiation therapy, surgery, and the psychological effects and societal discrimination of chronic illness have protean effects on the survivors [4]. These effects encompass the realms of medicine, psychology, education, and social service and will undoubtedly play a major role far into adulthood in these patients. In order to help deal with the wide-reaching secondary events, late-effects clinics are being developed in most large oncology programs, staffed by practitioners and other personnel with interest and expertise in this area [5]. Even today the very late effects to be encountered in the mature adult survivors are unknown [5,6].

Although findings vary significantly in different series, there is an indication of increased mortality compared to matched controls in adults previously treated for childhood malignancy. One series has suggested that this increase occurs primarily in patients who suffered a relapse of their primary disease before five years from diagnosis [7]. However, another series demonstrated an increased age-adjusted death rate in adult survivors continuing for more than five years after diagnosis, even excluding deaths from the primary cancer [8] (figure 2). Factors associated with increasing mortality rates included primary diagnosis, female sex, increased intensity of therapy, numbers of modalities of

D.O. Walterhouse and S.L. Cohn (eds), DIAGNOSTIC AND THERAPEUTIC ADVANCES IN PEDIATRIC ONCOLOGY. Copyright © 1997. Kluwer Academic Publishers, Boston. All rights reserved.

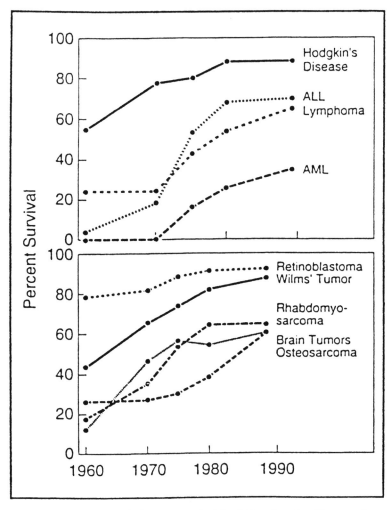

Figure 1. Cancer-specific trends in five-year survival for chldren less than 15 years of age.

treatment, and increasing chronologic age after therapy [9]. In this series, there was a greater risk in survivors of Hodgkin's disease and central nervous system (CNS) tumors, relative to other diagnoses.

At the present time, the spectrum of late effects is still evolving and will undoubtedly continue to change. Treatment modalities, chemotherapeutic agents, surgical techniques, and aggressiveness of therapy continue to develop, making the prediction of long-term problems based on historical controls difficult [5]. Nonetheless, there is an ever-increasing knowledge about the nature of these late events and their impact on patient survival and quality of life. We have only scratched the surface, however, in dealing with the impact of effects on the next generation, the progeny of present survivors [2,10–13].

344

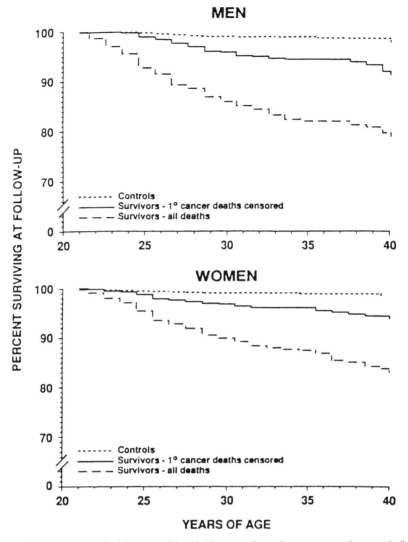

Figure 2. Estimated survival between 21 and 40 years of age for cancer survivors and sibling control subjects (finely dashed line) by sex. For survivors, two curves are show; all deaths are shown in one curve (dashed line), and in the second curve (solid line), only deaths from causes other than primary cancer are shown.

2. Nature of late effects

When one considers the modalities of treatment used, it is obvious that there are several different categories of late effects to be considered. First are the direct physical/anatomic changes engendered in the patient. Surgical resection may result in the loss of organs or limbs that have been resected/amputated for

345

the purpose of removing tumor. Thus, patients may have to adapt to a variety of changes in physical appearance and function, including alteration in skeletal structure, colostomy, cystectomy, nephrectomy, partial pneumonectomy, etc. These changes necessitate specific adaptive behaviors and the use of prostheses or appropriate medical supplies.

Irradiation therapy may likewise alter body habitus, particularly in the growing organism, and may result in assymetric appearance or discrepancies in the development of one side of the body, as in limb-length discrepancy [14] or scoliosis secondary to truncal assymetry [15,16]. Furthermore, radiation damage to bone or soft tissues may result in significant deformity, pathologic fracture, necrosis, and infection of structures, which can even necessitate further surgical resection [17,18].

Further physical problems may result from physiological/functional impairment secondary to surgical resection of organs and the combined effects on organs of chemotherapy and irradiation. Resultant organ damage may yield a variety of disabilities that may require medical therapy and/or alterations in life-style and quality of life. For example, cardiac dysfunction secondary to primary treatment may cause symptomatic heart disease, may necessitate limitation in certain physical activities, or may require active medical intervention for maximal function [19–22]. In addition, the physiologic effects of cancer treatment may even lead to the development of additional malignancies (second malignant neoplasms or SMNs), in themselves requiring further therapy [23,24]. Beyond this, gonadal effects of therapy can lead to alteration of reproductive function [25–27] with ramifications on the social and psychological function of survivors [28] and potentially on future generations [11,13,29]. Central nervous system effects of treatment can lead to neurological dysfunction and cognitive problems as well [30–32].

Of no lesser consequence are the psychosocial ramifications resulting from treatment. As mentioned above, cognitive difficulties may result from central nervous system therapy, leading to educational difficulties and subsequent problems with employment [33]. Furthermore, the simple consequences of chronic illness in childhood may lead to frequent school absences, with additional educational requirements and problems. Additionally, societal reaction to 'disabled' persons may create additional hurdles such as employment bias and insurance limitation [33–35].

3. Factors impacting on late effects

The nature of late effects is dependent on several factors. These include specific modalities of treatment, interaction between multiple treatment modalities, era of treatment, specific anatomic areas affected and consequently treated, disease-specific genetic associations, intensity and number of different treatments used, and age of the patient at the time of therapy. In the ensuing discussion, we will attempt to highlight these areas to assist in the prediction of effects for individual patient subgroups.

The effects alluded to above are also impacted by the interaction of different treatment modalities. Thus, certain chemotherapeutic agents may inhibit wound healing or decrease resistance to infections, thus increasing surgical morbidity. On the other hand, disruption of the blood–brain barrier by surgical intervention, by the tumor itself, or by irradiation in patients with brain tumors may increase sensitivity to and consequences of chemotherapy [36,37]. In addition, certain drugs are radiation sensitizers, increasing the local skin and tissue damage resultant from irradiation [38]. Of even greater concern is the interaction between chemotherapy and irradiation therapy, causing increased organ toxicity to heart, lung, liver, skin, kidney, bladder and central nervous system [39–41]. Although attempts are made to take these interactions into account during therapy, late and sometimes unanticipated consequences can result.

Genetic predispositions may also impact on the development of late effects. For example, children with Down's syndrome have an inherent increased sensitivity to methotrexate [42,43], resulting in increased immediate toxicity and potential for late toxicities as well. Certain genetic conditions such as Ataxia telangiectasia, Fanconi's anemia, and Bloom's syndrome result in faulty DNA repair mechanisms, increasing both the sensitivity of these patients to radiation therapy and their potential for secondary neoplasia [44–46]. Likewise, children from families with genetic cancer syndromes, such as the Li–Fraumeni syndrome, have increased incidence of secondary cancers [47].

The age of the child is another determining factor for the development of secondary consequences. The younger child with immature organ function may have enhanced toxicity from chemotherapy because of altered metabolism, thus increasing the risk of serious side effects, such as anthracycline cardiotoxicity at relatively lower doses [48]. Furthermore, the young child with significant growth potential will have a greater likelihood of developing physical problems related to further growth, such as short stature from spinal irradiation or leg-length discrepancy from surgical or radiation-induced interruption of the growth plate [49,50]. Likewise, the younger child is more likely to demonstrate cognitive difficulties after brain irradiation because of the continuing brain development in the normal young child [51]. On the other hand, for unclear reasons, peripheral neuropathies that may create long-term disabilities are more common in the older adolescent and in the adult. Likewise, gonadal effects resulting in fertility problems occur more commonly in postpubescent patients [52–54].

Intensity of treatment and number of relapses, both of which impact on the number of therapeutic regimens used in therapy, have obvious implications on late effects. Thus, for example, in evaluating the late effects resulting from bone marrow transplantation procedures, it is also important to review the prior therapy given, because of cumulative toxicities. In general, the more therapy, the greater the risk for early and late morbidity, and the patient suffering relapses is more likely to receive additional courses of treatment [7,10,55].

Finally, the era of treatment is another factor in the consideration of late effects [4]. Over the years, new chemotherapeutic agents have been developed, subjecting children to late morbidity that might not have occurred previously. Furthermore, the overall intensity of treatment has increased dramatically over the past 30 years [7,10]. On the other hand, supportive care measures have concurrently improved, minimizing some of these effects. Also, as we learn more about the nature of late morbidity, regimens are modified accordingly to try to decrease these effects. Certain disease entities are actually being treated with shorter courses of chemotherapy, as a result of enhanced survival and knowledge about potential damage from prolonged therapy, and with exclusion of radiation therapy [56]. In addition, radiation therapy techniques and equipment have improved significantly over the years, allowing increased tissue sparing [57]. Thus, for example, the marked scoliosis seen in Wilms' tumor patients 30 years ago is a lesser problem today [16,58]. In fact, with increased efficacy of chemotherapy, some patients who might previously have received radiation therapy are now treated without radiation or at least with lower treatment doses. Likewise, surgical techniques have vastly improved. Currently, the ability to perform limb-salvage procedures for certain children with limb sarcomas has obviated the necessity for amputation, thereby improving life-style [59]. Improved chemotherapy and radiation therapy protocols have decreased the utilization of mutilating surgery. As treatment protocols evolve, the spectrum of late effects changes. In addition, advances in other areas of medical care, such as heart and liver transplantation and modern reproductive technologies, may ameliorate some of the late effects, thereby improving survival and quality of life for survivors.

4. Modality-sepecific late effects

4.1. Surgery

In general, when one thinks of late effects of cancer therapy, one is likely to concentrate on the consequences of chemotherapy and radiation therapy. However, surgery remains a major modality in the treatment of pediatric cancers and may also impact on later quality of life. The results of cancer surgery are obviously related to the anatomic structures involved and in some instances may result in secondary effects as well. Postoperative complications may increase the severity of late effects [60].

The results of neurosurgery involving the brain can be easily deduced by an understanding of neuroanatomy. In addition to anticipated neurologic deficits, the presence of tumor and/or the surgical approach can result in serous endo-

crinologic sequelae such as permanent diabetes insipidus and other disturbances of the pituitary–hypothalamic axis [61]. In earlier years, it was common
to remove the eye and/or to perform orbital exenteration in patients with
retinoblastoma or orbital rhabdomyosarcoma [62]. Aside from the obvious
resultant loss of vision, this procedure led to facial deformities as the operated
orbit failed to grow [63]. Modern prosthetic devices have improved this situation. The majority of other head and neck tumors in children were usually
treated primarily with nonsurgical modalities. Radical neck dissections and
nasopharyngeal surgeries commonly performed in adults with carcinoma are
rarely done in children.

Resection of musculoskeletal structures results in obvious orthopedic disturbances. In addition, commonly performed limb-salvage surgeries, which are
prominent in the management of patients with bone tumors, may result in
asymmetric growth because of interruption of the growth plate or complications such as fracture or infection of the graft. Resection of paraspinal masses
with laminectomy, which was more commonly done in earlier years for treatment of impending cord compression and major truncal muscle resection for
sarcomas, may lead to assymetry and spine instability [64] and consequent
scoliosis, which may be very significant. In fact, significant thoracic scoliosis
may also impact on lung function.

Beyond this, the obvious impact of organ resection may have serious consequences for later function. Certain surgeries, such as unilateral nephrectomy,
partial hepatectomy, and (less commonly) resection of lung tissue if not extensive, appear to be tolerated with minimal long-term effects [65]. Other surgeries, however, have a very significant impact on quality of life. Splenectomy
results in increased risk of late sepsis, with life-long necessity for bacterial
prophylaxis [66]. The consequences of bowel resection vary with the level and
extent of resection and also vary concerning the possibility of reanastomosis.
When primary anastamosis is not possible, externalization of bowel may be
necessary [67]. In certain instances, specific malabsorption syndromes may
result. Similarly, bladder resection, which used to be commonly performed for
bladder–prostate rhabdomyosarcoma, is now less commonly done but still
occurs in some situations. This procedure may lead to nephrostomy,
ureterostomies, or an ileal conduit with impact on quality of life [68]. Furthermore, in some instances, these diversions may lead to frequent urinary tract
infections, with potential impairment of renal function. Retroperitoneal lymph
node dissection is uncommonly performed in children but may result in retro-
grade ejaculation [69]. Finally, removal of reproductive organs like treatment
with chemotherapy or irradiation, more commonly in females than males,
will impact on fertility, sexual function, and hormone levels, with resultant
premature menopause and necessity for hormone replacement therapy [70].

Currently, most treatment programs tend to utilize more conservative surgery with preservation of organ function, minimizing these effects. Nonetheless, it is essential to understand the potential consequences of surgery for
anticipatory guidance and counseling, as well as appropriate monitoring.

Radiation therapy itself can cause significant long-term sequelae. Certainly, treatment regimens have changed over time with attempts to decrease total dose, to shrink down portals, or in some cases to eliminate irradiation. And technology has immensely improved to provide greater accuracy of treatment, less scatter, and relative tissue sparing. In general, higher total dose and individual radiation fractions and younger age of the child at the time of radiation increase the risk for long-term sequelae [14,71]. Follow-up of survivors of childhood cancer means understanding the implications over time of the effects of radiation therapy.

Radiation therapy plays an important role in the treatment of pediatric brain tumors. Survival has increased over the last 20 years due to advances in surgery and chemotherapy as part of treatment [72]. Long-term effects of central nervous system (CNS) therapy have been studied extensively, and neurologic, neuropsychologic, and endocrinologic dysfunctions have been noted.

Radionecrosis of the brain is usually seen six months to two years following treatment and is related to a total dose of approximately 5000 cGy and a dose per fraction of 180–200 cGy [71]. Spontaneous brain and spinal cord hemorrhage has been infrequently reported 4 to 5 years following radiation therapy for a primary CNS malignancy [73,74]. Focal signs or signs of increased intracranial pressure can be seen, mimicking a structural lesion, and must be distinguished from recurrent tumor. The pathophysiology of this development is unclear [74].

Leukoencephalopathy is a late complication of treatment from radiation and certain chemotherapy, notably methotrexate [71,72]. Clinically, it is characterized by dementia, ataxia, focal motor deficits, coma, and death. Its pathological hallmark is white matter destruction. CT findings of leukoencephalopathy were first reported in 1978 by Peylan-Ramu and colleagues in patients with leukemia [72]. It has also been reported in children with brain tumors treated with radiation without chemotherapy.

Learning disabilities secondary to treatment and tumor-induced brain injury are frequently described but are difficult to quantitate. In general, children who received more than 2400 cGy suffer from more learning disabilities and a decline in IQ scores over time [72]. Children with brain tumors, who may receive 2 to 3 times the radiation dose of those with leukemia (4000–6000 cGy vs. 1800–2400 cGy), have generally more severe intellectual dysfunction. Age at the time of treatment (younger than 4 to 5 years), location of the tumor (hemispheric tumors), more rapidly growing tumors, the use of adjuvant methotrexate, higher total dose, and higher dose per radiation fraction, as well as the presence of hydrocephalus at the time of presentation, appear to be risk factors for increased neuropsychologic dysfunction [72].

Endocrinopathies affect not only children who have had radiation to the brain but also those who have had direct thyroid irradiation, as well as those who have received abdominal, spinal, or pelvic radiation with scatter to the ovaries or testes. These problems tend to be the most amenable to therapy. The most common complication of radiation is growth failure. Cranial irradiation will cause growth hormone deficiency in up to 80% of children with brain tumors and precocious puberty in some patients [74]. There is an immediate suppressive effect of radiation on the hypothalamic pituitary axis at a minimum total dose of approximately 2500 cGy [72].

Primary hypothyroidism may be seen as a late effect of radiation to the pituitary–hypothalamic axis or directly to the thyroid from cervical spine or neck radiation. Damage occurs usually when the dose exceeds 2000 cGy [14,75].

Gonadal dysfunction will affect males and females depending on the stage of pubertal development at the time of treatment and on the total dose of radiation. Reduced sperm production in postpubertal males has been seen with radiation scatter associated with pelvic therapy even with scrotal shielding [76]. Prepubertal testicular germ cells also appear to be radiosensitive to scatter from abdominal radiation [14,77]. Leydig cell toxicity with resulting inadequate production of testosterone will occur with direct exposure at higher dosage, as indicated from experience from children with testicular leukemia [78].

Assessment of effects on female hormonal and reproductive function is more difficult. Despite this uncertainty it is known that age and total dose of radiation are dependent factors. Delayed menarche, primary ovarian failure, or early menopause can result from abdominal, pelvic, spinal, or total body irradiation [67].

Radiation therapy can commonly cause functional and cosmetic disabilities involving bone, teeth, muscle, and other soft tissues. These are reported in 11% to 38% of pediatric cancers, primarily solid tumors [79]. Changes include scoliosis, impairment of soft tissue, and muscle and bone growth. Scoliosis is seen most commonly in Wilms' tumor patients treated with 1800 to 3500 cGy to the tumor bed, even when including the entire width of each vertebra in the field [67], and has also been observed in other solid tumors where the spinal column has been radiated [80]. The incidence and severity of scoliosis have decreased with the use of modern radiation equipment and field planning [16,80].

Atrophic or hypoplastic soft tissue, muscle, or bone will occur with radiation with severity related to the age of treatment of the child and the total dose of radiation. Tissues will become fibrosed, hair may not grow, skin may develop pigmentary changes, eyes may develop cataracts, hearing may be impaired. Growing bones may not grow or may develop avascular necrosis, osteoporosis, multiple fractures, or a second malignancy. Dentition may be delayed or arrested in development, or may have an increased propensity for malocclusion and caries when higher total doses are used (i.e., 4500–6000 cGy to the nasopharynx) [81,82].

Abnormalities that have been attributed to radiation-induced or radiation-

351

associated cardiopulmonary diseases have been well summarized [21,25,26]. Delayed effects include acute pericarditis and pericardial effusions, pericardial fibrosis, pancarditis, valvular defects, conduction defects, coronary artery disease, and chronic restrictive pulmonary fibrosis. A report from Stanford University retrospectively reviewed the records of 635 patients treated for Hodgkin's disease before 21 years of age. The authors concluded that mediastinal radiation of 4000 to 4500 cGy increases the risk of death from coronary artery and other cardiac diseases, with the greatest risk within five years of radiation [27].

Direct irradiation of the ocular apparatus can be avoided by shielding. Effects on the retina and the lacrimal glands are rare. The lens, however, is very radiosensitive. It can be affected by scattered doses even with shielding [71]. Cataract formation can be seen at a minimum dose of 200 cGy (approximately 400 cGy for hyperfractionated radiation) [83].

Chronic radiation otitis may occur with irradiation to the ear in doses greater than 5000 cGy. Radiation-induced deafness appears to be rare [71].

Fibrosis and enteritis are the most common late pathologic abnormalities of the gastrointestinal tract. They can occur anywhere from the esophagus to the rectum and are often associated with adhesions or stricture formation, which may be progressive or recurrent. The incidence of problems may increase with the concomitant use of certain chemotherapies and abdominal surgery. Fibrosis of the liver secondary to radiation is probably underreported because the incidence of subclinical hepatitis is unknown [67]. Similarly, hyposplenia or asplenia resulting from direct splenic irradiation occurs, but the true incidence is unknown [46].

Radiation dose exceeding 2300 cGy is a well-known cause of chronic nephritis [67]. Cystitis is also seen following radiation at an incidence of 5% of patients at doses less than 4000 Gy — an incidence that increase with distal urinary tract obstruction, infection, or the concurrent use of radiomimetic agents [67].

One of the most dreaded late effects is second malignancy. Acute nonlymphocytic leukemias have been observed, as well as bone tumors, melanomas, and breast tumors in the field of radiation [3,84,85].

Strategies for avoiding these late complications have focused on refining radiation techniques and on limiting radiation dosages by intensifying chemotherapeutic regimens.

4.3. Chemotherapy

The generally anticipated effects of chemotherapy, like radiation therapy, are related to the age of the child during the exposure and to dose and schedule. Chemotherapy, however, unlike radiation therapy and surgery, is most likely to result in acute toxicities, which are usually transient but occasionally persist. Because most chemotherapeutic agents are cell cycle dependent, their acute toxicites can be related to the proliferation kinetics of individual cell populations. Most susceptible are those tissues or organs with high cell turnover rates, such as the bone marrow, gastrointestinal mucosa, testes, epidermis, and liver. Least susceptible are those cells that replicate slowly or not at all, i.e., neurons, muscle cells, and connective tissue. Most chemotherapeutic agents do not directly affect linear growth, although there are exceptions to this statement and growth may also be affected indirectly.

Alkylating agents in common use are nitrogen mustard, cyclophosphamide, ifosfamide, busulfan, and procarbazine. This class of drugs is most lethal to rapidly dividing cells. These drugs can cause gonadal changes, including ovarian failure and damaged, decreased, or absent spermatogonia that may or may not be reversible depending on the total dose received [86,87]. Prepubertal gonads appear to be relatively resistant to injury, i.e., there is greater impact in patients in more advanced stages of sexual development [87–89].

Acute leukemias as a second malignancy neoplasm (SMN) related to alkylating agents have been noted up to 20 years after treatment, with the highest risk during the first two years posttreatment. The patient may present in a myelodysplastic phase. Cytogenetic analysis reveals an abnormal karyotype in up to 96% of patients, with the classic observation being loss of part or all of chromosome 5 or 7. The leukemia is most frequently FAB subtype M1 or M2 acute nonlymphocytic leukemia [85]. Other SMNs secondary to alkylating agents include lymphomas and bladder carcinomas. The mechanism by which chemotherapy induces an SMN is unknown but may be associated with the ability of these drugs to alter DNA. In 1995, Travis et al. found a significant (4.5-fold) risk of bladder cancer following cyclophosphamide therapy. The risk was dependent on cumulative dose and was most significant for a total dose of greater than 20 Gy [90].

Cyclophosphamide itself is associated with hemorrhagic cystitis, with about a 10% incidence [90]. There are occasional cases occurring decades after therapy. With ifosfamide, a cyclophosphamide analogue, the incidence may be as high as 45%, but the incidence is presumably reduced by use of prophylaxis with vigorous hydration and Mesna administration [91]. Ifosfamide, as well, can cause dose-related Fanconi's renal disease that may or may not be reversible. Risk factors for development of this syndrome include higher total dose, younger age of the patient, exposure to agents that also cause renal tubular defects, and presence of only one kidney [92].

Nitrogen mustard alone in this class can cause skin and tendon contractures from drug extravasation, resulting acutely in severe tissue necrosis and sloughing and subsequently in late soft tissue contractures.

The class of agents known as antibiotics (dactinomycin, doxorubicin, daunomycin, and bleomycin) have a diverse number of late effects. All except bleomycin are vesicant drugs similar to nitrogen mustard. Dactinomycin can cause late hepatotoxicity but usually only if there is evidence of acute toxicity. Bleomycin can result in pulmonary fibrosis at a higher total dose [93]. This drug may also play a role in the development of vasoocclusive disease and premature coronary artery disease [94]. A side effect specific to the

353

anthracyclines doxorubicin and daunomycin is dose-related cardiotoxicity, generally seen at a total dose in excess of $200\,mg/m^2$. However, age of the child during treatment and additional therapy including radiation therapy may be compounding factors, and cardiac toxicity, although dose related, is not consistently predictable [95]. Furthermore, cardiac damage continues to occur for at least 15 to 20 years after exposure, and the risk even at lower doses is not yet known. Anthracyclines, in the absence of radiation, have been associated with late echocardiographic abnormalities in 65% of survivors of childhood leukemia [20]. In 1992, Larsen studied survivors of childhood cancer [77]; patients who received anthracyclines alone (24 radiation therapy alone, and 27 who received both modalities). An increased frequency of electrocardiographic changes (QTc prolongation, supraventricular premature complexes, supraventricular tachycardia, ventricular premature complexes, couplets, and ventricular tachycardia) were noted in all groups when compared with age-matched controls. Serious ventricular ectopy has been noted in patients with a cumulative anthracycline dose of greater than $200\,mg/m^2$ [96].

The late effects of antimetabolites (methotrexate, 6-mercaptopurine, 6-thioguanine, 5-fluorouracil, and cytosine arabinoside) are usually a result of toxicity during therapy — for example, hepatic or renal toxicity [97,98]. However, leukoencephalopathy (described above in section 4.2) from intrathecal or high-dose intravenous methotrexate (MTX) may not be seen until years later and is most commonly seen when MTX is used in combination with radiation therapy [71,72].

The plant alkaloids vincristine and vinblastine are vesicants. Late persistent neurotoxicity — specifically, peripheral neuropathies — can be observed in children receiving multiple doses of vincristine. Older children and adolescents, as well as patients with unrecognized neurologic diseases such as Charcot-Marie-Tooth [99], tend to be more sensitive to vincristine.

The platinum drugs cis-platinum and carboplatinum are both ototoxic and renal toxic and can cause peripheral neuropathies. Cis-platinum effects, however, at standard therapy doses are more severe. Cis-platinum renal toxicity occurs in 50%–75% of patients and appears to be dependent on the individual dose intensity as well as the total cumulative dose. Renal failure from chemotherapy generally represents persistence of acute toxicity and does not usually develop in patients who had no problems during or shortly after therapy. However, late-onset hypomagnesemia and other electrolyte abnormalities can be seen despite normal or recovered levels at termination or early after therapy. Cis-platinum ototoxicity is also therapy related but may worsen over time. It has also been noted that high-dose cranial irradiation within 10 months of cis-platinum therapy increases the sensitivity to ototoxic effects [71]. Peripheral neuropathies seen more commonly in adults may be reversible [100].

Hormones such as estrogens, androgens, progestins, and corticosteroids have multiple late effects. Obesity, avascular necrosis [101], osteporosis, and cataracts are usually seen with prolonged and/or high-dose exposure.

Epidophylototoxins include etopiside (VP-16), tenoposide (VM-26), and topotecan. Therapy-related secondary acute nonlymphocytic leukemia, commonly with chromosomal translocation at the 11q23 locus, may occur after exposure to VP-16 and VM-26. This SMN appears to be related to the dose and schedule [94]. It is not yet clear whether the same phenomenon will occur with related topoisomerase II inhibitors.

5. Overview of late effects

While it is helpful to understand the late effects induced by specific modalities of therapy, as discussed previously, one must approach the patient in a more unified fashion. Therefore, it is important to consider, by systems, the nature of late events that may occur in order to plan an approach to health care maintenance in these patients. In general, most clinics have devised a systematic approach to the screening of survivors of childhood cancers based on the currently understood probabilities of certain adverse events. Thus, although this information may be contained elsewhere in this chapter, we will now attempt to outline by organ systems the consequences of therapy that can be anticipated.

5.1. Integument (skin, soft tissue, and mucous membranes)

Surgery may result in cosmetic defects; certain chemotherapeutic agents may lead to hyperpigmentation; and chronic graft-versus-host disease following bone marrow transplantation may cause scleredermatous changes in the skin and subcutaneous tissues [102,103]. However, radiation effects are far more prominent and may lead to significant hypoplasia of skin and underlying tissues. Likewise, radiation to the head and neck may cause atrophy of the salivary and/or lacrimal glands, with resultant sicca syndromes [82]. Chemotherapy alone, and radiation effects on salivation as well as direct effects on the teeth, particularly in children with preerupted permanent teeth, can cause permanent dental discoloration, hypoplasia, absence of secondary teeth, enamel changes, and increased incidence of dental caries [81,82,104]. Furthermore, the lack of saliva production impairs taste sensation and creates problems with eating and swallowing that may result in serious nutritional deficits [105]. Likewise, dry eyes may adversely effect the cornea. In addition, irradiation of the eye(s) can also lead to microphthalmia and cataract formation [106]. Furthermore, skin irradiation and chemotherapy may predispose later to second malignant neoplasms and benign melanocytic nevi [107–109].

5.2. Musculoskeletal and soft tissue

Surgical effects on bone and soft tissues have obvious consequences, depending on the nature of the surgery. Chemotherapy may affect the skeleton

355

through renal impairment, which may lead to altered mineral metabolism and rachitic changes in bone [110] or may directly cause skeletal changes such as osteporosis due to methotrexate [111] or aseptic necrosis from steroids [101]. Similarly, hormonal changes such as premature menopause may predispose to the development of osteoporosis [101].

Here also, the consequences of radiation therapy are particularly prominent. Chest wall irradiation in the growing child may inhibit later breast growth and may also predispose to development of mammary cancer [3,112]. Hypoplasia of muscle and soft tissue may lead to skeletal deformities and to scoliosis when the area irradiated involves the axial skeleton. Furthermore, irradiation of growing bones may inhibit growth, leading to limb asymmetries and short stature, or may cause direct osteonecrosis [113] or slipped capital femoral epiphysis [114].

5.3. Cardiovascular and pulmonary

All modalities of therapy may affect the heart, lungs, and vessels directly or indirectly. Anthracyclines and related drugs can cause decreased ventricular function and overt heart failure months to many years following therapy [115]. Ventricular arryhthmias can also be seen, and sudden cardiac decompensation during pregnancy has been observed [116,117]. Irradiation can independently cause or exacerbate these effects and may also cause fibrosis of cardiac muscle, pericardial effusions with tamponade, or vascular effects on the coronary arteries [118,119].

Other chemotherapies, such as bleomycin and potentially cisplatin, may cause arterial changes in small peripheral vessels and may potentially affect the coronary arteries [94], although this outcome has not been well documented. Additional cardiovascular effects may result from hypertension consequent to renal toxicities.

Pulmonary effects, whether induced by chemotherapy, irradiation, or surgery, may result in pulmonary hypoplasia and pulmonary fibrosis and insufficiency [120]. Particularly in children receiving chest irradiation at a young age, subsequent pulmonary development may be impaired, resulting in insufficient pulmonary volume to deal with increased demands secondary to subsequent patient growth [121].

All the cardiovascular effects may naturally be worsened by exposure to cigarette smoke. Patients may be further at risk because of inappropriate lifestyles such as inactivity, poor diet, or excessive anaerobic exercise [122].

5.4. Renal

Unilateral nephrectomy seemingly does not lead to significant renal problems, even with subsequent growth [123]. However, subsequent resection or toxicity to remaining renal tissue may lead to renal insufficiency. Furthermore, both irradiation and certain chemotherapeutic agents may cause substantial renal problems. Irradiation, for example, may lead to nephritis with deterioration of glomerular function [124]. Certain chemotherapeutic agents likewise can cause renal failure with increasing creatinine and the expected consequences [125], sometimes leading to chronic renal failure and the need for dialysis or transplant. Effects on renal vasculature, usually radiation induced, may cause systemic hypertension. Furthermore, several drugs cause tubular damage with renal Fanconi-like syndromes. These necessitate chronic mineral replacement therapy and may cause growth failure and skeletal changes secondary to renal rickets [26]. Additionally, hyperammonemic encephalopathy and hyperchloremic acidosis may result from ureteral diversions [68,126].

5.5. Gastrointestinal and hepatic

Gastrointestinal effects may occur anywhere from the mouth to the anus. Effects on oral function were mentioned above. Esophagitis may result from irradiation, chemotherapy, and infection and may result in swallowing difficulties and/or stricture with inability to aliment through the oral route [127]. Surgery at any level may rarely lead to the necessity for externalization. Uncommonly, as a result of combinations of therapy, there may be malabsorption that requires supplementation or even parenteral nutrition. More commonly, bowel irradiation may cause chronic colitis or proctitis and sometimes rectal incontinence [9,128].

While irradiation may damage the liver, it is more common to see hepatitis as a result of chemotherapy and/or infection that may emerge years later. Hepatic fibrosis is a much less common late effect and may be the result of multiple factors [98,129,130].

5.6. Genitourinary

GU tumors, most commonly rhabdomyosarcomas, necessitate chemotherapy and irradiation and sometimes bladder resections. Thus, late hemorrhagic cystitis with the possibility of secondary bladder cancers [92] or structural abnormalities of the urinary tract requiring diversion and/or externalization [131] may occur. These patients subsequently are at risk for urinary tract infections that, if not vigorously addressed, may actually lead to renal impairment.

6.7. Endocrine

Endocrine effects may involve the pituitary axis, thyroid gland, and gonads. In significant percentages of patients, neck irradiation may lead to hypothyroidism, necessitating life-long supplementation. Furthermore, thyroid cancer is also a risk in these patients, so careful monitoring is essential.

Central nervous system effects, most commonly due to cranial irradiation, increase in incidence with increasing dosage and may lead to growth hormone

357

deficiency and consequent growth failure [132] or to inhibition of releasing factors causing end-organ failure [133], including hypothyroidism and gonadal failure.

Reproductive organs may also be affected by treatment of pelvic disease. In the case of cancers involving the female genital tract, surgery may lead to loss or alteration of uterine, cervical, or vaginal structures, with resultant potential for altered sexual or reproductive capacity. Resection of testicular tumors, usually unilateral, may cause cosmetic alterations that may be extremely problematic for pubertal males.

Pelvic irradiation and certain chemotherapies may also cause gonadal atrophy with lack of appropriate hormone production, resulting in absent sexual maturation, infertility, and sexual dysfunction [132–134].

5.8. Genetic implications

Genetic effects on offspring appear, fortunately, to be uncommon. At present, late effects of chemotherapy to men or nonpregnant women do not appear to cause an increase in fetal abnormalities [2]. Effects on the rates of miscarriage are difficult to determine but likewise do not seem to be excessive. However, there are some studies suggesting a slightly increased incidence of fetal malformations, spontaneous abortion, and prematurity in the offspring of patients receiving irradiation and chemotherapy [135,136]. Malignancy in the progeny of survivors of childhood cancer can occur at slightly increased rates because of genetic predispositions, as in the Li–Fraumeni syndrome, but this outcome does not appear to be directly treatment related.

Genetics in long-term survivors of cancer have been and will continue to impact research, education, and clinical care of patients. In certain well-studied situations, genes that predispose to childhood cancer may also predispose to other malignancies in the patient or offspring [12]. Retinoblastoma has provided the model for genetic studies in long-term survivors.

Patients with bilateral retinoblastoma have been found to transmit the disease to their offspring in 50% of cases, regardless of the family history. A small number of unilateral retinoblastoma cases are also attributable to a germline mutation, though these usually have a family history, and thus there may be a risk of the disease in offspring [136].

Patients with retinoblastoma have also taught us another lesson with respect to genetic predisposition. Long-term survivors of the heritable form of retinoblastoma have been found to have a high risk of second tumor, primarily osteosarcoma, but also sarcomas, melanomas, and an array of other adult carcinomas. In a 12–18-year follow-up of heritable retinoblastoma patients, Draper et al. demonstrated a projected cumulative risk of second malignancy to be 8%–9% over 18 years. The risk was highest in those treated with radiation therapy [56].

The best-known description of a familial pattern of diverse neoplasms, not necessarily following an overt predictable autosomal-dominant inheritance, is the classic Li–Fraumeni syndrome. Since their initial studies in 1969, Li and Fraumeni have reported an unusually high risk of cancer — particularly sarcomas and carcinomas of the breast, lung, and prostate — in family members of patients with childhood soft tissue sarcomas [137,138]. In 1993, Strong studied 159 survivors and families of patients with childhood soft tissue sarcoma. The risk of cancer in relatives of patients who had a second malignancy was significantly greater than in those relatives of patients who did not have additional cancers [12]. A more detailed description of genetics and childhood cancer can be found in the relevant chapter of this book.

5.9. Neuropsychiatric

The majority of effects on the nervous system are secondary to cranial radiation, or to a lesser extent neurotoxic chemotherapeutic agents, particularly methotrexate. There are some drugs (e.g., vina alkaloids, platinum analogues) that cause peripheral neuropathies that may persist after discontinuation of the drug [100]. These neuropathies are more commonly seen in adults. On the other hand, alterations in cognition and intellectual function, including learning disabilities and attentional problems with consquent impact on school performance, are fairly common in children receiving treatment that is toxic to the neuroaxis. Overt leukoencephalopathy [139,140] and delayed cerebral necrosis [141,142] are the most devastating disabilities seen and fortunately occur in the minority of patients. With recognition for these syndromes, most modern treatment approaches attempt to minimize dosage and/or delay irradiation of the brain in the very young child.

5.10. Secondary malignancy

There is an increased incidence of secondary malignancy in patients treated in childhood for a primary cancer, with a cumulative risk of 1.3% to 20% at 20 years [143,144]. This incidence appears to start approximately five years after treatment and continues to increase over time for more than 25 years after initial diagnosis [145]. The ultimate incidence of secondary malignancy is not yet known because of the relatively short period of follow-up in effectively treated patients with childhood cancer. Furthermore, genetic factors that predisposed to the first cancer may also predispose to further malignancy, particularly in patients with known familial cancer syndromes [3,144]. The nature and timing of the secondary tumors is dependent on the genetic predisposition and the modalities and drugs included in the initial treatment regimen. Thus, irradiation, alkylating agents, and topoisomerase inhibitors will lead to secondary nonlymphocytic leukemias and myelodysplastic syndromes [146,147]. Irradiation therapy, on the other hand, may also lead to sarcomas in the irradiation field and skin cancers [148,149], mainly in irradiated tissues in the period 5 to 10 years following treatment, with carcinomas predominating in later years [3,145] (figure 3).

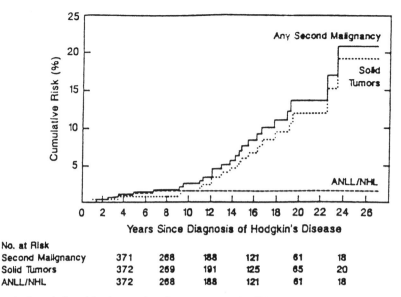

No. at Risk						
Second Malignancy	371	268	188	121	61	18
Solid Tumors	372	269	191	125	65	20
ANLL/NHL	372	268	188	121	61	18

Figure 3. Cumulative risk of second malignancy, second solid tumor, or second ANLL/NHL following therapy for Hodgkin's disease. The second CML was included in the second malignancy but not in the second hematologic malignancies (ANLL/NHL).

5.11. Psychosocial

In dealing with all the consequences of therapy, it is vital to recognize the hidden, nonphysical late effects of cancer in the growing organism. Occurrence of a chronic, life-threatening illness, associated with serious alteration in body image as well as accompanying social isolation and school absences, may have serious psychological ramifications affecting the patient and family that may persist long after the primary problem is resolved [28,150]. Furthermore, the secondary effects alluded to above may also have an impact on psychological well-being and social adjustment. Reports vary on the impact of surviving childhood cancer on psychosocial adjustment. Although problems clearly exist, survivors also may benefit psychologically from their experience [28,150] In addition, these patients must deal with a degree of insecurity about the future [151] in terms of physical problems, possibility of secondary malignancy, questions about fertility and future generations, and the response of society to their past medical problems. These problems are obviously impacted also by the social milieu, which may add further stresses related to the ability to obtain employment and insurance [148]. Although efforts are being made to combat discrimination, currently survivors of cancer encounter problems in obtaining health and life insurance. Similarly, problems remain in obtaining equal opportunities for employment and military service.

Obviously, all these points underscore the need for careful surveillance, counseling, and intensive support of these patients. Recommendations for monitoring these children will vary according to primary disease, treatment modalities, initial toxicities, and genetic factors. Furthermore, specific recommendations may vary from center to center. Included in this chapter is a summary of our current approach to these patients. A disciplined, multiservice approach to the survivors of childhood cancer, organized and supervised at least initially by the treating center, with recommendations for future health care and health practices, will be essential for optimal medical care of this group of patients.

5.12. General follow-up

Very few survivors of childhood malignancy will be free of long-term problems relating to their initial disease and treatment; some problems may be life-threatening [26,152]. Therefore, follow-up of these patients is essential throughout their lives. Recognition of the spectrum of delayed consequences following cancer treatment is one aspect of the study of late effects. Another involves the actual tracking, monitoring, and ongoing medical care of patients. Pediatric oncology centers have established late-effects programs to study and monitor the late adverse physical and psychosocial sequelae of cancer treatment, as well as to provide therapeutic intervention and counseling. Most survivors will receive at least part of their care from nononcologic health care providers who are not experts in oncology and are frequently unaware of some of the potential late complications of childhood cancer treatment. It is important to educate pediatricians, internists, obstetricians, and family practitioners, as well as nurses, social workers, psychologists, and school personnel, about late effects and their significance.

Because many problems first appear many years after treatment or may progress over time, reevaluations should be done optimally every year or every other year for life. However, more frequent surveillance may be necessary during defined high risk periods, e.g., during adolescent growth spurt or pregnancy. Adverse consequences of engaging in unhealthy life-style habits are magnified in this population. Examples include smoking in a patient who received lung irradiation or alcohol abuse within a patient with hepatotoxicity [152].

The typical visit of a survivor to a long-term follow-up clinic will involve significant preplanning by the medical care team. The multidisciplinary team usually includes a physician, an advanced practice nurse, and a social worker and/or psychologist, with at least peripheral involvement of a radiation oncologist, cardiologist, endocrinologist, and orthopedist. Other important consultants may include dentists, opthalmologists, and physical therapists. A detailed summary of the medical records with a history of the patient's disease and therapeutic interventions can anticipate individual patient problems, necessary screening tests, and counseling interventions.

At each visit, an interim history should focus on intercurrent illnesses, problems, review of systems, medication, education, employment, insurance status, marital history, menstrual and reproductive history, interpersonal relationships, sexual activity, and family history (specifically for cancer diagnoses). It may be important to update records or residence and participating health care providers for tracking and communication purposes. A complete physical examination, including height and weight, that looks for late effects is routine.

Recommendations for laboratory or other diagnostic tests are individualized according to clinical findings and past history. The extent of systematic screening of asymptomatic individuals remains controversial and varies significantly from clinic to clinic. It is clear, however, that health care providers should be knowledgeable about surveillance for delayed toxicities of treatment and should be sensitive to early, sometimes subtle signs and symptoms that may indicate treatment complications. Prompt evaluation and care of symptomatic disease is essential. Table 1 shows one schema for minimal screening targeted to prior treatment modalities.

Assessment of overall quality of life should be part of regular follow-up of a childhood cancer survivor. Many children seem to cope well despite their disabilities. However, in some systematic studies of childhood cancer survivors, disabilities that significantly alter quality of life have been detected in up to 40% of patients [26]. To maximize patient compliance with follow-up efforts, the importance of late effects should be emphasized while the patient is still undergoing therapy. This education may include suggestions for individualized life-style modifications, as well as consideration of other psychosocial issues such as employment, insurance, or interpersonal relationships.

Patients who received anthracycline therapy with or without mediastinal radiation should be cautioned about initiating strenuous physical activity or becoming pregnant without adequate evaluation. Individuals deemed to be at increased risk for an SMN should be counseled regarding the importance of regular surveillance and, where appropriate, the potential role of genetic predisposition, so that an early diagnosis can facilitate a second cure. Scrupulous oral hygiene, including flossing and fluoride supplementation to minimize dental abnormalities, may be necessary for survivors at high risk for oral pathology. Counseling and intervention concerning neurologic sequelae should begin early in therapy when risk is high in order to maximize patient function. Education concerning the quality of patient outcomes is important to help the family facilitate and plan for careful educational and vocational interventions.

The main goal of treatment of childhood cancer has been to cure the patient, permitting normal development to occur and resulting in a useful and productive adult life. Approximately 80% of children under the age of 15 years with cancer can now be expected to be cured of their disease [153]. Cure of malignancy is clearly important but may not be a sufficient endpoint for determining protocol success.

Table 1. Schema for minimum screening for late effects of prior treatment modalities

Treatment	Known late effects	Screening and diagnostic tests	Frequency of follow-up	Intervention
Chemotherapy				
I. Antitumor antibiotics (anthracyclines) & related drugs	Cardiotoxicity	Echocardiogram Physical exam	ECHO frequency is dose dependnt. Total anthracycline dose: — 150–300mg/m² every 5 years if normal — 300–450mg/m² every 3–4 years if normal — 450mg/m² or above, every 2 years if normal. More frequent if pt. rec'd mediastinal XRT or was <3 years at exposure.	Referral to cardiologist for abnormal studies
• Idarubicin				
• Adriamycin (doxorubicin)				
• Daunomycin (daunorubicin)				
• Mitoxantrone				
• Actinomycin D		Routine physical exam		
• Bleomycin	Chronic pulmonary fibrosis • (increased risk with concurrent lung irradiation) • Pt. to avoid high concentrations of O_2 administration pre & post op	Pulmonary function tests as indicated clinically CXR as indicated clinically	PRN	
II. Alkylating agents All alkylating agents	Infertility, changes in gonadal function	LH, FSH, estradiol; testosterone for males, semen analysis if pt. interested, and clinically indicated	PRN	If menses irregular, for difficulty achieving pregnancy, or for fertility screening if desired, refer to endocrinology or ob/gyn
• Mechlorethamine (nitrogen mustard)	Second malignant neoplasms, most commonly ANLL (acute non-lymphocytic leukemia)	CBC, physical exam	Yearly	

363

Table 1 (continued)

Treatment	Known late effects	Screening and diagnostic tests	Frequency of follow-up	Intervention
• Cyclophosphamide (cytoxan)	Hemorrhagic cystitis Bladder fibrosis; ↑ risk with XRT	Urinalysis	Yearly	Urology referral for persistent or unexplained hematuria
• Ifosfamide	Chronic hemorrhagic cystitis; bladder fibrosis Renal Fanconi's syndrome Renal rickets Renal insufficiency	Urinalysis BUN, Cr, lytes with CO_2, Ca, PO_4, Mg	Yearly q 2–3 years if normal	Urology referral for persistent, unexplained hematuria Nephrology referral for renal insufficiency or persistent electrolyte abnormalities Electrolyte supplements as needed
III. Antimetabolites (folic acid antagonists) • Methotrexate (MTX) Intrathecal	Leukoencephalopathy • Progressive white matter loss or deterioration (manifestations include severe cognitive impairments, dementia, ataxia, spasticity, seizures, coma and/or death) Cognitive defects • Increased risk if cranial irradiation was given	CT/MRI scan if symptomatic Psychological evaluation for learning or attention problems		Supportive care Educational evaluation and assistance
• Methotrexate (MTX) — I.V. or p.o.	— Hepatic fibrosis/cirrhosis — Leukoencephalopathy (as with intrathecal MTX) — Cognitive defects (I.V. only) (as with intrathecal MTX) — Osteoporosis (rare)	LFTs Hepatitis screen CT/MRI scan if symptomatic Psychological evaluation PRN learning problems X-Rays; bone mineral density PRN	q 5 years × 2 if normal q 5 years × 2 if normal PRN symptoms PRN symptoms	GI referral PRN Supportive care Educational evaluation and assistance
• 6-Mercaptopurine 6-Thioguanine	— Chronic lung disease (rare)	PFTs, CXR PRN symptoms		

364

IV. Plant alkaloids				
• Vincristine	Peripheral neuropathy • generalized weakness • localized weakness • lack of coordination • tingling and numbness	Neurologic exam	Yearly and PRN	Referral to physical therapy
• Etoposide (VP-16) Teniposide (VM-26)	Second malignant neoplasms	Physical exam CBC	Yearly	
V. Miscellaneous agents				
• Cisplatin	Sensorineural hearing loss • Cranial radiation in conjunction enhances effect, ↑ in pts with brain tumors • High-frequency hearing loss • Tinnitus • Vertigo Renal damage • Tubular dysfunction • Mg$^+$ wasting • Renal insufficiency Peripheral neuropathy	Conventional pure tone audiogram Urinalysis BUN, Cr, Lytes, CO_2, Ca, PO_4, Mg Neurological exam	Baseline & q 3–4 years if normal Yearly Baseline & q 2–3 years if normal × 3–4 Yearly and PRN	If abnormal, refer to ENT or audiology for amplification Electrolyte supplements Refer to nephrology PRN
• Carboplatin (paraplatin)	Small potential for renal damage, hearing loss	BUN, Cr, Lytes, CO_2, Cat PO_4, Mg Audiogram	Baseline & q 3–4 years if normal ×2 Baseline, PRN	As for cisplatin
Radiation All Fields	Secondary tumors in radiation field	Physical exam X-ray	Yearly PRN	
Cranium and nasopharynx	Thyroid dysfunction	T4, TSH	5 years after diagnosis; if normal, q 3–5 year intervals	If abnormal, refer to endocrinology or give replacement
	Leukoencephalopathy, CNS necrosis Secondary gonadal dysfunction • Doses >5500 cGy cause Hypothalamic damage	Hx, physical exam, CT or MRI Testosterone levels, LH, FSH, estradiol	PRN As clinically indicated or when patient needs fertility information	Endocrine or gyn referral PRN

Table 1 (continued)

Treatment	Known late effects	Screening and diagnostic tests	Frequency of follow-up	Intervention
	Chronic sinusitis	Sinus films or CT	PRN	
	↓ Salivation, dry mouth Dental and maxillofacial changes 2000–4000 cGy head or neck	Dental F/U	q 6 months	Meticulous dental care
Orbital	Cataracts Orbital asymmetry		Yearly PRN	Ophthalmologic consultation Plastic surgery
Neck	Thyroid dysfunction Decreased secretions	T4, TSH Dental exam	5 to 10 years from diagnosis; if normal q 3–5 years for doses >2000 cGy	Meticulous dental care
Mediastinum; chest wall	Cardiotoxicity • Thickening of the atrioventricular valves (AV) and pericardium • Disposition to early atherosclerosis • Damage to RV & myocardial fibrosis	Echocardiogram History and physical exam	q 3–5 years if normal	Referral to cardiology if abnormal
	Scoliosis	PE, spine films	PRN	Orthopedic referral PRN
	Breast cancer Lack of breast development	Mammogram	Baseline at 25 years, then every 5 years if normal	
	Pulmonary fibrosis • Seen when >2000 cGy delivered to more than 50% of lung volume	CXR Pulmonary function tests	PRN	
Whole lung	Pulmonary fibrosis Breast cancer	CXR PFT Mammogram	PRN Baseline at 25 years old, then q 5 years if normal	
Abdominal	Renal insufficiency	BUN, Cr, creatinine clearance (PRN), urinalysis	q 3–5 years if kidney was irradiated Yearly	Nephrology referral if abnormal
	Colitis, GI malignancy	Stool for occult blood	Yearly if bowel irradiated	
• Splenic	• Increased susceptibility to infection			Prophylactic PenVK 250 mg p.o. b.i.d.

Pelvis	Aseptic necrosis of femoral head	X-rays	Orthopedic referral
	Pelvic asymmetry		
	Gonadal insufficiency	LH, FSH, prolactin, estradiol, testosterone	PRN	Endocrine referral
	Bladder fibrosis, cancer	Urinalysis; voiding history	Yearly	Urology referral
	Proctitis, rectal carcinoma	Stool guaiac; endoscopy	Yearly PRN	
Spine	Gonadal insufficiency	LH, FSH, estradiol, testosterone	PRN	Endocrine referral
	Vertical compression fracture	Spine films	PRN	Orthopedic referral
	Scoliosis	Spine films	PRN	
Testes	Gonadal insufficiency–sterility 400–600 cGY azoospermia may be reversible	LH, FSH, testosterone, semen analysis	PRN	Endocrine or fertility referral PRN
	>600 cGy azoospermia permanent			
	>2000 leydig cell damage atrophic testes			
Surgery			
Splenectomy	Increased susceptibility to infection			Prophylactic PenVK 250 mg p.o. b.i.d.
				Empiric antibiotics covering encapsulated organisms with febrile illness
Amputations		Orthopedic follow-up		Prosthetic device
Enucleations		Ophthalmologic follow-up		Prosthetic device
Nephrectomy		Urinalysis	Yearly	
		BUN, CR	q 2–3 years	
Thoracotomy	Chest asymmetry	Pulmonary function tests	PRN	
Lobectomy	Pulmonary insufficiency	PFTs, CXR	PRN	

Note: Some screening studies such as PFTs are recommended PRN but may in the future be recommended on a regular schedule if early interventions are developed.

6. Ramifications of the study of late effects

Obviously, with an estimated one in 900 young adults being a survivor of childhood cancer, late effects of treatment are and will continue to be a significant public health issue. Furthermore, over time there may be an increase in the manifestations of cancer treatment as survivors become mature and elderly adults. The superimposition of early treatment of cancer onto the normal health problems that accompany aging is likely to result in additional, as yet unforeseen problems. These problems, furthermore, will be treated not by pediatricians or pediatric oncologists but by internists, obstetricians, gynecologists, general practitioners, surgeons, and geriatric specialists. Therefore, as previously mentioned, it is imperative that these practitioners be educated about the potential for late effects and that communication about later health problems be communicated back to the pediatric oncologists.

Multidisciplinary late effects clinics are increasingly incorporated into the comprehensive care of children with cancer. The role of such clinics is multifactorial and includes health maintenance, counseling, surveillance and monitoring of late effects, dealing with psychosocial issues, and communication to other oncologists and practitioners of adult medicine. Habits that may affect health in all young people, such as smoking, alcohol and drug abuse, exercise and diet, and medical surveillance, need to be discussed with the patients with emphasis on the necessity for good health practices.

Obviously, anticipatory guidance and education of other practitioners can only be as good as the information available. It is therefore essential to learn more about late effects, occurring not only during youth but also throughout adulthood. All this is essential in order to permit the health care team to find means of improving the quality of life of our survivors.

Knowledge about late effects will assist practitioners to be advocates for their patients in areas such as insurance, employment, and military service. Furthermore, with time and increased follow-up, we will add to the information about genetic effects, which will be vital for counseling.

Finally, additional data will be essential for pediatric oncologists as front-line and salvage protocols continue to be devised and refined.

References

1. Boring CC, Squires TS, Tong T, Montgomery S. 1994. Cancer statistics, 1994. Cancer 44:7–26.
2. Li FP, Fine W, Jaffe N, Holmes GE, Holmes FF. 1979. Offspring of patients treated for cancer in childhood. J Natl Cancer Inst 62:1193–1197.
3. Meadows AT, Baum E, Fossati-Bellani F, et al. 1985. Second malignant neoplasms in children: an update from the Late Effects Study Group. J Clin Oncol 3:532–538.
4. Garre ML, Gandus S, Cesana B, et al. 1994. Health status of long-term survivors after cancer in childhood. Results of an uniinstitutional study in Italy. Am J Pediatr Hemat Oncol 16:143–152.
5. DeLaat CA, Lampkin BC. 1992. Long-term survivors of childhood cancer: evaluation and identification of sequelae of treatment (review) [see comments]. Cancer 42:263–282.

6. Neglia JP. 1994. Childhood cancer survivors. Past, present, and future (editorial). Cancer 73:2883–2885.

7. Green DM, Zevon MA, Reese PA, Lowrie GS, Michalek AM. 1994. Factors that influence the further survival of patients who survive for five years after the diagnosis of cancer in childhood or adolescence [see comments]; published erratum appears in Med Pediatr Oncol 1996 Jan;26(1):72]. Med Pediatr Oncol 22:91–96.

8. Robertson CM, Hawkins MM, Kingston JE. 1994. Late deaths and survival after childhood cancer: implications for cure. Br Med J 309:162–166.

9. Beer WH, Fan A, Halsted CH. 1985. Clinical and nutritional implications of radiation enteritis. Am J Clin Nutr 41:85–91.

10. Nicholson HS, Fears TR, Byrne J. 1994. Death during adulthood in survivors of childhood and adolescent cancer. Cancer 73:3094–3102.

11. Hawkins MM, Draper GJ, Winter DL. 1995. Cancer in the offspring of survivors of childhood leukaemia and non-Hodgkin lymphomas [see comments]. Br J Cancer 71:1335–1339.

12. Strong LC. 1993. Genetic implications for long-term survivors of childhood cancer. Cancer 71:3435–3440.

13. Green DM, Zevon MA, Lowrie G, Seigelstein N, Hall B. 1991. Congential anomalies in children of patients who received chemotherapy for cancer in childhood and adolescence [see comments]. N Engl J Medicine 325:141–146.

14. Potter R. 1993. Late side effects of pediatric radiotherapy (review). Recent Results Cancer Res 130:237–249.

15. Neuhauser EB, Willenborg MH, Berman CZ, Cohen J. 1952. Irradiation effects of roentgen therapy on the growing spine. Radiology 59:637–650.

16. Rate WR, Butler MS, Robertson WW Jr, D'Angio GJ. 1991. Late orthopedic effects in children with Wilms' tumor treated with abdominal irradiation (see comments). Med Pediatr Oncol 19:265–268.

17. Katzman H, Waugh T, Berdon W. 1969. Skeletal changes following irradiation of childhood tumors. J Bone Joint Surg 51A:825–849.

18. Marcus RB, McGrath B, O'Conner K, Scarborough M. 1994. Long term effects on the musculoskeletal and integurmentary systems and the breast. In Schwartz CL, Hobbie WL, Constance LS, Ruccione KS (eds.), Survivors of Childhood Cancer. Assessment and Management. Mosby-Year Book.

19. Steinherz LJ, Steinherz PG, Tan CT, Heller G, Murphy ML. 1991. Cardiac toxicity 4 to 20 years after completing anthracycline therapy. JAMA 266:1672.

20. Lipshultz SE, Colan SD, Gelber RD, Perez-Atayde AR, Sallan SE, Sanders SP. 1991. Late cardiac effects of doxorubicin therapy for acute lymphoblastic leukemia in childhood [see comments]. N Engl J Med 324:808–815X.

21. Stewart JR, Fajardo LF. 1984. Radiation-induced heart disease: an update (review). Prog Cardiovasc Dis 27:173–194.

22. Trueschell S, Schwartz CL, Clark E, Constance LS. 1994. Cardiovascular effects of cancer therapy. In Schwartz CL, Hobbie WL, Constance LS, Ruccione KS (eds.), Survivors of Childhood Cancer. Assessment and Management. Mosby-Year Book.

23. Breslow NE, Takashima JR, Whitton JA, Moksness J, D'Angio GJ, Green DM. 1995. Second malignant neoplasms following treatment for Wilms' tumor: a report from the National Wilms' Tumor Study Group. J Clin Oncol 13:1851–1859.

24. Scaradavou A, Heller G, Sklar CA, Ren L, Ghavimi F. 1995. Second malignant neoplasms in long-term survivors of childhood rhabdomyosarcoma. Cancer 76:1860–1867.

25. Jakacki RI, Schramm CM, Donahue LR, Haas F, Allen JC. 1995. Restrictive lung disease following treatment for malignant brain tumors: a potential late effect of craniospinal irradiation. J Clin Oncol 13:1478–1485.

26. Meadows AT, Hobbie WL. 1986. The medical consequences of cure. Cancer 58:524–528.

27. Hancock SL, Donaldson SS, Hoppe RT. 1993. Cardiac disease following treatment of Hodgkin's disease in children and adolescents [see comments]. J Clin Oncol 11:1208–1215.

28. Mulhern RK, Wasserman AL, Friedman AG, Fairclough D. 1989. Social competence and

behavioral adjustment of children who are long-term survivors of cancer. Pediatrics 83:18–25.

29. Nicholson HS, Byrne J. 1993. Fertility and pregnancy after treatment for cancer during childhood or adolescence (review). Cancer 71:3392.

30. Packer RJ, Meadows AT, Rorke LB, Coldwein JL, D'Angio G. 1987. Long-term sequelae of cancer treatment on the central nervous system in childhood (review). Med Pediatr Oncol 15:241–253.

31. Duffner PK, Cohen ME, Thomas PR, Lansky SB. 1985. The long-term effects of cranial irradiation on the central nervous system. Cancer 56:1841–1846.

32. Glauser TA, Packer RJ. 1991. Cognitive deficits in long-term survivors of childhood brain tumors (review). Childs Nerv Sys 7:2–12.

33. Hays DM, Landsverk J, Sallan SE, et al. 1992. Educational, occupational, and insurance status of childhood cancer survivors in their fourth and fifth decades of life. J Clin Oncol 10:1397–1406.

34. Hearing on discrimination agains cancer victims and the handicapped; hearing on HR 192 and HR151 6; before the Subcommittee on Employment Opportunities of the House Commission on Education and Labor, 100th Congress 1st sessio 28:1987(statement) of Representative Morio Bragge, 31–33 and statement of Barbara Hoffman. 1987. National Coalition for Cancer Survivorship, pp. 41–53.

35. Koocher GP, O'Malley JE. 1982. The Damocles Syndrome: Psychological Consequences of Surviving Childhood Cancer. New York: McGraw Hill.

36. Moore IM, Packer RJ, Karl D, Bleyer WA. 1994. Adverse effects of cancer on the central nervous system. In Schwartz CL, Hobbie WL, Constance LS, Ruccione KS (eds.), Survivors of Childhood Cancer. Assessment and Management. Mosby-Year Book.

37. Cohen BH, Packer RJ. 1992. Adverse neurologic effects of chemotherapy and radiation therapy. In Berger BO (ed.), Neurologic Aspects of Pediatrics. Boston: Butterworth-Heinemann, pp. 567–594.

38. Nixon DW, Pirozzi D, York RM, Black M, Lawson DH. 1981. Dermatologic changes after systemic cancer therapy. Cutis 27:181–2, 186–188.

39. Rubin P. 1984. The Franz Buschke lecture: late effects of chemotherapy and radiation therapy: a new hypothesis (review). Int J Radiat Oncol Biol Phys 10:5–34.

40. Philips TL. 1989. Chemical modifiers of normal-tissue radiation injury (review). Front Radiat Ther Oncol 23:177–184.

41. Stewart FA. 1991. Keynote address: modulation of normal tissue toxicity by combined modality therapy: considerations for improving the therapeutic gain (review). Int J Radiat Oncol Biol Phys 20:319–325.

42. Peeters M, Poon A. 1987. Down syndrome and leukemia: unusual clinical aspects and unexpected methotrexate sensitivity. Eur J Pediatr 146:416–422.

43. Ueland PM, Refsum H, Christensen B. 1990. Methotrexate sensitivity in Down's syndrome: a hypothesis. Cancer Chemother Pharmacol 25:384–386.

44. Deschavanne PJ, Debieu D, Fertil B, Malaise EP. 1986. Re-evaluation of in vitro radiosensitivity of human fibroblasts of different genetic origins [published erratum appears in Int J Radiat Biol 1986 Dec;50(6):1129]. Int J Radiat Biol 50:279–293.

45. Gotoff SP, Amirmokri E, Liebner EJ. 1967. Ataxia telangiectasia. Neoplasia, untoward response to x-irradiation, and tuberous sclerosis. Am J Dis Child 114:617–625.

46. Cunlift PN, Mann JR, Cameron AH, Roberts KD, Ward HN. 1975. Radiosensitivity in ataxia–telangiectasia. Br J Radiol 48:374–376.

47. Malkin D, Jolly KW, Barbier N, et al. 1992. Germline mutations of the p53 tumor-suppressor gene in children and young adults with second malignant neoplasms [see comments]. N Engl J Med 326:1309–1315.

48. Pratt CB, Ransom JL, Evans WE. 1978. Age-related adriamycin cardiotoxicity in children (review). Cancer Treat Rep 62:1381–1385.

49. Silber JH, Littman PS, Meadows AT. 1990. Stature loss following skeletal irradiation for childhood cancer. J Clin Oncol 8:304–312.

50. Anderson M, Green WT, Messner MB. 1978. The classic. Growth and predictions of growth in the lower extremities by Margaret Anderson, MS, William T, Green MD, and Marie Blail Messner AB, from the Journal of Bone and Joint Surgery, 45A:1, 1963. Clin Orthopaed Related Research 7–21.

51. Silber JH, Radcliffe J, Peckham V, et al. 1992. Whole-brain irradiation and decline in intelligence: the influence of dose and age on IQ score [see comments]. J Clin Oncol 10:1390–1396.

52. Byrne J, Mulvihill JJ, Myers MH, et al. 1987. Effects of treatment on fertility in long-term survivors of childhood or adolescent cancer. N Engl J Med 317:1315–1321.

53. Ash P. 1980. The influence of radiation on fertility in man (review). Br J Radiol 53:271–278.

54. Brauner R, Caltabiano P, Rappaport R, Leverger G, Schaison G. 1988. Leydig cell insufficiency after testicular irradiation for acute lymphoblastic leukemia. Horm Res 30:111–114.

55. Van Leeuwen FE, Somers R, Taal BG, et al. 1989. Increased risk of lung cancer, non-Hodgkin's lymphoma, and leukemia following Hodgkin's disease. J Clin Oncol 7:1046–1058.

56. Draper GJ, Sanders BM, Kingston JE. 1986. Second primary neoplasms in patients with retinoblastoma. Br J Cancer 53:661–671.

57. Thomas PR, Griffith KD, Fineberg BB, Perez CA, Land VJ. 1983. Late effects of treatment for Wilms' tumor. Int J Radiat Oncol Biol Phys 9:651–657.

58. Riseborough EJ, Grabias SL, Burton RI, Jaffe N. 1976. Skeletal alterations following irradiation for Wilms' tumor: with particular reference to scoliosis and kyphosis. J Bone Joint Surg 58:526–536.

59. Simon MA, Aschliman MA, Thomas N, Mankin HJ. 1986. Limb-salvage treatment versus amputation for osteosarcoma of the distal end of the femur. J Bone Joint Sur 68:1331–1337.

60. Baumann M. 1995. Impact of endogenous and exogenous factors on radiation sequelae. In Dunst J, Daver R (eds.), Late Sequelae in Oncology. Springer-Verlag, pp. 3–12.

61. Packer RJ, Sposto R, Atkins TE, et al. 1987. Quality of life in children with primitive neuroectodermal tumors (medulloblastoma) of the posterior fossa. Pediatr Neurosci 13:169–175.

62. Heyn R, Ragab A, Raney RB Jr, et al. 1986. Late effects of therapy in orbital rhabdomyosarcoma in children. A report from the Intergroup Rhabdomyosarcoma Study. Cancer 57:1738–1743X.

63. Osborne D, Hadden OB, Deeming LW. 1974. Orbital growth after childhood enucleation. Am J Ophthalmol 77:756–759.

64. Punt J, Pritchard J, Pincott JR, Till K. 1980. Neuroblastoma: a review of 21 cases presenting with spinal cord compression. Cancer 45:3095–3101.

65. Laros C, Westerman C. 1987. Dilatation, compensatory growth or both after pneumonectomy during childhood and adolescence. Cardiovasc Surg 93:570.

66. Krivit W, Giebink GS, Leonard A. 1979. Overwhelming postplenectomy infection. Surg Clin North Am 59:223–233.

67. Blatt J, Bleyer A. 1989. Late effects of childhood cancer and its treatment. In Pizzo P, Poplack DG (eds.), Principles and Practice of Pediatric Oncology. Philadalphia: J.B. Lippincott, pp. 1003–1026.

68. Zinchke H, Segura JW. 1975. Ureterosigmoidostomy: critical review of 173 cases. J Urol 113:324–327.

69. Javadpour N, Moley J. 1985. Alternative to retroperitoneal lymphadenectomy with preservation of ejaculation and fertility in stage I nonseminomatous testicular cancer. A prospective study. Cancer 55:1604–1606.

70. Nicosia SV, Matus-Ridley M, Meadows AT. 1985. Gonadal effects of cancer therapy in girls. Cancer 55:2364–2372.

71. Donahue B. 1992. Short- and long-term complications of radiation therapy for pediatric brain tumors (review). Pediatr Neurosurg 18:207–217.

72. Duffner PK, Cohen ME. 1991. The long-term effects of central nervous system therapy on children with brain tumors (review). Neurol Clin 9:479–495.

73. Chung E, Bodensteiner J, Hogg JP. 1992. Spontaneous intracerebral hemorrhage: a very late delayed effect of radiation therapy. J Child Neurol 7:259–263.

74. Allen JC, Miller DC, Budzilovich GN, Epstein FJ. 1991. Brain and spinal cord hemorrhage in long-term survivors of malignant pediatric brain tumors: a possible late effect of therapy. Neurology 41:148–150.

75. Oberfield SE, Allen JC, Pollack J, New MI, Levine LS. 1986. Long-term endocrine sequelae after treatment of medulloblastoma: prospective study of growth and thyroid function. J Pediatr 108:219–223.

76. Shapiro E, Kinsella TJ, Makuch RW, et al. 1985. Effects of fractionated irradiation of endocrine aspects of testicular function. J Clin Oncol 3:1232–1239.

77. Shalet SM, Beardwell CG, Jacobs HS, Pearson D. 1978. Testicular function following irradiation of the human prepubertal testis. Clin Endocrinol 9:483–490.

78. Sklar CA, Robison LL, Nesbit ME, et al. 1990. Effects of radiation on testicular function in long-term survivors of childhood acute lymphoblastic leukemia: a report from the Children Cancer Study Group. J Clin Oncol 8:1981–1987.

79. Blatt J, Copeland DR, Bleyer WA. 1997. Late effects of childhood cancer and its treatment. In Pizzo P, Poplack DG (eds.), Principles and Practice of Pediatric Oncology, 2nd ed Philadelphia: J.B. Lippincott.

80. Makipernaa A, Heikkila JT, Merikanto J, Marttinen E, Siimes MA. 1993. Spinal deformity induced by radiotherapy for solid tumours in childhood: a long-term follow up study. Eur J Pediatr 152:197–200.

81. Jaffe N, Toth BB, Hoar RE, Ried HL, Sullivan MP, McNeese MD. 1984. Dental and maxillofacial abnormalities in long-term survivors of childhood cancer: effects of treatment with chemotherapy and radiation to the head and neck. Pediatrics 73:816–823.

82. Fromm M, Littman P, Raney RB, et al. 1986. Late effects after treatment of twenty children with soft tissue sarcomas of the head and neck. Experience at a single institution with a review of the literature. Cancer 57:2070–2076.

83. Merriam GR, Focht EF. 1957. A clinical study of radiation cataracts and the relationship to dose. Am J Roentgenol 77:759–785.

84. Hawkins MM, Wilson LM, Stovall MA, et al. 1992. Epipodophyllotoxins, alkylating agents, and radiation and risk of secondary leukaemia after childhood cancer. Br J Med 304:951–958.

85. Ellis M, Ravid M, Lishner M. 1993. A comparative analysis of alkylating agent and epipodophyllotoxin-related leukemias (review). Leuk Lymphoma 11:9–13.

86. Schilsky RL, Sherins RJ. 1982. Gonadal dysfunction. In Devita VT Jr, Hellman S, Rosentberg SA (eds.), Cancer: Principles and Practice of Oncology. Philadelphia: J.B. Lippincott, pp. 1713–1719.

87. Sherins RJ, DeVita VT Jr. 1973. Effect of drug treatment for lymphoma on male reproductive capacity. Studies of men in remission after therapy. Ann Intern Med 79:216–220.

88. Sherins RJ, Olweny CL, Ziegler JL. 1978. Gynecomastia and gonadal dysfunction in adolescent boys treated with combination chemotherapy for Hodgkin's disease. N Engl J Med 299:12–16.

89. Whitehead E, Shalet SM, Jones PH, Beardwell CG, Deakin DP. 1982. Gonadal function after combination chemotherapy for Hodgkin's disease in childhood. Arch Dis Child 57:287–291.

90. Travis LB, Curtis RE, Glimelius B, et al. 1995. Bladder and kidney cancer following cyclophosphamide therapy for non-Hodgkin's lymphoma. J Nat Cancer Inst 87:524–530.

91. Klein HO, Wickramanayake PD, Coerper C, Christian E, Pohl J, Brock N. 1983. High-dose ifosfamide and mesna as continuous infusion over five days — a phase I/II trial. Cancer Treat Rev 10(Suppl A): 167–173.

92. Stillwell TJ, Benson RC Jr, Burgert EO Jr. 1988. Cyclophosphamide-induced hemorrhagic cystitis in Ewing's sarcoma. J Clin Oncol 6:76–82.

93. Jules-Elysee K, White DA. 1990. Bleomycin-induced pulmonary toxicity (review). Clin Chest Med 11:1–20.

94. Edwards GS, Lane M, Smith FE. 1979. Long-term treatment with cisdichlorodiam-

372

mineplatinum(II)–vinblastine–bleomycin: possible association with severe coronary artery disease (letter). Cancer Treat Rep 63:551–552.

95. Arsenian MA. 1991. Cardiovascular sequelae of therapeutic thoracic radiation (review). Prog Cardiovasc Dis 33:299–311.

96. Larsen RL, Jakacki RI, Vetter VL, Meadows AT, Silber JH, Barber G. 1992. Electrocardiographic changes and arrhythmias after cancer therapy in children and young adults. Am J Cardiol 70:73–77.

97. Dahl MG, Gregory MM, Scheuer PJ. 1971. Liver damage due to methotrexate in patients with psoriasis. Br Med J 1:625–630.

98. McIntosh S, Davidson DL, O'Brien RT, Pearson HA. 1977. Methotrexate hepatotoxicity in children with leukemia. J Pediatr 90:1019–1021.

99. Neumann Y, Toren A, Rechavi G, et al. 1996. Vincristine treatment triggering the expression of asymptomatic Charcot-Marie-Tooth disease. Med Pediatr Oncol 26:280–283.

100. Hansen SW, Helweg-Larsen S, Trojaborg W. 1989. Long-term neurotoxicity in patients treated with cisplatin, vinblastine, and bleomycin for metastatic germ cell cancer. J Clin Oncol 7:1457–1461.

101. Redman JR, Bajorunas DR, Wong G, et al. 1988. Bone mineralization in women following successful treatment of Hodgkin's disease. Am J Med 85:65–72.

102. Sullivan KM, Agura E, Anasetti C, et al. 1991. Chronic graft-versus-host disease and other late complications of bone marrow transplantation (review). Semin Hematol 28:250–259.

103. Shulman HM, Sullivan KM, Weiden PL, et al. 1980. Chronic graft-versus-host syndrome in man. A long-term clinicopathologic study of 20 Seattle patients. Am J Med 69:204–217.

104. Maguire A, Craft AW, Evans RG, et al. 1987. The long-term effects of treatment on the dental condition of children surviving malignant disease. Cancer 60:2570–2575.

105. Marcial V. 1989. The oral cavity and oropharynx. In Moss WT, Cox JD (eds.), Radiation Oncology. St. Louis: Mosby-Year Book.

106. Brady LW, Shields J, Augusburger J, Markoe A, Karlsson UL. 1989. Complications from radiation therapy to the eye. Front Radiat Ther Oncol 23:238–250.

107. Hughes BR, Cunliffe WJ, Bailey CC. 1989. Excess benign melanocytic naevi after chemotherapy for malignancy in childhood. Br Med J 299:88–91.

108. Green A, Smith P, McWhirter W, et al. 1993. Melanocytic naevi and melanoma in survivors of childhood cancer. Br J Cancer 67:1053–1057.

109. Meadows AT, Fenton JG. 1994. Follow up care of patients at risk for the development of second malignant neoplasms. In Schwartz CL, Hobbie WL, Constine LS, Ruccione KS (eds.), Survivors of Childhood Cancer: Assessment and Management. St. Louis: Mosby-Year Book, pp. 319–328.

110. Skinner R, Pearson AD, Price L, Coulthard MG, Craft AW. 1990. Nephrotoxicity after ifosfamide. Arch Dis Child 65:732–738.

111. Ragab AH, Frech RS, Vietti TJ. 1970. Osteoporotic fractures secondary to methotrexate therapy of acute leukemia in remission. Cancer 25:580–585.

112. Rosenfield NS, Haller JO, Berdon WE. 1989. Failure of development of the growing breast after radiation therapy. Pediatr Radiol 19:124–127.

113. Libshitz HI, Edeiken BS. 1981. Radiotherapy changes of the pediatric hip. AJR 137:585–58X.

114. Dickerman JD, Newberg AH, Moreland MD. 1979. Slipped capital femoral epiphysis (SCFE) following pelvic irradiation for rhabdomyosarcoma. Cancer 44:480–482.

115. Laurel J, Steinhertz L, Steinhertz P. 1988. Cardiac failure more than six years post anthracylcines (abstract). Am J Cardiology 62:505.

116. Davis LE, Brown CE. 1988. Peripartum heart failure in a patient treated previously with doxorubicin. Obstet Gynecol 71:506–508.

117. Billingham ME, Mason JW, Bristow MR, Daniels JR. 1978. Anthracycline cardiomyopathy monitored by morphologic changes. Cancer Treat Rep 62:865–872.

118. Martin RG, Ruckdeschel JC, Chang P, Byhardt R, Bouchard RJ, Wiernik PH. 1975. Radiation-related pericarditis. Am J Cardiol 35:216–220.

119. McReynolds RA, Gold GL, Roberts WC. 1976. Coronary heart disease after mediastinal irradiation for Hodgkin's disease. Am J Med 60:39–45.

120. Gross NJ. 1977. Pulmonary effects of radiation therapy (review). Ann Intern Med 86:81–92.

121. Wohl ME, Griscom NT, Traggis DG, Jaffe N. 1975. Effects of therapeutic irradiation delivered in early childhood upon subsequent lung function. Pediatrics 55:507–516.

122. Ali MK, Ewer MS, Gibbs HR, Swafford J, Graff KL. 1994. Late doxorubicin-associated cardiotoxicity in children. The possible role of intercurrent viral infection. Cancer 74:182–188.

123. Bhisitkul DM, Morgan ER, Vozar MA, Langman CB. 1991. Renal functional reserve in long-term survivors of unilateral Wilms tumor. J Pediatr 118:698–702.

124. Van Slyck EJ, Bermudez GA. 1968. Radiation nephritis. Yale J Biol Med 41:243–256.

125. Vogelzang NJ. 1991. Nephrotoxicity from chemotherapy: prevention and management (review). Oncology 5:97–102.

126. Kaufman JJ. 1984. Ammoniagenic coma following ureterosigmoidostomy. J Urol 131:743–745.

127. Hays DM. 1989. General principles of surgery. In Pizzo PA, Poplack DC (eds.), Principles and Practice of Pediatric Oncology. Philadelphia: J.B. Lippincott, pp. 207–232.

128. Wellwood JM, Jackson BT. 1973. The intestinal complications of radiotherapy. Br J Surg 60:814–818.

129. Tefft M, Mitus A, Das L, Vawter GF, Filler RM. 1970. Irradiation of the liver in children: review of experience in the acute and chronic phases, and in the intact normally resected. AJR 108:365–385.

130. Vernant JP. 1986. Hepatitis B and non-A-non-B hepatitis after allogeneic bone marrow transplantation in leukemia. Bone Marrow Transplant 1:183–184.

131. Raney B Jr, Heyn R, Hays DM, et al. 1993. Sequelae of treatment in 109 patients followed for 5 to 15 years after diagnosis of sarcoma of the bladder and prostate. A report from the Intergroup Rhabdomyosarcoma Study Committee. Cancer 71:2387–2394.

132. Brown IH, Lee TJ, Eden OB, Bullimore JA, Savage DC. 1983. Growth and endocrine function after treatment for medulloblastoma. Arch Dis Child 58:722–727.

133. Constine LS, Woolf PD, Cann D, et al. 1993. Hypothalamic–pituitary dysfunction after radiation for brain tumors [published erratum appears in N Engl J Med 1993 Apr 22;328(16):1208; see comments]. N Engl J Med 328:87–94.

134. Lushbaugh CC, Casarett GW. 1976. The effects of gonadal irradiation in clinical radiation therapy: a review. Cancer 37:1111–1125.

135. Holmes GE, Holmes FF. 1978. Pregnancy outcome of patients treated for Hodgkin's disease: a controlled study. Cancer 41:1317–1322X.

136. Vogel F. 1979. Genetics of retinoblastoma (review). Hum Genet 52:1–54.

137. Li FP, Fraumeni JF Jr. 1969. Soft-tissue sarcomas, breast cancer, and other neoplasms. A familial syndrome? Ann Intern Med 71:747–752.

138. Li FP, Fraumeni JF Fr. 1969. Rhabdomyosarcoma in children: epidemiologic study and identification of a familial cancer syndrome. J Natl Cancer Inst 43:1365–1373.

139. Li FP, Winston KR, Gimbrere K. 1984. Follow-up of children with brain tumors. Cancer 54:135–138.

140. Tamareff M, Saliven R, Miller DR. 1984. Compaison of neuropsychologic performance in children treated for acute lymphoblastic leukemia with 1800 rads cranial radiation plus intrathecal methotrexate or intrathecal methotrexate alone (abstract). Proc Am Soc Clin Oncol 3:198.

141. Sheline GE, Wara WM, Smith V. 1980. Therapeutic irradiation and brain injury (review). Int J Radiat Oncol Biol Phys 6:1215–1218.

142. Pizzo PA, Poplack DG, Bleyer WA. 1979. Neurotoxicities of current leukemia therapy (review). Am J Pediatr Hematol-Oncol 1:127–140.

143. Hawkins MM, Draper GJ, Kingston JE. 1987. Incidence of second primary tumours among childhood cancer survivors. Br J Cancer 56:339–347.

374

144. Li FP, Corkery J, Vawter G, Fine W, Sallan SE. 1983. Breast carcinoma after cancer therapy in childhood. Cancer 51:521–523.

145. Beaty O, Hudson MM, Greenwald C, et al. 1995. Subsequent malignancies in children and adolescents after treatment for Hodgkin's disease [see comments]. J Clin Oncol 13:603–609.

146. Tucker MA, Meadows AT, Boice JD Jr, et al. 1987. Leukemia after therapy with alkylating agents for childhood cancer. J Natl Cancer Inst 78:459–464.

147. Pui CH, Hancock ML, Raimondi SC, et al. 1990. Myeloid neoplasma in children treated for solid tumors. Lancet 336:417–421.

148. Springfield DS, Pagliarulo C. 1985. Fractures of long bones previously treated for Ewing's sarcoma. J Bone Joint Surg 67:477–418.

149. Heyn R, Newton WA, Ragab A. 1987. Second malignant neoplasms in patients treated on the Intergroup Rhabdomyosarcoma Study I-II (abstract). Proc Assoc Soc Clin Oncol 5:215.

150. Wasserman AL, Thompson EI, Wilimas JA, Fairclough DL. 1987. The psychological status of survivors of childhood/adolescent Hodgkin's disease. Am J Dis Child 141:626–631.

151. Mullen F. 1984. The educational needs of the cancer survivor. Health Educ Q (Suppl) 10:88–94.

152. Mulhern RK, Tyc VL, Phipps S, et al. 1995. Health-related behaviors of survivors of childhood cancer. Med Pediatr Oncol 25:159–165.

153. Bleyer WA. 1990. The impact of childhood cancer on the United States and the world. Cancer 40:355–367.

Index

Nerve growth factor receptor, in
    neuroblastoma, 140–141
Neuroblastoma, 125–151
    anatomic sites of, 127
    angiogenesis in, 143
    bone marrow transplantation in, 147–149
    CD44 in, 143
    cerebellar encephalopathy in, 129–130
    chemotherapy in, 146–149
    chromosome 1 abnormalities in, 139–140
    clinical presentation of, 127–130
    clinical prognostic factors in, 134
    diagnosis of, 130–131
    diarrhea in, 128–129
    differential diagnosis of, 132
    disseminated, 146, 147–149
    embryology of, 126–127
    etiology of, 126
    extension of, 131–132
    familial, 126
    flow cytometry in, 139
    genomic imprinting in, 21
    histology of, 134–135
    HOX gene expression in, 14
    hyperbaric oxygen treatment in, 149
    hypertension in, 128
    imaging evaluation of, 131–132
    immunotherapy of, 150
    incidence of, 125
    localized, 145
    MDR1 gene in, 142–143
    131supI MIBG treatment in, 149–150
    monoclonal antibody treatment of, 150
    multidrug-resistance-associated protein
        in, 142–143
    MYCN amplification in, 135–139
    nerve growth factor receptor defects in,
        140–141
    pentetreotide treatment in, 150
    P-glycoprotein in, 142
    ploidy in, 139
    prognosis for, 134–143
    regional, 146–147
    regression of, 146
    retinoic acid treatment of, 150–151
    screening for, 144
    sites of, 127
    stage 4, 146, 147–149
    stage 4S, 146
    staging of, 132–134
    surgical treatment of, 145
    treatment of, 144–149
    TrkA gene in, 141

tumor markers in, 131, 134, 135
Neurofibromatosis (von Recklinghausen's
    disease)
    genetics of, 82–84
    Wilms' tumor in, 113
Neuropathy, chemotherapy-associated,
    354
NF1 gene, 83–84
NF2 gene, 84
Non-Hodgkin's lymphoma
    in acquired immunodeficiency
        syndrome, 51–54
    in immune deficiency states, 40–41

O

Osteoma, familial adenomatous polyposis
    and, 76
Osteosarcoma, 215–242
    alkaline phosphatase in, 228, 230
    angiogenesis inhibitors in, 238–239
    biological response modifiers in,
        238–239
    biopsy of, 228
    cell cycle dysregulation in, 220
    chemotherapy in, 230, 231, 233–238,
        240–242
    cisplatin toxicity after, 241
    clinical presentation of, 223–225
    complications of, 240–242
    cytogenetics of, 217–218, 232
    diagnosis of, 225–229
    differential diagnosis of, 228–229
    dominant-acting oncogenes in, 220–221
    doxorubicin-related cardiotoxicity
        after, 241
    epidemiology of, 215, 216
    etiology of, 215–217
    fluoride and, 217
    fos genes in, 220–221
    growth hormone antagonists in, 238
    histology of, 222–223, 231
    interferon in, 238
    of jaw, 222
    jun genes in, 220–221
    lactate dehydrogenase in, 228, 230
    in Li-Fraumeni syndrome, 219–220
    magnetic resonance imaging of, 225,
        226–227
    metastatic, 225, 227, 239–240
    molecular biology of, 218–221

X

X chromosome, in CNS germ cell tumors, 190

Xl-fli gene, in embryonic development, 25

X-linked lympholiferative disease, in immune deficiency states, 41

Y

Yolk sac tumor. See *Endodermal sinus tumor.*